HUMAN SAFETY AND RISK MANAGEMENT

HUMAN SAFETY AND RISK MANAGEMENT

A. Ian Glendon
Aston Business School, Aston University, UK

and

Eugene F. McKenna
University of East London, UK

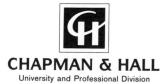

CHAPMAN & HALL
University and Professional Division

London · Glasgow · Weinheim · New York · Tokyo · Melbourne · Madras

Published by Chapman & Hall, 2–6 Boundary Row, London SE1 8HN, UK

Chapman & Hall, 2–6 Boundary Row, London SE1 8HN, UK

Blackie Academic & Professional, Wester Cleddens Road, Bishopbriggs, Glasgow G64 2NZ, UK

Chapman & Hall GmbH, Pappelallee 3, 69469 Weinheim, Germany

Chapman & Hall USA, One Penn Plaza, 41st Floor, New York, NY 10119, USA

Chapman & Hall Japan, ITP-Japan, Kyowa Building, 3F, 2-2-1 Hirakawacho,, Chiyoda-ku, Tokyo 102, Japan

Chapman & Hall Australia, Thomas Nelson Australia, 102 Dodds Street, South Melbourne, Victoria 3205, Australia

Chapman & Hall India, R. Seshadri, 32 Second Main Road, CIT East, Madras 600 035, India

First edition 1995

© 1995 A. Ian Glendon and Eugene F. McKenna

Typeset in 10/12 pt Times by Gray Publishing, Tunbridge Wells

Printed in Great Britain by Hartnolls Ltd, Bodmin, Cornwall

ISBN 0 412 40250 5

A catalogue record for this book is available from the British Library

CONTENTS

PREFACE

There are two strategic origins for this book. One is risk management (RM) – specifically, those aspects of RM relevant to human risk components such as motivation, attitudes, perception and behaviour. The other orientation is psychological aspects of managing human resources – in this case those aspects concerned with risks relating to human activities. As chartered psychologists, we bring a primarily, though not exclusively, psychological focus to managing risks which relate to human resources. Organizational problems cannot be fitted into traditional discipline-based categories. Increasingly, an overview approach is required in which the whole picture is informed by problem-solving activities which incorporate many varieties of human behaviour. Thus, there are both micro (individual, psychological) and macro (managerial, organizational) as well as intermediate (group, team) levels to be managed by professionals and line managers with responsibility for managing and developing human resources.

A problem identified in a paper on the role of occupational psychologists in business (Anderson and Prutton, 1993) is that occupational psychologists are not considered by senior managers to make a significant contribution to strategic decision-making processes. Rather they were seen as providers of technical services, particularly psychometric tests (chapter 6, pp. 149–155) – a relatively small part of the total possible range of the professional offerings from this group. To enable occupational and other applied psychologists to offer more strategic inputs, more strategically oriented frameworks are required for identifying and evaluating topics and processes which are relevant to organizations.

This book seeks to offer a potential framework for some of the major psychological issues which may be subsumed under a human resource management (HRM) heading – one which is oriented towards risk management (RM). One of our objectives is to stretch psychology from a basis of existing empirical and theoretical knowledge, into some new areas. For example, in the UK government white paper *Health of the Nation* (1992), major agenda items at a political and strategic level include mental health and accidents – issues which can be validly and usefully informed by input from applied psychological knowledge. This book highlights areas of relevance to such issues.

This book reflects the changing nature of approaches to managing risk as it applies to individuals and other social units. In essence, it attempts to bring relevant components of applied behavioural science within the managerial philosophies of human resource management (HRM) and risk management

(RM). The linking philosophy is that by applying emergent principles of HRM and RM to different aspects of human behaviour within a safety and risk context, more effective management of human resources in this field will result. In compiling this book, we have opted to concentrate upon an essentially psychological approach which reflects our own discipline. The first chapter considers the structure of the book, its target audiences and present-ational style.

ACKNOWLEDGEMENTS

Several people have helped us with the preparation of this book and a number merit specific mention. Special thanks are due to Professor Andrew Hale who reviewed an early draft – his perceptive remarks led us to revise many of our views and approaches to topics. We also particularly thank Professor Peter Waterhouse and Dr Alan Waring who read complete drafts of the book at a later stage and for whose helpful insights and valuable advice we are most grateful. Other colleagues read and made very useful comments on drafts of individual chapters, for which our appreciation is due to: Professor Richard Booth, Dr Tony Boyle, Sue Glendon, Dr Gerry Matthews and Dr Neville Stanton. On behalf of these colleagues we of course submit to the usual disclaimer that any remaining errors are entirely our responsability.

For being able to use material from their publications, we acknowledge permissions granted from: Professor Richard Booth, Dr Sara Lichtenstein and colleagues, Dr Paul Slovic and colleagues, Dr Michel Pérusse, American Psychological Association, Saville & Holdsworth Ltd, TMS (UK) Ltd, Cambridge University Press, Butterworth-Heinemann Ltd, Elsevier Science Publishers, Pergamon Press.

By no means least, we would like to thank both our publishers for their patience in waiting for the manuscript and our families for tolerating our efforts to produce it.

PART ONE
Introduction

1 AUDIENCE AND STRUCTURE

❏ This chapter serves the function of introducing the book, identifying those who might be its audience and outlining the structure in respect of the parts of the book and the focus of each chapter. An objective of this chapter is to explain the primary, though not exclusively psychological, orientation of the book in respect of safety and risk issues.

INTRODUCTION

Although not an academic monograph, this book does have roots in theoretical approaches to its subject material. As far as the interplay between theory and application is concerned, we have adopted the principle that it is necessary to have at least a minimal appreciation of theory in order to judge whether recommended applications are valid and appropriate – that is, a degree of transparency is required. However, theory without application is interesting, while applications devoid of theoretical basis may be groundless. The main orientation is psychological, although not exclusively so. In presenting the human side of safety and risk management, the book draws out applied psychological knowledge into new directions.

AN AUDIENCE FOR THIS BOOK

The intended audience is all those who have professional or applied interests in managing human resources as a vital component of risk management (RM). This means strategic as well as day-to-day involvement in decision-making and is likely to include present and aspiring personnel managers, human resource managers and risk managers as well as health, safety and risk professionals. Increasingly, individuals in all these roles are being required to adopt a strategic orientation in their professional roles.

As far as the audience for this book is concerned, we were obliged to derive a satisfactory generic title which would be acceptable to all those likely to read it – not an easy task. Because we are seeking to reach a wide spectrum of those involved in safety and risk matters – be they practitioners or students (in the broadest sense) of the subject area, the term had to encompass all these groups. We decided upon the generic term 'safety and risk professional' to indicate inclusion of all those working in the field or who had jobs or aspirations which incorporate any aspect of health, safety or risk – either directly in an occupational (e.g. workplace) setting, or in some other role, for example advisory, enforcement, teaching, research, consultancy or support. Although everyone has concerns about aspects of safety and risk in their everyday lives, not everyone has a professional concern over these matters. As is usual, it is to be understood that within the term 'safety' we include such concepts as health (especially mental health) and welfare, while the expression 'risk' is also taken to include reference to terms such as 'hazard' and 'danger', even though it is recognized that these terms do have distinct meanings (see chapter 10, pp. 315–322, especially figure 10.1 for a review of definitions and relationships between these concepts).

In adopting an overview perspective of the organizations for which safety and risk professionals have some responsibility, a thorough knowledge of the 'nuts and bolts' of safety, or even of the legal requirements pertaining to a workplace, is less and less likely to be sufficient. While much health and safety and other employment legislation is relevant to topics in this book, very little reference is made to legislation on the grounds that this is intended as a human behaviour text and not one which addresses legislative issues.

In accepting members for entry to its Professional Register, the Institution of Occupational Safety and Health (IOSH) – the main UK professional body for health and safety professionals – requires evidence of expertise across a broad range of topics, essentially oriented towards a strategic approach to managing workplace risks, including those associated with human behaviour.

For many years, students of safety and risk management as well as health and safety professionals have needed a book about safety and risk aspects of human behaviour which will be of practical assistance to them in their work. The general purpose of the book is to make available to those who do not necessarily have a social science background, essential psychological components of workplace safety and risk. Specifically, this book aims to improve understanding of ways in which human behaviour on the one hand influences, and on the other can be shaped by, effective management of workplace safety and risk.

Thus, the material is presented for a practitioner audience as well as for students of health, safety and risk management in the broadest sense. With its unique coverage of psychological aspects of safety and risk, elements of this field are made available between the covers of a single book for the first time. Safety and risk professionals, particularly those taking National Examination Board in Occupational Safety and Health (NEBOSH) Risk Management courses, will find that this book addresses essential parts of the NEBOSH syllabus using relevant examples. However, the book does not adhere slavishly to any syllabus, but addresses psychological topics with particular relevance to safety and risk management. References are provided for following up particular topics. Our aim is to present a contemporary view. Where older works are cited, often these are classic studies or important milestones in the relevant area and we have been selective in the presentation of referenced material.

Trainers and teachers in safety, risk and related areas will discover here a book which deals with behavioural aspects of health and safety in a straightforward way which students will be able to relate to. Students on courses which involve any safety and risk input – including: Ergonomics, General Management, Human Resource Management, Personnel Management, Risk Management, Psychology, Engineering, Environmental Health, Occupational Hygiene, Occupational Health and Safety – will find that this book offers a sensible path through individual, group and organizational aspects of risk-related behaviour. In particular, tutors and students on undergraduate and postgraduate courses which are devoted specifically to occupational health, safety and risk issues will discover that the chapters deal comprehensively with the human side of safety and risk. Over 20 higher education institutions in the UK alone offer courses in safety, risk and related areas, including the universities of: Aston, Bournemouth, Brighton, Cranfield, Glamorgan, Glasgow Caledonia, Greenwich, King's College London, Leeds Metropolitan, Loughborough, Nottingham Trent, Paisley, Portsmouth, St Andrews, Salford, Sheffield, South Bank, Surrey, Thames Valley, UMIST, West of England. Doubtless others will follow these institutions as well as the many colleges and other bodies which offer NEBOSH courses and other courses in this expanding field.

General readers with an interest in safety and risk issues, perhaps from reading about disasters in which management or human behaviour played an important part, will find insights into everyday safety and risk issues alongside psychological explanations for such behaviour.

Written by social scientists with many years' experience in teaching, researching and consultancy in psychological aspects of safety and risk management, the book expands an earlier outline of behavioural science contributions to accident control offered by one of the authors (Glendon, 1987a) who identified three main areas for future progress. These were:

1. cognition (mental processes) – including risk perception, development and learning, hazard perception and labelling, attributing responsibility, cause and blame;
2. behaviour – including accident causation, responding to hazards, making and correcting errors;
3. environment – including valid indicators of risk exposure, safety culture, training, education and communication.

This book expands and develops these and other important areas.

When writing a book for both student and practitioner audiences, it is easy to 'fall between two stools' and offer a text which is not entirely suitable to either. In an attempt to overcome this particular problem, the book has been organized so that the student can turn next to chapter 2 and work through what is intended to be a logical progression of topics to the end of the book. The alert practitioner on the other hand, may choose to begin with chapter 11 – the action framework, and then proceed to select those chapters and sections which are relevant to addressing the question 'why do you say this?' while reading the sections in chapter 11. This format also reflects the view that 'theory' and 'practice' are not two distinct entities, but are part of the same learning process – a process which is outlined in chapter 2 (p. 15 ff., especially figure 2.4). Frequent cross-referencing between chapters and sections throughout the book is intended to illustrate the mutual interdependence of much of the subject material.

STRUCTURE OF THE BOOK

There are four parts to the book. Part I (Introduction) comprises this chapter and the next – on training strategy for safe performance. Chapter 2 explains the importance of a strategic approach to managing risk as it applies to human resources. Training and development processes are central in this approach because they represent the principal expression of **investment** in human resources.

Part II is concerned with **individual** factors, primarily though not exclusively at work, and begins with a chapter on a central concept in psychology, that of motivation and the associated factor of reward. As well as underlying training and other efforts to change behaviour, motivation is also the key link between management action in this area and the individual factors considered in the following three chapters on: attitudes and attitude change (chapter 4), perception and risk perception (chapter 5) and personality (chapter 6). The topics in each of these chapters are considered in a way that makes a contribution to managing health and safety risks.

In Part III of the book, the focus turns to the work **environment** and aspects of this are dealt with in the three chapters comprising this part. Chapter 7 focuses upon groups and teams; chapter 8 is concerned with psychological health issues – particularly stress and stress management. Chapter 9 deals with human error and human factors more generally – including ergonomics. In each case, the orientation is again aligned with the contribution which each can make to managing human aspects of health and safety risks.

In Part IV, chapter 10 deals with the critical issue of **managing** human risks, specifically through a logical approach which accords with risk management principles of identifying, evaluating, controlling and monitoring risks within a positive safety culture. The final chapter (chapter 11) draws together the main lessons from the book as a basis for action and further understanding of relevant problems. It summarizes essential points from each chapter and may be used as supportive material for safety and risk professionals in their work. The emphasis throughout is upon the **use** of strategic and theoretical approaches in the service of applications. To this end, relevant examples are selected to illustrate salient points. The structure of the book is summarized in figure 1.1.

As well as identifying the major relations (represented by the solid lines) between the different topics, figure 1.1 also includes some of the cross linkages between topics – the dashed lines. However, even a diagram which includes all these topics cannot reflect the total complexity of this fascinating area.

To assist the reader, the textual material in this book has been broken up so that much of it is displayed in the form of illustrations (figures) or in boxes.

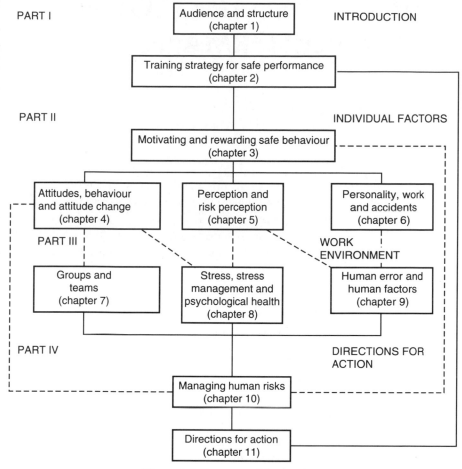

Figure 1.1 Structure of the book.

The boxes perform two main functions:

- outlining material which is not central to the text – for example, descriptions of theories;
- presenting illustrative case studies or experiments.

All the boxed material and figures are referred to at appropriate places in the text. The reader may opt to skip some of the theoretical descriptions and case illustrations. However, some of these may prove useful for training interventions such as a basis for class discussions or for developing health and safety applications in respect of human behaviour.

2 TRAINING STRATEGY FOR SAFE PERFORMANCE

❑ This chapter offers a strategic perspective for the important topic of safety training, including training decisions that have to be made, illustrated by a typical training sequence. Learning principles are discussed as a basis for training and the interesting topic of behaviour modification is reviewed. It is pointed out that in human resource terms, training is an investment not a cost. The chapter leads to a consideration of motivation issues in chapter 3.

INTRODUCTION

The objective of this chapter is to provide a strategic context for safety training principles and practices. The aim is to provide a framework for developing effective safety training policy and for considering relevant research evidence for safety training applications. Although a variety of bodies is involved in providing safety training, a substantial amount is conducted by employers and it is primarily to them that this chapter is directed. It is assumed that the safety and risk professional will be involved at all stages of the safety training process.

This chapter considers safety training from a variety of perspectives. Initial discussion focuses upon the importance of a strategic approach in which safety training is developed as a key component of risk management and human resource strategies, and how decisions on safety training can be made. The issue of a logical training sequence is next addressed before a consideration of learning principles – which provide a sound basis for training practices. Discussion then turns to the forms that safety training might take, using a simple model of the different levels of human performance that are addressed by training. A review section on studies of behaviour modification in the safety field is followed by a discussion of safety training in the context of safety culture – a topic which is reviewed in greater detail in chapter 10 (pp. 291–5) – and conclusions to the chapter. The chapter will indicate that although there is no one correct way of carrying out safety training, a systematic approach is always appropriate. An underlying assumption is that training, including safety training, is critical to optimal organizational functioning.

A STRATEGIC PERSPECTIVE

Like any aspect of business, training – including safety training – should have a coherent basis. This is provided by considering how training contributes to business goals, i.e. the extent to which it is regarded as an investment in the organization's human resources rather than a cost. Two strategic bases for training and development in health and safety (hereafter 'safety training') can be identified. The first originates in an organization's corporate objectives, for example growth and profitability – for a private sector organization, and devolves through the various managerial divisions (marketing, finance, human resources, etc.) to the training support function. This, in turn can be divided into different training programmes (induction, organization development, safety, etc.), each of which may have knowledge, skills, attitudinal and other components. This corporate human resource basis for training is illustrated in figure 2.1.

A strategic human resource management approach, which views safety training as a contributor to the organization's overall business or public accountability objectives, can be complemented by another strategic approach in which safety training is viewed as a component of risk management. In this approach, risk management is devolved into: hazard identification, risk evaluation, development and implementation of controls, and monitoring or feedback. Safety training, in its various forms, has relevance to all aspects of the risk management sequence. For example, it is among the controls which can be developed to manage risk. In this context, training given may be either technical (e.g. relating to specific job skills) or procedural – relating to managing risk through policy, legislative or organizational requirements. It may be

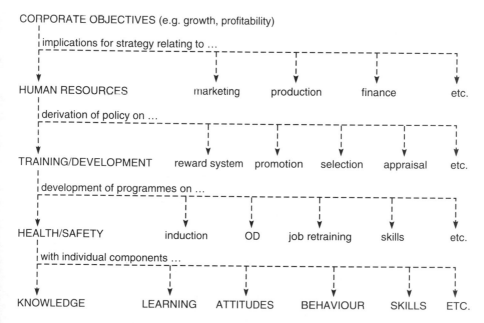

Figure 2.1 Deriving safety training from corporate objectives.

conceived as addressing either the organization as a whole or specific individuals or groups. Figure 2.2 outlines a risk management approach to safety training.

These two strategic approaches to safety training may be combined so that safety training takes account of strategic human resource objectives as well as addressing risk management criteria. Summary text 2.1 shows illustrative safety training objectives derived from both these strategic bases.

From the discussion so far, an important principle of safety training will have become apparent. It is important to be concerned not only with training individuals and groups, but also to ensure that the organizational environment within which those parties operate is consistent with training provision. Training needs to meet the needs of both individuals or groups and those of the organization. A strategic approach should ensure that training matches organization development.

It is important to set a strategic agenda for safety training so that its contribution to the organization's objectives can be appreciated – this largely determines what is included in a training programme. It is also essential to establish a methodology for safety training – for example as supplied by a risk management approach – as this provides guidance for training components.

THE DECISION-MAKING SEQUENCE

Once strategic issues have been addressed, a training programme can be established to incorporate objectives set for both individuals and the

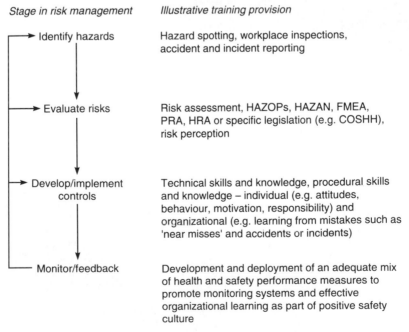

Stage in risk management	Illustrative training provision
Identify hazards	Hazard spotting, workplace inspections, accident and incident reporting
Evaluate risks	Risk assessment, HAZOPs, HAZAN, FMEA, PRA, HRA or specific legislation (e.g. COSHH), risk perception
Develop/implement controls	Technical skills and knowledge, procedural skills and knowledge – individual (e.g. attitudes, behaviour, motivation, responsibility) and organizational (e.g. learning from mistakes such as 'near misses' and accidents or incidents)
Monitor/feedback	Development and deployment of an adequate mix of health and safety performance measures to promote monitoring systems and effective organizational learning as part of positive safety culture

Figure 2.2 A strategic approach to safety training from risk management.

Summary text 2.1 Illustrative objectives for safety training from corporate strategy and risk management

Organizational
- continual attention to safety culture – e.g. in deriving functional strategy from corporate objectives;
- develop ability of the organization to learn – e.g. institute systems for analysing and monitoring accident/incident/near miss data as a basis for developing appropriate controls;
- achieving and maintaining genuine commitment by senior management to safety – e.g. by accountability procedures for health and safety provision at all levels;
- reduce losses (damage, compensation, claims, lost time, etc.) from accidents, incidents, absences, etc. – e.g. by establishing and monitoring safe systems of work;
- increase participation throughout organization – e.g. in safety committees, safety auditing, safety inspections.

Individual
- improve skills base – e.g. hazard identification, risk assessment;
- incorporate safety within other training programmes (e.g. induction, OD);
- increase understanding of risks (perception, knowledge, etc.);
- develop responsibility and motivation in respect of safe attitudes and behaviour.

---

organization. To obviate the possibility that safety training might be conducted on an ad hoc basis, it is important to establish a logical sequence for it. Various techniques may be used to establish priorities for training. For example, a skills audit can be used to determine what skills the organization currently has. A review is also needed of the skills required to meet organizational objectives. The gap between these two assessments represents the deficit to be made up. Reference should be made to the organization's human resources policy parameters (budget, objectives, constraints, etc.) for guidance on addressing any deficit. For example, a policy of no compulsory redundancies may mean that a retraining programme is appropriate. If an industry is contracting, then the necessity for internal change may be an opportunity to restructure departments and functions in response to changes in the external environment. Training may then be offered as an alternative to redundancy or as a reward for continuing employment. There are many variations on these possibilities. Another scenario is that the organization can determine its human resources policy on the basis of job-related criteria. This may provide it with an opportunity to establish the most appropriate approach to any particular skills need which has been identified. An example will help to illustrate the decision-making sequence.

At present, there is considerable development within the field of health and safety software (see for example, Kibblewhite, 1988; Glendon *et al.*, 1992). In order to evaluate the potential utility of this range of software, organizations need to acquire or access relevant expertise which will provide sound advice and guidance in respect of:

- whether the organization should acquire such software (for accident/incident analysis, safety auditing, etc.) at all;
- if it does use health and safety software, what form should the management

of the new software take and over what time period should it be planned;
* who should be involved in the decision-making process – to advise and
  influence such decisions as: buy in proprietary software or develop in-house,
  costs and benefits of each option, which brand to purchase, etc.

Organizations have the option of developing relevant expertise in-house or
of purchasing it externally, for example through consultants, or a combination
of both. To facilitate this process, a logical sequence may be identified for
establishing whether this is a matter for training or for selection or for both.
Summary text 2.2 outlines the illustrative case.

A simple representation of the decision-making sequence for determining
whether the acquisition of expertise required to evaluate safety software is
one of training or selection, as shown in summary text 2.2, is important. This
is because making the wrong decision at an early stage can later prove to be
expensive. A simple view of the essential questions to be asked can reveal the
optimum decision for acquiring a given skill to address a particular problem.

THE TRAINING SEQUENCE

Having established strategic and decision-making bases for training, it is
important to follow a logical series of steps in carrying out the training. This is
by now a well-established sequence (e.g. Patrick, 1992) and again will be illustrated with an example, in this case health and safety advisers. The outline
sequence, taken from Glendon (1987a), is shown in figure 2.3.

It is important to acknowledge that training can only be expected to achieve

---

Summary text 2.2 Sequence for deciding whether to select or to train for expertise

1. **Set objectives for task** – (acquisition of skills to) evaluate health and safety software for use by organization; then ask ...
2. **Are some individuals significantly better than others at the task?** If the answer is
   'no' and current performance, for example of the safety adviser and line managers, is adequate then they should be able to do the task. If the answer is 'yes',
   then ask ...
3. **Can enough already capable people be found on the market?**
   If the answer is 'yes' and they can be identified satisfactorily and cheaply enough,
   then they can be selected on acquired or innate skill – either as consultants or new
   employees. If they are either not available or too costly to acquire, then ask ...
4. **Can the required skills be taught adequately?**
   If the answer is 'no' then the original task must be redesigned. If people can be
   trained to evaluate safety software (which it can be assumed is the case), then ask ...
5. **Do individuals differ in their trainability?**
   In most cases people will differ in their ability to undertake a wide range of tasks
   and there are ability and other tests as well as other devices which may be used
   to identify such differences. Thus, individuals would normally be selected on the
   basis of their ability to acquire, in this case, basic computing skills as well as
   appropriate knowledge of the organization's health and safety function and
   current computing policy and usage.

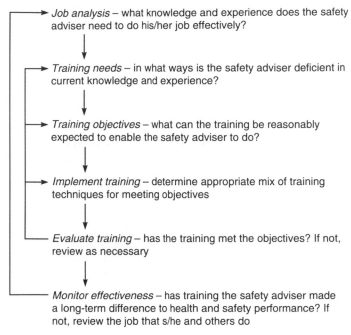

Job analysis – what knowledge and experience does the safety adviser need to do his/her job effectively?

Training needs – in what ways is the safety adviser deficient in current knowledge and experience?

Training objectives – what can the training be reasonably expected to enable the safety adviser to do?

Implement training – determine appropriate mix of training techniques for meeting objectives

Evaluate training – has the training met the objectives? If not, review as necessary

Monitor effectiveness – has training the safety adviser made a long-term difference to health and safety performance? If not, review the job that s/he and others do

Figure 2.3 Illustrative sequence for training a safety adviser.

certain types of objectives and that relevant experience may be the only way of acquiring some types of abilities. A useful distinction can be made between knowledge in the traditional sense of knowing about something – for example, facts about health and safety legislation (referred to as 'declarative knowledge' because it can be recited – or declared) and experiential knowledge, for example, knowing ways and means of successfully implementing workplace health and safety legislation, including the likely constraints and problems to be overcome. This latter type of knowledge is sometimes referred to as 'procedural knowledge' because it relates to a person's ability to do things – hence procedural – and is likely to be based upon long-term experience – including training.

An organization may use the difference between the health and safety skills revealed as being available by a skills audit and those that are deemed to be required by the organization as the basis for determining requirements for any particular job – for example, that of a safety adviser. The first step is to establish what the safety adviser has to know in order to do his/her job. This can be done by means of job/task analysis, on which various texts may be consulted (e.g. McCormick, 1976a; Drury, 1983; Shepherd, 1985). A more detailed discussion of task analysis is provided in chapter 9 (pp. 275–7). The safety adviser's current skills and knowledge can then be compared with the job requirements to determine present deficiencies. This establishes the training needs. A study of training needs of safety advisers was carried out by Dawson and her colleagues (Dawson, 1986; Dawson *et al.*, 1984) and the main findings from this work are shown in summary text 2.3. Such research is useful in identifying skills and knowledge required for safety advisers in general and for guiding organizational assessments of training needs for individual safety advisers. Individual safety advisers who already possess the relevant skills and knowledge would not benefit from the training. Another example of training needs analysis, in this case for UK government health and safety inspectors, is given by Hale (1978).

Training needs are used as a basis for determining training objectives – expressed as a statement of what the safety adviser should be able to do afterwards. These help to identify the training to be undertaken – including an appropriate mix of techniques, timescale, in-house or external, etc. DeJoy (1990) notes the importance of deriving training objectives for employees that are specific to workplace hazards behaviour.

The next stage is the one most likely to be omitted, yet is crucial and that is to evaluate the training. A useful text on training evaluation is Hamblin (1974). In an important review, Hale (1984) highlights the problematic nature of conclusions in the safety training field, due to the dearth of research into safety training evaluation. The evaluation process assesses the training provided against the objectives, for example in respect of adding appropriately to the safety adviser's skills and knowledge. If evaluation shows that the training has not (fully) met the objectives, then it may mean that training provision has not been linked with organizational objectives, and therefore that the organization is unable to make effective use of the new skills and knowledge resource. It will then be necessary to review not just training provision, but the whole training sequence, including objectives and training needs. Most of the evaluation studies that have been reported have been concerned with safe behaviour modifications (pp. 25–7).

Evaluation also extends to the long term in that it is important to monitor training effectiveness in carrying out the job. This means answering the question, 'In the long term, has training the safety adviser made a detectable difference to the organization's safety performance?' This may be a very difficult question to answer with confidence. However, it is very useful to be able to do so, for example by setting appropriate criteria in advance against which performance may be measured – such as increasing safety audit scores

---

Summary text 2.3 Training needs of safety advisers (after Dawson, 1986)

- skill at handling interdisciplinary concepts at interface of technology, science and society
- hazard identification and control skills
- knowledge of legal requirements
- appreciation of organizational position of the safety adviser, especially relation with line management and multi-disciplinary team member
- analytical skills as important as substantive knowledge to deal with changes in the working environment and to solve problems related to future hazards

across the organization by a certain amount within a given time period (chapter 10, pp. 298–312 on this topic). If this question is answered in the negative, then it may prompt a review of the job carried out by the safety adviser in relation to others within the organization – for example, those of line managers. It may raise issues of which task, such as safety auditing, is best carried out by which managerial or staff function.

LEARNING PRINCIPLES AS THE BASIS FOR TRAINING

Learning is a natural human function which involves both mental (cognitive) activity and behaviour (verbal and non-verbal). Because it is a complex process, it is helpful to have a coherent picture of what learning comprises. One of the best-known models for describing the learning process is that of Kolb (1984), whose basic argument is that people learn by testing their understandings (i.e. personal theories) against their experiences and modify their understandings as a result. Kolb developed the notion of a 'learning cycle' in which our experiences are the basis for learning. These are followed by reflecting on the experiences and by making generalizations from these reflections, which are then tried out in new situations. To help explain Kolb's learning cycle, figure 2.4 shows this together with a safety example.

Kolb's model of learning is an example of a system which provides feedback to the individual which can result in modified behaviour and thought patterns. The importance of feedback in learning is discussed later in this section. The model also illustrates the interplay between attitudes (cognitions) and

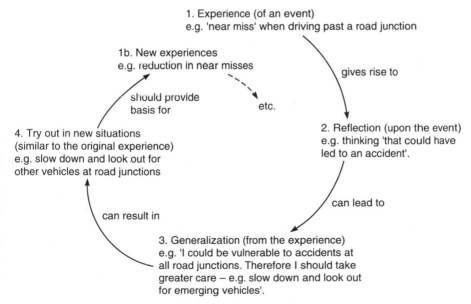

Figure 2.4 The learning cycle (after Kolb, 1984) with a safety example.

behaviour (actions), considered in chapter 4 (especially pp. 76–84).

Using Kolb's ideas as a basis, Honey and Mumford (1986) developed the notion that individuals have their own preferred styles of learning and that preferences could be related to different stages of the learning cycle. Thus, some people might have a preference for learning through active experience, others would prefer to spend a lot of time reflecting upon their experiences and so forth. The best learners have preferences for all components of the learning cycle. Honey and Mumford's ideas on learning styles are reviewed in summary text 2.4.

Although individuals differ in their preferred learning styles (summary text 2.4) and these may have a bearing upon training methods which are selected, there are a number of general features of the training context which are likely to influence learning, irrespective of individual preferences. A substantial psychological literature on the principles of learning exists (for example, Hill, 1980; Bower and Hilgard, 1981; Stammers, 1987) and a number of learning principles are regularly incorporated into effective training provision. Among the most important is motivation, covered in more detail in chapter 3. Trainees need to be motivated in order to learn. Motivation may be intrinsic, that is be generated internally by a trainee's desire to learn, or extrinsic – derived from the training environment, for example a trainer's enthusiasm. Training can of itself provide motivation, for example by demonstrating that an organization is interested in developing an individual's skills and knowledge (extrinsic), or because the trainee finds the subject matter and its application fascinating (intrinsic). Summary text 2.5 summarizes key competencies required by trainers.

A second crucial aspect of learning which should be incorporated within training is feedback or knowledge of results. To learn effectively, trainees need to be able to measure their own progress over time. They may also seek to compare their progress with that of their peers. Sessions which incorporate a test or exam on which trainees receive feedback are an example of how this learning principle can be put into practice. Another example is the immediate feedback which can be given to first-aid trainees who practise cardiopulmonary resuscitation (CPR) on a recording manikin which provides an immediate print-out of their CPR performance (Glendon *et al.*, 1988). Trainees can adjust their subsequent practice towards a goal of performance optimization.

A related learning principle for use in training is that of positive reinforcement – provided as some form of reward. Rewards for performance during training sessions, used in combination with feedback (which also constitutes reinforcement) contribute to motivational effects (see also chapter 3). Rewards may take the form of verbal encouragement from a trainer or the satisfaction of passing a test or exam and receiving a certificate. Rewards are also necessary during training to sustain interest and motivation. Petersen (1989), following behaviourist reinforcement principles, argues the advantages of reinforcing safe behaviour over reprimanding unsafe behaviour, citing a number of studies that have used reinforcement principles to improve

Summary text 2.4 Individual learning styles (Honey and Mumford, 1986)

There are various ways of describing the different ways in which individuals learn. One way of measuring these differences was devised by Honey and Mumford (1986), who developed the learning styles questionnaire. Results from completing the questionnaire enable a person to determine their preferred combination of learning styles. Advantages of having this information about your preferred learning style(s) are that you can then:

• increase awareness of learning opportunities which are (in)congruent with your preferred learning style(s);
• make more informed choices among learning opportunities to improve performance;
• identify where less preferred learning styles can be improved;
• develop ways to improve specific learning skills.

The four learning styles identified by Honey and Mumford are: activist, reflector, theorist and pragmatist. There are links between these types and personality dimensions – discussed in chapter 6 (particularly pp. 142–9) – as well as with stages of Kolb's learning cycle. Each learning style is described briefly below in respect of its main strengths and weaknesses.

Activist strengths – flexible and open minded, happy to 'have a go', happy to be exposed to new situations, optimistic about anything new, unlikely to resist change;
Activist weaknesses – tend to take immediately obvious action without thinking, often take unnecessary risks, tend to do too much themselves and hog the limelight, rush into action without sufficient preparation, get bored with implementation/consolidation.
Reflector strengths – careful, thorough and methodical, thoughtful, good at listening to others and assimilating information, rarely jump to conclusions;
Reflector weaknesses – tendency to hold back from direct participation, slow to make up their minds or to reach a decision, tend to be too cautious/not take enough risks, not assertive or forthcoming – no 'small talk'.
Theorist strengths – logical thinkers, rational and objective, good at asking probing questions, disciplined approach;
Theorist weaknesses – restricted in lateral thinking, intolerant of uncertainty, disorder and ambiguity, intolerant of subjectivity or intuition, full of 'shoulds' and 'musts'.
Pragmatist strengths – keen to test things out in practice, practical, down to earth and realistic, business-like, get straight to the point, technique orientated;
Pragmatist weaknesses – tend to reject anything without an obvious application, not very interested in theory or basic principles, tend to seize on first expedient solution to a problem, impatient with 'waffle', tend to be task oriented rather than people oriented.

For each of the four styles described there are situations in which individuals learn best and least well. Ideally, training situations should take account of individual differences in learning styles so as to maximize training effectiveness. However, it can be argued that once individuals become aware of their preferred learning style(s), they should take greater responsibility for their own development and seek out situations – experience as well as training – which are most likely to improve their own skills and knowledge.

work practices and reduce workplace hazards and reported injuries.

Another important feature of learning, particularly in respect of tasks or jobs which are undertaken infrequently, or which may never be used at all

---

Summary text 2.5 Key competencies required by trainers/agencies

1. Identify needs, customers and markets, involving ability to:
   - undertake needs analysis for individuals;
   - undertake needs analysis on basis of business/organizational profiles;
   - segment consumer markets;
   - market programmes effectively;
   - time and locate programmes effectively;
   - understand business/organization development processes.

2. Develop appropriate programmes, involving ability to:
   - develop range of programme typologies;
   - use relevant environment;
   - use existing materials and guides;
   - produce own material as required;
   - lay out attractive programme material.

3. Deliver programmes effectively, involving ability to:
   - adopt flexible teaching styles;
   - deliver enterprise skills training;
   - train in an enterprising fashion;
   - teach in a multi-disciplinary fashion;
   - counsel groups and individuals;
   - use invited speakers.

4. Evaluate and control, involving ability to:
   - assess, monitor and evaluate programmes.

(e.g. an emergency drill) is that of overlearning. In training terms, this means that the candidate practises a skill or sequence of actions until it becomes 'automatic'. The skill is then more resistant to forgetting and can be reinforced by occasional refresher training which uses the residual knowledge as a basis for bringing the skill up to the original level in a relatively short period of time. A good example again is CPR (Glendon *et al.*, 1988). Overlearning is a principle applied by professional performers such as musicians or actors and may be encapsulated in the phrase: 'an amateur practises until s/he gets it right; a professional practises until s/he can't get it wrong'.

A traditional debate within training is whether trainees should practise a task in separate parts and then link them together or practise the whole sequence from the start. Evidence tends to support the whole task option on the grounds that if the complete sequence is learned from the start then each step is more likely to remain embedded within it. If trainees learn parts of a task separately, then they have an additional series of tasks in linking the parts together and are more likely to omit steps in the sequence at a later date. This may be particularly important in times of stress – when errors are more likely, for example a control room emergency. Under such conditions, operators are less likely to omit crucial stages in a sequence of actions if they have been taught the sequence as a whole. As a performance *aide mémoire*, checklists or permit-to-work procedures may be used as a reference point for action sequences.

When being trained for a task or job, it is generally held to be preferable for trainees to be actively involved in the learning process, as opposed to being passive recipients of material. This is true whether we are dealing with acquiring skills (where 'hands on' is essential), rule-based behaviour (in which sequences need to be practised) or performance which is based upon knowledge (in which case, an active, questioning mind is required). Dale and Nyland (1985) propose a 'cone of learning' (summary text 2.6) which matches the degree of involvement that a trainee has with the extent to which material is remembered. For learning tasks which involve bodily movements, active trainee participation may take the form of practising a simple task or series of actions at one end of the spectrum, to highly complex and lengthy experience in a simulator – for example, as in pilot training. Those being trained for jobs which have a high thinking component also ben-efit from active learning involvement. For example, management trainees in assessment or development centres which incorporate group discussions, interview practice and 'in tray' exercises can derive great benefit from such events – providing that adequate feedback is given in the form of debriefing. It is a maxim of the theatrical profession that you should always rehearse even the simplest appearing actions on stage on the grounds that these can always encounter snags when carried out in practice. Thus it is with training and particularly so for tasks which have implications for safety – and most do. It is never likely to be sufficient to be told what to do, it is necessary to do it. Rehearsed action sequences provide a much firmer basis for subsequent behaviour than merely listening to a lecture or film. Once learned in such a way, subsequent mental rehearsal – i.e. going over a planned sequence in your mind – can then be a very effective way of refreshing the behaviour – and is analogous with overlearning discussed above.

Summary text 2.6 The 'cone of learning' (after Dale and Nyland, 1985)

Involvement level	*% likely to be remembered*
Active, doing – e.g. performing a job or task, simulating a real experience, doing a dramatic presentation.	90%
Active, receiving and participating – e.g. taking part in a discussion, giving a talk.	70%
Passive, visual receiving – e.g. seeing something being done, watching a demonstration, looking at an exhibit, watching a film.	50%
Passive, verbal – looking at pictures.	30%
– hearing words.	20%
– reading.	10%

Not all training is concerned with skilled behaviour in the traditional sense or with performance which is based upon a series of steps or rules. Other learning principles will be involved when there is a requirement for training in problem-solving activity for novel situations. In such instances, trainees may be encouraged to brainstorm possible solutions to a problem or to consult with others in seeking a solution. An important feature of problem-solving may be to have available ways of breaking the mental set of an individual or group, who may otherwise be inclined to reuse a previously successful strategy inappropriately. This approach is analogous with lateral thinking (De Bono, 1976) in which people are encouraged to think of fresh approaches to a problem. One antidote is to institute practices which are designed to promote a heterogeneity of inputs – i.e. from people with different skills, outlooks and backgrounds, to avoid the classic 'groupthink' phenomenon in which everyone in a group thinks along similar (and perhaps incorrect) lines (chapter 7, pp. 189–92). Alternatively, expert systems type methodology may be used to diagnose exhaustively the state of a system, an approach which is analogous with using checklists at the rules-based level. Summary text 2.7 summarizes training requirements for the three performance levels mentioned.

In the case of complex tasks, such as control room operation, work with detailed electrical or mechanical operations or piloting a ship or aeroplane, another vital aspect of training is to ensure that trainees have a good understanding of the system and how its components interlink. For most of us as drivers, there is little need for us to understand much about the workings of the car we drive apart from basic maintenance requirements. However, Formula One drivers need expert knowledge of the workings of their car in order to maximize the driver-car performance within safe limits and to make appropriate adjustments in the event of failures in system components, including track conditions. There are a number of examples of failures in which key operators did not have an adequate or accurate representation of the system which they were in charge of, for example Three Mile Island (Kemeny, 1979) and Herald of Free Enterprise (Department of Transport, 1987), although not all these can be attributed to training lapses. A case which has features which might more appropriately be attributed, at least in part, to training deficiencies is the Kegworth air crash (Department of Transport, 1990) where the pilots' training did not include an appreciation of the working of the automatic fuel distribution system which adjusted the flow of fuel to the two engines and which disengaged when they shut down the healthy engine, apparently solving the problem of the broken engine. Neither did their training include an appreciation of the accuracy of the new engine vibration gauges which, in combination with better design, could have alerted them to the true state of the system they were attempting to bring under control.

Training in circumstances in which humans are included in a system to sort out routine or unusual problems, should seek to alert trainees to be aware of situations which require a problem-solving approach – i.e. at the knowledge-based level, rather than to refer to rules and procedures – which may be inappropriate to the circumstances. This presents a stern challenge for safety

---

Summary text 2.7 Illustrative training requirements for different levels of performance

Performance level – skills
Involves routine repetitive tasks which may be performed 'automatically ' – e.g. operating a keyboard or familiar machine, riding a bicycle.

Illustrative training requirements
Repetition of the task sufficient times, with trial and error, in order to cement the skill as it should be performed. In the case of rarely used skills (e.g. emergency drills), training should be given to the extent of 'overlearning' the skill so that it is more likely to be retained when needed – e.g. under stressful conditions.

Performance level – rules
Involves following a sequence of steps which need to be learned as a complete task but which require thought to put into action – e.g. monitoring control operations, electrical switching sequence task, reading a map to find your way to a destination.

Illustrative training requirements
Teaching the complete sequence each time to reduce the likelihood that steps will be omitted (or repeated or new ones introduced). Also important to emphasize retention of **awareness** of sequence (so as not to revert to 'automatic' mode as in skills-based performance) as different process sequences will be required for different tasks and confusion can occur (chapter 9, especially pp. 244–61). Checklists can be useful as an aide mémoire for following sequences. Other aids to rule-following involve procedures such as are incorporated into safe systems of work, including lock-off and permits-to-work. Expert systems, if available, can be useful in cases where diagnostics are particularly important – e.g. identifying a problem by following a set of diagnostic rules – e.g. of the form 'if ... a symptom, then ... such and such is likely to be a problem'.

Performance level – knowledge
Involves learning something for the first time or encountering new situations – even if in familiar surroundings – e.g. being presented with a novel combination of symptoms when flying a plane or driving a car, implementing health and safety legislation, industrial relations problems.

Illustrative training requirements
Important to start from basic principles – take a broad approach. In problem-solving, involve as wide a constituency as possible. Take as much time as possible in order to reflect and have opportunity to come forward with alternative solutions (e.g. group brainstorming or individual 'lateral thinking'). Don't foreclose options too early (e.g. as in 'groupthink' – chapter 7, pp. 189–92). Take stock and evaluate on the basis of as much information as possible. **Recognize** the problem as knowledge-based and don't attempt to apply rule-based solutions – i.e. what worked last time a similar looking problem occurred won't necessarily work this time.

---

training because it involves training for situations which cannot be foreseen and which it is therefore impossible to simulate or even to describe. Case studies, including examples of disasters from other industries, can be valuable as part of a problem-solving approach to complex safety issues. This is because participants can be directed towards analysing the situation – for example, from a risk management perspective, to imagine scenarios under which similar circumstances could befall their own organization and whether it would be adequately equipped to deal with them. This can then be developed into a consideration of ways in which their own organization is deficient in managing risk and determining personal and organizational plans to address the deficit.

A final important principle, which is particularly apposite to safety, is that of learning appropriately from experiences. One of the problems associated with this approach to learning is that in its 'raw' state, it takes the form of trial and error learning – not an efficient method, and one which can lead to disaster if you have not had an opportunity to try out an experience before you encounter it for real. This presents another challenge for safety training – how to maximize the utility of relevant experiences by incorporating them into the learning process. Training for many skills, such as flying an aeroplane or driving a car, often aims to provide trainees with the basics and then leaves them to learn the rest by experience – i.e. learning as you go. However, young male drivers who are 'unsafe' tend to perceive driving as essentially a skill-based activity (Rolls and Ingham, 1992). Such drivers then have to learn through experience (i.e. having accidents or 'near misses') that the time scale of decision-making in driving is longer than they first thought and that other types of abilities are involved – for example, planning and accurately perceiving risks in the environment. Training, for example using refresher courses, which involves the discussion of 'trial and error' or trainees' 'near-miss' experiences, can be a valuable way of increasing awareness of risk and improving safe behaviour. For examples of how this principle has been successfully used in training, see Lagerlöf (1982) on forestry workers, and Lewin (1982) on drivers. Learning exclusively from our own experiences is both less comprehensive and less efficient than learning from a larger sample of incidents, most of which have happened to other people. It is most likely that 'near-miss' incidents as well as case studies of accidents will come to be increasingly used in safety training. Their use in this context will depend upon their development and sophistication (for example, van der Schaaf *et al.*, 1991).

This section has reviewed some important features of learning which should be incorporated within most forms of training. It has also highlighted some special features of training for safe performance which make this form of training particularly challenging. We may be training not just for safe performance in the routine sense – as in skills which may be exercised daily and rules which provide sequences to be followed, but also delivering training which addresses high level cognitive processes which may need to be used to appraise accurately and to deal with a particular emergency never previously encountered, yet which, if wrongly handled, could turn into a disaster. In assessing this situation, it becomes evident that training cannot be the sole influence upon safe behaviour (a point made by Shaw and Sichel, 1971, in their study of accident proneness), nor as a cure for all safety problems within an organization (Everett, 1989), nor a substitute for health and safety practices which are inadequate. Rather, training for safety must be considered as

Summary text 2.8 Improving safe performance by training

Individual characteristics – can be improved by training

Characteristic	Illustrative examples
Knowledge	of health and safety legislation, understanding of nature of hazard and risk, of specific hazards
Skills	in relation to safe performance of a routine task
Attitudes	in respect of health and safety issues (chapter 4)
Behaviour	in relation to hazards and risk-taking and when interacting with others (e.g. seeking to improve their behaviour, either informally or through training, etc.)
Habits	at work and off-the-job in respect of doing things safely
Motivation	in respect of wanting to behave safely on the basis of understanding the need for such behaviour (chapter 3)

Environment – cannot be improved directly by training

Physical hazards	which translate into risks as a result of exposure – need to be managed (e.g. safety management can be improved by training)
Social factors	group norms and peer pressure which may/not favour safe behaviour (chapter 7, particularly pp. 177–80)
Background	e.g. – cultural differences in risk perception from family or peers (chapter 5, particularly pp. 121–30)
Organization	e.g. – structural factors, safety culture, communication (chapter 10, particularly pp. 290–5)

one component of a system which also addresses commercial, organizational, design and other ergonomic issues as part of a strategic programme for safety. Summary text 2.8 summarizes the main individual characteristics which can be improved by training and environmental factors which cannot.

Although environmental factors cannot be changed directly by training, a case study of how an organization was able to use a disaster as a stimulus for developing a safety training programme is given in summary text 2.9. It is to be hoped that other organizations can learn from such experiences.

Summary text 2.9 A lesson learned through a disaster

A large chemical company experienced an explosion in a work area. Such was the force of the explosion that all five employees who were working in that area at the time were killed. Furthermore the damage was so extensive that the accident investigation team that conducted a study of the site were unable, even after thorough investigations, to arrive at a conclusion as to what caused the explosion. This outcome failed to satisfy the enforcing authority, who commenced their own investigation of the disaster. After a painstaking investigation and with the full cooperation of the company, they too were obliged to deliver an open verdict as to the cause of the explosion.

An independent research team learned of the outcome of these investigations and offered to carry out their own study; the offer being accepted by the company. The research team spent time investigating the management and organizational procedures in place and also searched through personnel records relating to the individuals who had been working in that part of the plant when the explosion occurred. They also established what job each was doing on the day of the explosion. While the research team was no more successful than either of the previous two accident investigations in arriving at a conclusion regarding the actual cause of the accident, they were able to point out that none of the five workers could have been regarded as being fully trained for the jobs that they were doing on that particular day.

The team made recommendations in respect of training, particularly safety training, for all personnel working in the company; recommendations which were subsequently taken up by the organization, which went on to achieve a high standard of safety in later years.

WHAT FORM SHOULD SAFETY TRAINING TAKE?

Reviews of the literature on safety training (e.g. Hale, 1984) point to the large variety of inputs and methods which have been given the heading 'safety training'. In view of the corresponding variety of needs and objectives for safety training, this is probably unsurprising. However, what is of greater concern is whether the substance and process of safety training matches the requirements of those for whom it is designed. This is an important, though difficult area to address. One way in which it may be approached is through the application of a systematic model of the processes involved.

One approach is to consider the different levels at which safety knowledge or skill is required, for which there are well-established models available. One such, that of Bloom (1956) is shown in summary text 2.10, along with examples of health and safety objectives at each of the six levels of this model. One problem with using such a model is that it is very generalized and may not be an exact fit for any particular safety training problem. Nevertheless, such models do provide a useful guide as to whether the appropriate level of input is being supplied in a training programme. A safety training application of the Bloom model is provided by Waring (1990).

An alternative to basing a safety training programme on a generalized model of training is to use a model which is specifically concerned with an outcome of safety training, for example enhancing ability of an individual or

---

Summary text 2.10 Six levels of skill for training objectives (after Bloom, 1956) with health and safety examples

1. Knowledge – e.g. recall facts of health and safety legislation
2. Comprehension – e.g. provide examples of different types of hazard
3. Application – e.g. outline possible solutions to safety problems at a general level
4. Analysis – e.g. explain why something is a hazard
5. Synthesis – e.g. plan a detailed solution to a particular safety problem
6. Evaluation – e.g. compare risks and benefits of different solutions to a safety problem

---

group to address danger situations appropriately. One such model is that of Hale and Glendon (1987), who propose a model formulated as a series of questions about the nature of danger and a party's response to it. Stages of the model correspond with the skills, rules and knowledge levels of functioning and can be considered as a series of questions, each of which needs to be answered in the affirmative for danger to be positively influenced by the human(s) in the system. Summary text 2.11 shows outline steps in the model and reviews the type of training to be undertaken at each level as well as the limitations of such training.

BEHAVIOUR MODIFICATION

To secure long-term positive changes in safety practices it is necessary to change both behaviour and attitudes and this topic is explored in more depth in chapter 4 (in particular pp. 76–84 and 93–7). Changing attitudes is a necessary but not a sufficient condition for changing behaviour. However, compared with most approaches to safety training, for example those based upon cognitive (e.g. attitude change) or knowledge-based (examination, assessment and authorization – for example Health and Safety Commission, 1990b), that which goes under the heading of behaviour modification is perhaps more readily appraised. Thus, it is unsurprising to find a profusion of studies in this area. As these have been extensively reviewed elsewhere, only some examples from illustrative studies will be outlined. In most of these studies, links between learning and training, for example through behaviour modification, and motivation (chapter 3) emerge strongly. Sulzer-Azaroff's (1982) review of some two dozen studies is mirrored by that of McAfee and Winn (1989) who report findings from the same number of studies which examined the effectiveness of positive reinforcement and feedback and found that all revealed some success in improving safety or reducing accidents. Petersen (1989) reviewed 26 studies, many of them the same as those in McAfee and Winn (1989). Becker and Janz (1987) undertook a comparable review of studies of health risk appraisal, and advocate feedback of health-related information, for example in the form of counselling, as part of a programme of cognitive and behavioural interventions. Weiss *et al.* (1991) describe a number of health promotion programmes. Glendon (1991) reviews three studies of safe behaviour

Summary text 2.11 Using a model of behaviour in the face of danger (after Hale and Glendon, 1987) to identify training objectives and limitations

Using a logical model, in this case comprising a series of steps in recognizing and controlling danger (whether in the form of potential long-term health damage or a short-term safety emergency), it is possible to identify operator requirements and corresponding training objectives as well as training methods and limitations in outline for each performance level represented by types of external triggers. To illustrate this process, examples at each of the three performance levels (see summary text 2.7) are given.

Performance level – skill-based.
External trigger – programmed or insistent danger signals (e.g. an alarm).
Individual/operator requirements – recognize signals, execute response correctly.
Illustrative training objectives – recognize danger signals from background noise; separate danger from non-danger signals; execute correct response when required, but not at other times; not execute incorrect response.
Illustrative training methods – laboratory training (e.g. vigilance tasks); simulation; behaviour modification; CAL; on-the-job experience.
Training limitations – humans are imperfect and will occasionally make mistakes (chapter 9, pp. 244–61); and thus, for critical tasks, system back-up will be required – especially under high stress conditions.

Performance level – rules-based.
External trigger – obvious warning (e.g. burning smell – safety warning; high blood pressure – health warning).
Individual/operator requirements – know correct procedure; accept responsibility for implementing procedure; choose correct procedure; execute correct procedure.
Illustrative training objectives – know correct procedure and when to take personal responsibility for implementing this; choose and execute correct procedure.
Illustrative training methods – use of diagnostic checks; use of PTW system; expert system (if available); feedback from personal health programme; demonstration; job instruction; video instruction; programmed learning; job rotation (planned experience).
Training limitations – humans can make errors when following sets of rules (chapter 9, pp. 244–61); interruptions can disrupt even well-learned sequences.

Performance level – knowledge-based.
External trigger – need to test for danger known (e.g. understanding nature of possible harm that could occur as a threat to health or safety – i.e. correct danger labelling).
Individual/operator requirements – responsibility for testing accepted; correct test chosen; test correctly executed; need for action recognized; responsibility for action accepted or allocated; correct plan or procedure chosen; plan or procedure correctly executed.
Illustrative training objectives – ensure that managers, supervisors and operatives understand their health and safety responsibilities, can formulate appropriate plans and procedures in respect of health and safety and can execute these plans and procedures as appropriate.
Illustrative training methods – individual coaching; assignments and projects; lectures; group discussion, exercise, games, role-playing, etc.; 'discovery method'.
Training limitations – breadth of potential knowledge to be covered is so great as to mean that some aspects will inevitably be missed for at least some trainees. Thus, there is the possibility that latent – or system – errors (chapter 9, pp. 244–61) or 'resident pathogens' (Reason, 1990) will remain. Training must be supplemented by adequate management operating systems.

modification, as does Zohar (1980b), all of the latter involving increasing use of ear plugs, two using a token reward system (in which tokens are given as secondary reinforcers which could be exchanged for goods or services) and the other using feedback.

Studies of safety behaviour modification include those by: Smith *et al.* (1978) and Zohar *et al.* (1980), both of which used information feedback as a powerful reinforcer to overcome barriers associated with PPE use. Sulzer-Azaroff and De Santamaria (1980) used supervisor feedback and found that hazard frequencies dropped by 60%. Komaki *et al.* (1980) showed workers slides of safe and unsafe behaviour to demonstrate the importance of providing feedback after training and that knowledge (of hazards) alone is not enough. In Chhokar's (1987) study, training consisted of showing slides depicting safe and unsafe behaviour. Motivation was provided by periodic feedback on performance and praise from supervisors. However, the initial increase in safety performance returned to previous levels when feedback was discontinued. Haynes *et al.* (1982) used a combination of daily feedback on accident-free driving, team competition and frequent low-cost incentives (cash, free passes for relatives, free fuel) to reduce accidents among urban transit operators in a US city. They indicated that, although the variables were confounded, it might be possible to phase out the incentives, leaving feedback and competition as an effective long-term strategy. Hopkins *et al.* (1986) used simple on-the-job training and maintenance procedures to change the behaviour of workers exposed to styrene. Warg's (1990) use of feedback techniques to change risk behaviour successfully in a slaughter-house indicates that safe behaviour modification techniques continue to be reported.

A number of authors have provided overviews of safe behaviour modification (also referred to as behavioural safety programmes or applied behaviour analysis). Chhokar (1987) describes the essence of this approach as being the observation, analysis and measurement of behaviour and how it changes. Reber *et al.* (1989) describe the stages of a behavioural safety programme as being:

1. identify safe and unsafe acts;
2. train employees to recognize each of these;
3. motivation – e.g. goal setting with feedback or incentives.

Summarizing requirements for success of safety training, Cohen *et al.* (1979) consider these to be:

1. positive approaches that stress the learning of safe behaviours – not the avoidance of unsafe acts;
2. suitable conditions for practice that ensure their resistance to stress, etc.;
3. include the means for evaluating training effectiveness, including feedback.

More detailed reviews are provided by Petersen (1984), Krause *et al.* (1990a) and, more specifically on safety training, ReVelle (1980).

Although a large number of studies have now reported successful behaviour change interventions in respect of health and safety risk behaviours, it can still be argued that such interventions are likely to be less cost-effective than engineered controls. This point is considered in greater detail in chapter 10, pp. 298–312 (in particular summary text 10.4).

SAFETY TRAINING AND SAFETY CULTURE

Just as there is a strategic context for the overall objectives and thrust of safety training within an organization, so there must be strategic direction to the shape, format and methods of safety training. Once it has been established what role safety training will play within the organizations's overall strategy, the components can be planned. The principles and objectives of safety training may be enshrined within a good safety policy, although this may not be sufficiently detailed to provide guidance for the structure and format of safety training. Warburton (1986) identifies a number of features of safety training which are associated with good safety (and other) performance:

- identification of training needs and target groups;
- feedback of accident and inspection data into safety training programme design;
- periodic monitoring/review of training for effects (i.e. evaluation);
- provision for updating amendment;
- assessment of training providers' ability;
- involvement/consultation of employees/representatives in development/evaluation;
- management commitment to safety training clearly stated in safety policy.

The importance given to, and the effectiveness of, safety training are among the key aspects of safety climate (Glennon, 1980, 1982; Zohar, 1980a), although the term 'safety culture' is now more generally used and is discussed in more detail in chapter 10, pp. 291–5. To open their first report on training and related matters, The Advisory Committee on the Safety of Nuclear Installations Study Group on Human Factors expressed the view that, 'The main priority for training so far as safety is concerned is the creation of a "Safety Culture"' (HSC, 1990). In practice this may mean a variety of things (chapter 10, pp. 292–3). The safety culture of an organization comprises the combination of employee attitudes, values and behaviours which reflect the commitment and actions of its management to safety.

An important component of a positive safety culture is top management commitment to safety. One way of expressing management commitment to safety training is for them to be involved, both as participants and as trainers. This might be done through a hierarchical or cascade approach to safety training. For example, in one large organization, as part of a realignment of safety culture, all senior managers – from the chairman down – were required to attend a three-day strategic safety management course, the 30 or so initial courses taking a year to complete. Each course concluded with a one-hour exam and workbook assessment, both of which trainees were required to pass, and input from a board member or other senior manager. On successful

Summary text 2.12 Using accident data to help formulate safety training strategy

This case example relates to the assessment of training needs over the employment life cycle and illustrates how one of the features identified by Warburton (1986) – see text – may be used as the basis for a safety training programme. The graph shown in the figure is derived from the all-accident rate (per 1000 employees) for a large UK organization averaged over two years. The data reveal a classic pattern of accidents over the population employed there. Accident rates are highest for the youngest – aged up to 24 years – workers, before falling at first fairly steeply and then more steadily to their lowest point – the 40–44 years age group – with a brief upward excursion along the way. They then start to rise again to retirement age, although never reach the rate of the youngest groups. A similar pattern, with variations, may be found in most industry sectors, where there are sufficiently large numbers of employees to calculate meaningful accident rates.

Graph showing 2 years' accident rates for different age groups in a large organization

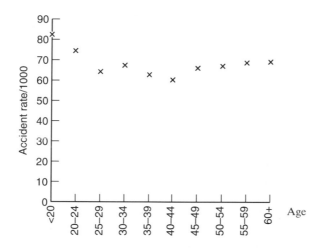

How might these data be used as an ingredient in devising a safety training strategy? A first step would be to divide the data into a number of sections, depending upon what is happening to the figures. An argument could be made for a division into 5 groups. The paragraphs below briefly review the broad descriptions of each of these age groups and possible training implications (in italics). Clearly, these are generalizations which would not apply to all individuals within each group, but which can provide useful guidance on safety training strategy for each group.

Group 1: Up to 24 years, accident rates are at their highest, as is shown in a number of studies (for a review, see Hale and Hale, 1986). Workers here are characterized by relative ignorance of hazards, immaturity and inexperience.

Induction training is critical, backed up by careful supervision to ensure that young workers do not attempt to replicate too early the skills – and perhaps poor work habits – exhibited by older colleagues.

Group 2: For the 25–29-year-old group, there is a relatively sharp decline in the accident rate as workers acquire the necessary skills and risk perception to work relatively more safely.

Summary text 2.12 (continued)

A strategic implication would be to consider involving workers in this age group in training younger workers. This would help to consolidate the skills and knowledge which they have now acquired as well as helping to alert them to the dangers of complacency with respect to hazards.

Group 3: The accident rate swings temporarily upward again for the 30–34 years age group – a typical mid-career 'blip', possibly due to complacency with respect to hazards which workers are now getting used to as well as testing their skills to the limit, perhaps to compete with younger workers.

This is an opportunity for refresher training in safety matters, perhaps using case studies and near miss incident reports as an aid to guard against complacency and as a reminder of continuing workplace hazards.

Group 4: For the 35–44 years age group, the accident rate reaches its lowest point as workers achieve positions of responsibility with maturity and greater knowledge.

Opportunities are likely to exist at this stage of involving workers in supervision and training of younger workers to pass on valuable experience and knowledge.

Group 5: Accident rates at the final stage of the career cycle (45+ years) rise again, although fairly gradually perhaps as physical and mental facilities decline with advancing years.

Retraining for changed work tasks and refresher training as well as involvement in training others are all likely to have a place here. Sensitive training and counselling for graceful degradation of faculties is also likely to be appropriate.

---

completion of this course, managers could then select from a range of other modules according to their particular needs, for example: risk analysis, hazard management, and management of contractors. Other managers and supervisors were required to take a safety management foundation course. This is an example of an organization taking a structured approach to safety training. Another example, in this case of how an organization might use input from its accident data as a guide to safety training policy, is given in summary text 2.12. The example accords with Hale's (1984) indication that a systematic basis for safety training can help to reduce accident rates.

CONCLUSIONS

It is important for employers to consider training, including safety training, as an investment in effective use of human resources and not as a cost. In this context, training requires a strategic framework for proper implementation. As for any training, it is important to set realistic, credible, achievable and measurable objectives for safety training and to realize the importance of a logical sequence within which safety training is incorporated. Several frameworks for determining the provision of training have been proposed – for example, corporate strategy, risk management, models of the accident process or individual differences such as age, as well as a more pragmatic approach (what has worked for others) or a combination of approaches. One of the most demonstrably successful approaches to safety training in terms of positive evaluation from controlled studies, is that of behaviour modification, which like other aspects of safety training, is closely linked with motivation (chapter 3).

Although individuals have preferred combinations of learning styles, application of general learning principles to training is likely to enhance outcomes. These principles include: motivation (intrinsic and extrinsic), feedback (e.g. knowledge of results), positive reinforcement, overlearning (of skills), whole task training (as for rule following sequences), brainstorming or lateral thinking (for original or novel solutions to new problems), active trainee involvement (including rehearsal), understanding as a basis for learning about a system, and incorporating learning from experience – both direct and indirect (e.g. using case studies).

Although training, education and development may have different time scales and objectives, there is considerable overlap between them. For many purposes they may be regarded as elements of the same continuum and all are aspects of learning and the acquisition of competencies in health and safety. It may be useful to distinguish between longer-term training – for example for the health and safety profession, and short-term, for example to develop or enhance a particular skill. Different training requirements will exist at the different performance levels – skills, rules and knowledge – and different methods and limitations are also likely to apply at the different levels.   Most aspects of health and safety should be addressed with reference to safety training, which should be considered as part of safety culture (chapter 10, pp. 291–5). However, safety training cannot be a substitute for good safety policies and practices, but rather should support these. Thus, it is important to be aware of the limits of any form of training and of what it can and cannot reasonably be expected to achieve.

PART TWO
Individual Factors

3 MOTIVATING AND REWARDING SAFE BEHAVIOUR

❏ This chapter considers meanings of the term 'motivation' and discusses the various approaches to it that have been advanced by psychologists over the years. Attention is then directed at the specific topic of work motivation before motivating for safety is addressed in a focused way. Key concepts and examples are given in this important section. The chapter opens the door to a consideration of attitudes, perception and personality in the following three chapters on individual factors.

INTRODUCTION

The objectives of this chapter are to:

- explain what human motivation is;
- outline the main approaches to motivation and reward;
- demonstrate the relevance of different approaches to motivation to safety and risk management;
- synthesize principles in providing guidance for safety motivation as a component of risk management programmes.

The early part of the chapter reviews motivation as psychologists and others have studied it. It is relevant to have some grasp of the different perspectives because this helps understanding of the various meanings of the term 'motivation'. The later part of the chapter draws upon this material to derive practical health and safety applications.

Motivation is the basis for nearly all human behaviour. This means that most of our actions are governed, or at least strongly shaped, by our motives. Exceptions include occasions when our actions are genuinely involuntary – as when we react to the experience of intense pain (or pleasure) or move quickly to avoid imminent danger. Even such responses as these – sometimes called 'instinctive' – can be suppressed by a determined person. In such cases, we might consider that the person is motivated not to reveal their 'natural' reaction to pain (as a footballer or boxer might do so as not to give advantage to an opponent) or to combat their personal fear of danger (it has been alleged that the truly brave are not those who are 'fearless' but rather those who feel fear but who strive to overcome it). Motives which shape these behaviours include self-esteem or ego defence (acts designed to defend ourselves against real or imagined threats). Thus, human motivation is a powerful force, taking many forms and expressions.

Because of the centrality of motivation to human behaviour, it is important that everyone who has an interest – either as students (in the broadest sense) or as practitioners – in understanding why people behave as they do should have some awareness of the range of human behaviour which is influenced by motivation. Specifically, if we are to understand how motivation and reward factors operate in the field of risks to health and safety, then some appreciation of the routes by which motivation has come to its present status is useful.

WHAT IS MOTIVATION?

Advertisements frequently appear in the safety press, stating for example that 'Opportunities exist for self-motivated health and safety professionals...'. Can health and safety professionals – or any employees – be 'self-motivated'? What does this term mean? What can theories of motivation tell us about accident likelihood? What about reducing the likelihood of accidents using motivational techniques such as incentive programmes or the manipulation of rewards and expectations? This chapter considers these and related issues.

Motivation, like 'personality' or 'intelligence', is a term which has a number of meanings. We shall consider psychological approaches to motivation and concentrate upon those aspects which have greatest relevance to the management of safety and risk. However, a number of dictionary meanings for motivation exist.

First, there is the notion of **movement** – essentially to do with behaviour. Second, motivation embodies the idea of **energy**, implying direction or focus. Together, these two components comprise the concept of **motive force** – to get up and **do** something. However, another meaning for the term is that of **self-interest**, that we are motivated to do some things but not others because of the benefits which this will bring to us – implying a purposeful or cognitive (meaning knowing or 'of the mind') component. Finally, there is the notion of **volition** – behaviour which is driven by particular needs but which is engaged in voluntarily. Could it be a combination of all these meanings which the advertisement is seeking in applicants?

These everyday meanings for motivation are parallelled by research and theorizing by psychologists and others and are discussed in this chapter. Motivation is a central concept in psychology (first used in the 1880s) and is a key to understanding human behaviour. Links between motivation and other human attributes (some of these are discussed in other chapters) are shown in figure 3.1.

As a rule of thumb, we will treat motivation as being 'what makes people tick'. In doing so, we will review the concept of motivation in four overlapping phases. The first of these phases is the **mechanistic** and refers to early ideas about motivation. Central to mechanistic approaches to motivation is the

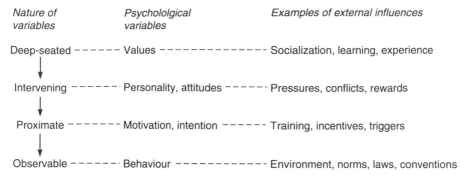

Figure 3.1 Psychological variables and influences.

notion that motivational states, primarily **instinct**, are **inborn** and that, as a consequence, individuals are the victims of uncontrollable inner forces and urges.

The second major phase, the **behaviourist**, continues to exert considerable influence upon motivation. This may be seen in a number of behaviour modification studies in workplace safety which were considered in chapter 2 (pp. 25–7). In behaviourist parlance, behaviour is motivated by **drive reduction** and individual motivation is fuelled by tension to reduce drives and thence to **satisfy basic needs**. Other motivational concepts associated with behaviourist approaches to motivation are **habit**, **reinforcement**, **reward** and **punishment**.

The most recently developed approach to human motivation is the **cognitive** (relating to knowing or understanding). This approach to understanding human behaviour is the main alternative to the behaviourist way of thinking. The essence of the cognitive approach to motivation is that human behaviour is **purposeful** and that the mainspring is human desire to master the environment rather than to be controlled by it – as in the behaviourist approach, or to be at the mercy of deep seated emotions as in the mechanistic tradition. Concepts which are central to the cognitive approach to motivated behaviour are concerned with **predicting** what will happen and thereby exerting some individual **control** over important events.

Finally, traversing both behaviourism and cognition, there is an important **applied** tradition in motivation in which central concepts are **change** and **influence** over behaviour. Applied approaches seek to understand specific cases of motivated behaviour. A good example of a specific orientation to motivation is that of the work environment. Another is the study of purchase motivations in consumer behaviour – why people buy particular goods and brands. Other examples include individual cognitive differences in motivation as well as motivation in learning and development (relevant to training applications – chapter 2). A final example, which is the focus of this chapter, is motivated behaviour in the field of safety and risk-taking.

Before turning to the safety environment and some of the findings which have shaped thinking in this field, we consider briefly the traditions which have influenced current stances on motivation. More comprehensive reviews can be found in texts on motivation (for example, Weiner, 1992).

THE MECHANISTIC TRADITION

We devote little space to this approach to motivation, although it is relevant to record that remnants of its influence continue to pervade our thinking and language, sometimes inappropriately. For example, a football commentator talks about a goalkeeper making an 'instinctive save'. This is incorrect because humans do not have an inborn predisposition to prevent footballs from entering nets – any more than they do for kicking, throwing, placing or striking them with a variety of objects so that they reach a specified target. What is actually being referred to in this case is highly skilled behaviour which has been **learned**, and this is an important distinction.

What is instinctive – in humans and in other animals – is the propensity to avoid painful or noxious stimuli, such as temperature extremes, loud noises or choking gases. Behaviour which corresponds with these instincts may be observed in all humans (who have all their faculties and senses) when exposed to such stimuli. Thus, we all have a relatively small number of inborn 'harm avoidance' mechanisms which are designed to protect us from environmental excesses. A study which demonstrates the influence of such instinctive behaviour is that of the 'visual cliff' in which a crawling baby refuses to cross to its mother over a piece of strong glass through which it can see a drop of several feet (Gibson and Walk, 1960).

One interesting observation about instinctive behaviour is human capacity for over-riding aspects of it through learning experiences and the acquisition of certain skills. For example, fire-fighters develop skills which enable them to enter burning buildings, steeplejacks learn how to operate at heights, and workers in a wide range of occupations learn that it is possible to work in noisy or otherwise dangerous environments if the correct equipment is used. These are examples of how humans have developed ways of countering their instincts to fear or to avoid harmful stimuli. Occasionally, our learning becomes too sophisticated and we forget or disregard our original instinctive reaction – for example to heights – and this failure to respect natural dangers can result in behaviour which leads to death or other sad consequences (for an example, see summary text 3.1).

Thus, innate mechanisms which determine behaviour are the starting point for considering motivation. Instinct determines primitive forms of behaviour, which in turn can be overlaid by voluntary and intelligent behaviour. Thus, the notion of instinct, while retaining some influence (for example, in recognition of 'crimes of passion') has been overtaken by other approaches to motivated behaviour.

THE BEHAVIOURIST ERA

Behaviourist approaches to motivation emerged out of the mechanistic tradition and the term 'motivation' gained widespread acceptance by the 1930s. As

Summary text 3.1 A tragic event

One of the authors, while visiting another country during the summer of 1992, was watching (from the ground) bungee jumping – in which participants hurl themselves off a platform, perhaps 80–100 feet above the ground with an elasticated rope attached, usually to their ankles and feet, sometimes to the body. The rope – adjusted for the weight of the jumper – is designed to allow the person to end up swinging a few feet from the ground (or water). One would-be participant 'chickened out' on reaching the platform – his instinctive fear of heights had over-ridden his attempt to overcome that fear – motivated by a desire to impress his friends below. The 19-year-old assistant on the platform, wishing to demonstrate to the would-be bungee jumper that the jump would be quite safe, proceeded to attach the rope to his own ankles before leaping off the platform.

Unfortunately, the other end of the elasticated rope had become detached from its anchorage point and continued to play out so that the young man hurtled tragically to his death. In this case, the behaviour, motivated by a desire to show the would-be jumper that the experience would be safe – and to encourage others to follow so that the commercial basis of the venture would be sustained, omitted a critical step in the safety sequence. Assuming that, because he had jumped a number of times before and therefore had the required skill, and caught up in the immediate objective, the young man had over-ridden his instinctive fear which was designed to alert him to the danger.

with the approach to motivation through instinct, in the behaviourist approach thought processes were largely ignored and only simple behaviour was studied.

Early behavioural experiments on motivation were mainly carried out on animals – particularly rats and monkeys, largely responsible for the traditional image of the white-coated psychologist running laboratory white rats through a maze to a plate of food. Most of the studies were concerned with deprivation of food or water or with applying aversive stimuli – particularly electric shocks – and this popular stereotype of the behaviourist psychologist proved to be particularly resistant to extinction. The irony here is that one of the main dependent variables (outcomes which are measured by scientists) of these experiments was resistance of behaviour to extinction, i.e. how long an animal continued to engage in a behaviour when a reward such as food, which had been forthcoming before, was no longer in the expected place. Other dependent variables used in these studies included the amount of consummatory behaviour (e.g. eating, drinking or, if the animals were really lucky, sexual activity) and speed of learning.

Given the nature of early behaviourist research into animal behaviour, bordering as it did on the instinct approach, is it not surprising that this approach to motivated behaviour was dubbed the 'Four Fs' – feeding, fleeing, fighting and mating behaviour! Another suggestion was that organisms were motivated to engage in arousal-seeking behaviour, such as risk-taking, problem-solving and seeking adventure or excitement. The notion of optimal arousal level for performance is an important one and is summarized in figure 3.2. The concept of arousal is linked with that of stress, considered in chapter 8.

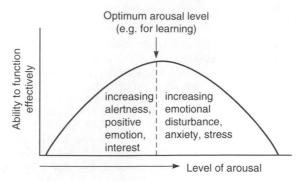

Figure 3.2 Ability to function effectively dependent upon level of arousal.

Skinner, a well-known behaviourist, urged a rigorous explanation for motivated behaviour. He defined the main behaviourist concepts thus:

- **drive** – the motivational factor that makes an activity occur;
- **reinforcer** – the incentive which determines behaviour;
- **goal direction** – observable, purposive aspects of behaviour.

Goals can be seen as reinforcers which shape responses – this constituted **learning** for behaviourists.

Positive reinforcers were things which increased the probability of response – e.g. expecting to find food after completing a task such as running a maze. Negative reinforcers were things which decreased the probability of response – e.g. receiving an electric shock if a lever is pressed reduces the likelihood that the lever will be pressed again. However, to avoid confusion between behaviour motivated by avoiding a negative stimulus (e.g. electric shock) and applying the same negative stimulus as a result of carrying out an action, an important distinction came to be made between negative reinforcement and punishment. Thus, negative reinforcement is now described as motivating behaviour to avoid a negative stimulus – e.g. climbing onto a platform to avoid an electric shock from the floor of a cage. Thus, negative reinforcers also increase the probability of response – and may act in concert with positive reinforcers – as in a 'carrot and stick' approach. Punishment is any unpleasant stimulus – e.g. inflicting pain – which occurs **after** a given behaviour.

This discussion of behaviourist attempts to explain motivation is of more than historical interest for it reveals the difficulty which early researchers had in understanding the concept of motivation and thus its complexity. It also highlights the difficulty which we have in discarding inadequate concepts and explanations for behaviour and our reluctance to consider new approaches and ways of looking at behaviour. Behaviourism has bequeathed a number of useful motivational concepts – particularly those of reinforcement, incentive and reward – which are much used in applied fields, such as safety and risk management and work motivation as well as learning (chapter 2, especially pp. 15–23 and 25–7). However, it has also revealed the inadequacy of studying animal behaviour if the ultimate goal is to understand the complexities of human behaviour and motivation. Thus, the onset of a more human-oriented approach to motivation (and learning) which took account of human factors such as intelligence, personality and perception, could not be forestalled indefinitely.

GENERAL THEORIES OF MOTIVATION

The roots of the cognitive approach to studying motivation and learning can be traced back to elements of earlier theorizing. For example, the notion of 'cognitive mapping' was developed by Tolman (1959) to explain the mechanism by which rats ran a maze. The idea was that the rat had a mental picture which it used to run the maze, in the same way as we have cognitive maps for our neighbourhood, workplace and other locations which we visit frequently and which we can find our way about in without difficulty. Thus, the notion that cognitions – such as perception, memory, learning and problem-solving – were important in motivated behaviour, was not new.

However, during the 1950s and 1960s, when the behaviourist approach was recognized as being inadequate but before cognitive theories had been sufficiently developed to replace it, there were a number of attempts to build general theories of human motivation. In a sense, these were in the Freudian tradition in that they were concerned with **human** (not animal) behaviour and they were general insofar as they purported to provide explanations for behaviour which were based upon a single central idea. However, unlike Freud's instinct-based theory of motivation, these were hybrid theories – with elements of behaviourism, cognition and occasionally even instinct within them.

Lewin's (1951) field theory had its origins in the Gestalt tradition (the idea of 'wholeness' as a guiding principle for perception or learning). Field theory held hedonistic (pleasure seeking) assumptions about motivated human behaviour and was probably more behaviourist than cognitive, but the essential equation was that:

$$Behaviour = f(person \times environment)$$

It thus diverged from the behaviourist tradition in recognizing the individual as an **active** agent in behaviour, while the cognitive dimension in field theory is represented by the idea of **life space** – which is the psychological field in which the individual operates. An example of this is shown in figure 3.3 and described in summary text 3.2.

The life space consists of a series of obstacles which the individual must overcome in order to achieve his or her goals. In traversing this life space, individuals encounter a number of choice points and these can involve three different types of conflicts. These are described in summary text 3.3.

While field theory contains ideas which appear to translate readily into everyday individual experience, it is not a complete theory of motivation because many aspects of behaviour cannot readily be incorporated within it. For example, it ignores arousal-seeking behaviour, so that day-to-day instances of problem-solving or risk-taking are excluded.

Summary text 3.2 Narrative for figure 3.3

Figure 3.3 shows diagrammatically the life space of a student of safety and risk management, whose ambition is to reach the dizzy heights of the Risk Manager's position. Our young trainee has a plan – like an extended cognitive map (see text for explanation) of his or her future – for achieving that ambition. This consists of passing the relevant exams next year before negotiating the hurdles of work experience and promotions over an estimated 15-year period before being in a position to apply for, and hopefully be selected for the Risk Manager's job. Could this be the meaning of the advertisement requiring 'self-motivated' individuals for the safety professional's post?

A person with ambition who can be motivated by the idea of their own career progression may well be considered to be self-motivated. In field theory terms, the *tension* multiplied by the psychological distance from the desired object (the Risk Manager's job) results in the desired object having a *valence* (incentive value). This creates a *force field* and the force (as in 'may the force be with you') acts upon the individual to move them towards the goal object. When the goal is attained, tension is released, the valence and force is reduced and behaviour towards the goal ceases (our subject retains the Risk Manager's job to retirement). However, there are individual differences so that some people would be satisfied while others would want to achieve still more. As George Bernard Shaw noted, 'There are two tragedies in life. One is to lose your heart's desire, the other is to gain it' (*Man and Superman*).

The next general theory of motivation to be briefly considered is that of Murray (1938). Showing the influence of Freud, Murray postulated a list of **needs** as the basis for human motivation. These were at two levels – the fundamental needs which were called viscerogenic and some 40 non-fundamental needs, termed psychogenic. This attempt to translate the idea of instincts into a need-driven theory of motivation might have remained in obscurity if it had not been developed by one of the best known motivation theorists – Abraham Maslow (1954).

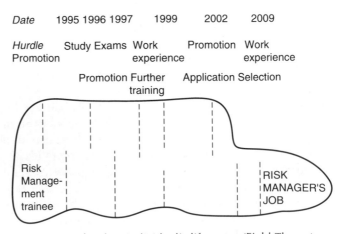

Figure 3.3 Example of an individual's life space (Field Theory).

Summary text 3.3 Conflicts in field theory

The first type of conflict is an approach–approach conflict. This consists of two equally desirable options – for example, while applying for promotion within the company, our subject also applies for other jobs to further his or her career and suddenly finds that s/he has the possibility of promotion within the present company and a job offer from another employer. Both options are attractive (hence approach–approach) but the situation is unstable – i.e. it cannot persist because one of the offers must soon be accepted – either to seek progression within a known environment or to broaden experience by seeking pastures new.

The second type of conflict is approach–avoidance and happens when an option has both pleasant and unpleasant aspects. For example, our subject take the job at the other company where pay and conditions are better but soon finds that the workload has increased to the point where considerable stress is being experienced. Some aspects of the job are enjoyable, but the work pressure is unrelenting. Nevertheless, with career prospects in mind, our subject sticks with the job on the grounds that such experience is probably necessary to future prospects and that to leave soon after taking the job would not look good on the cv. Thus, approach–avoidance conflicts are stable once a decision has been made about how to resolve them.

The third type of conflict is avoidance–avoidance, in which there are two equally unpleasant options. The new company has been taken over and is being radically restructured. The new regime looks threatening to our subject's position and it is very clear that a job in the newly structured company will be of a lesser status than the present one – thereby setting back career ambitions as well as reducing job satisfaction. Attempts to seek work elsewhere have not proved successful, although a small amount of redundancy money has been offered if s/he wishes to leave. The money would not last long and the prospect of unemployment with a young family, even if there is a chance of finding a job soon, is not at all appealing. Such avoidance–avoidance conflicts, while being hard to resolve, are stable because the individual continues to be torn between the options, even if one has eventually to be chosen.

Maslow's hierarchy of needs also shows the influence of the Gestalt school – seeking wholeness in explanation – as well as that of Freud in which needs exist because they serve a **function** for the individual. Its intuitive appeal has captured the imagination like no other theory of motivation and its all-embracing nature spans aspects of instinct, cognition and philosophy.

In Maslow's theory, the remnants of instinct reinforce basic needs, which in turn are overwhelmed by culture and learning. The cognitive aspect is revealed through individuals **choosing** their needs – thereby exerting some control over their life. Philosophically, the theory is within the humanist tradition of maintaining basic human rights and it is the only theory of motivation which admits to a normative basis – to seek a better world. Maslow, in his concern for individuals' psychological health, maintains that the possession and gratification of needs is essential in avoiding psychological illness.

Maslow acknowledges that there are determinants of behaviour other than needs and desires, for example cultural norms and expectations. In addition, the theory is developmental because it is concerned with individual growth and maturation. The hierarchy of needs is proposed on the basis of prepotency – so that in general, lower-order needs must be satisfied before higher-order needs become potent. However, it is recognized that ideals and values (e.g. for truth, beauty or for a religious or political cause) can over-ride all needs. Neither is the hierarchy immutable, for example some people may crave esteem from others in preference to having the ostensibly lower-order needs of love satisfied. Others may be capable of self-actualizing (the peak of the hierarchy, deemed to be the right of all but reached by few) despite a lack of basic needs being satisfied. Maslow's well-known hierarchy of needs is outlined in summary text 3.4, which also describes Alderfer's classes of needs.

While Maslow's theory is widely known and much cited, it is not without its criticisms. For example, Wahba and Bridwell (1976) identify a number of flaws in need theories such as Maslow's which mean that they are not useful for guidance on motivating individuals, for example at work. As with its predecessors, Maslow's theory lacks essential empirical verification, although some aspects have received support (Williams and Page, 1989). It is general to the extent that it can make no practical predictions for any given individual and there is thus a trade-off between the comprehensiveness of the theory and specifying predictions. Finally, it is culture-bound to individualistic style cultures such as those typical of Western capitalism in which the individual is the basic unit (as opposed to group or culture).

Another theory to be considered is the achievement-motivation theory of

---

Summary text 3.4 Maslow's hierarchy of needs

1. **Physiological needs** (drives) – e.g. hunger, thirst.
2. **Safety needs** – in the sense of stability, dependency, protection, freedom from fear, anxiety or chaos, etc. Need for structure, order, law, etc. – best seen in children. In adults, it may only be seen in emergencies or in certain forms of neurotic behaviour (e.g. obsessive). In healthy adults, knowledge, familiarity and personal skills serve to neutralize most dangers.
3. **Belongingness** – giving and receiving love.
4. **Esteem** – of two kinds, from:

   - **inside** the individual – represented as a desire for strength, achievement, adequacy, mastery, competence, confidence, independence and freedom (cognitive elements);
   - **outside** the individual – reputation, prestige, status, fame, glory, dominance, recognition, attention, importance, dignity and appreciation (influences: Adler, McClelland).

5. **Self-actualization** – desire for self-fulfilment; here are found the greatest individual differences; self-actualizers are held to be self-movers (i.e. self-motivated).

   According to Sugarman (1986), self-actualizing people have firm moral standards, are objective, creative, accepting of themselves and others, spontaneous, secure and autonomous, and have close relationships with and respect for others.

Alderfer (1972) proposed three classes of need:

- existence (equates to Maslow's levels 1 and 2);
- relatedness (belongingness and esteem from others);
- growth (self-esteem and self-actualization).

McClelland *et al.* (1953). This cognitive theory is at least partly behaviourist. Thus, **need achievement** (known as NAch) replaces the notion of drive, **expectancy** is instead of habit strength and **pay-off** substitutes for reinforcement. As in mainstream behaviourism, assumptions for behaviour are essentially hedonistic and there is a general lack of emphasis upon mental events.

Need achievement theory assumes that the likelihood of attaining a goal is mediated by the individual's perception of the task and the final achievement-related response. It maintains that achievement-related behaviour results from a conflict between hope of success (approach motivation) on the one hand and fear of failure (avoidance motivation) on the other. Resultant behaviour is explained by reference to the formula:

Behaviour = f(Achievement-related needs – e.g. NAch and failure anxiety **and** Expectancy of success and failure – e.g. probability estimates **and** Incentive value of success and failure – e.g. rewards and punishments).

Cassidy and Lynn (1989) describe need for achievement as comprising:

- work ethic – motivation to achieve based upon a belief that performance per se is 'good';
- pursuit of excellence – the desire to perform to the best of one's ability;
- status aspirations – desire to climb the status hierarchy and to dominate others;
- competitiveness – desire to compete with and to beat others;
- acquisitiveness – money/wealth;
- mastery – achieve competence against established standards.

Need achievement theory is also a primitive personality theory (chapter 6) because it also emphasizes individual differences – specifically that individuals differ in their need for achievement, some being high in NAch and others low. As Sir John Vanburgh wrote, 'The want of a thing is perplexing enough, but the possession of it is intolerable' (*The Confederacy*). A consistent finding is that high NAch individuals prefer tasks of intermediate difficulty with an approximately even chance of succeeding because of the challenge involved and the opportunity to test their skills and personal worth. Conversely, low NAch individuals prefer to tackle **either** easy **or** difficult tasks. Why should this be so? For an explanation, see summary text 3.5.

A four-country study undertaken by McClelland found that executives in sales and marketing were primarily characterized by high NAch, while those in production, engineering and finance were more likely to display low NAch characteristics. Whether safety and risk professionals have a tendency to one or the other may well depend upon what type of a role the individual perceives it is necessary to play. Is risk management to do with finding engineering solutions to problems or is it more akin to marketing those solutions? Most probably, it is a combination of these.

Most recently, Klein (1989) proposed control theory as a linking motivation framework which seeks to integrate the various approaches to motivation. Its

---

Summary text 3.5 High and low achievers

High NAch individuals are characterized by continual striving to test their skills and abilities. Therefore, tasks or jobs which they perceive to be within their range of competency will be sought out and undertaken so as to give maximum feedback on their skills and abilities. For low NAch people on the other hand, there is no such striving for testing or feedback and they select either easy tasks because of the high likelihood of success, or difficult tasks where the expectancy of failure is in any case high. Thus, neither situation is a real test of their skills or abilities. An epitaph to a low NAch might read:

> They said it couldn't be done,
> He said he'd go right to it,
> He tackled the thing that couldn't be done ...
> And couldn't do it.

There are also differences between high and low NAch people in respect of the differential effects of success and failure upon their motivation to perform a task. Thus, for high NAch individuals success **decreases** motivation – they have achieved something and now want to go on to do something else, the 'been there, done that' syndrome. However, failure for high NAch people **increases** motivation – stemming from the determination not to be beaten by a task, the 'if at first you don't succeed, try, try and try again' philosophy.

However, for low NAch individuals, success enhances motivation – even if this is at an easy task, whereas failure inhibits motivation – i.e. when difficult tasks are attempted. Thus, the composite picture is one of high NAch individuals continually seeking tasks to match and thereby test their competencies, while low NAch people are either aiming too high or too low in their activities because they have no need to, or have a fear of, testing their competencies. One of the significant aspects of this motivation theory is that it incorporates individual differences, albeit fairly crude ones. Could it be that it is a high NAch person that was being sought in the advertising copy cited earlier in this chapter?

---

basis is that a person assesses his/her present state and compares this with a desired state. If there is a discrepancy, then behaviour is motivated to reduce the discrepancy. The person also considers whether the discrepancy is due to internal (i.e. to do with the person) or external (e.g. to do with others or to the environment) factors, whether the cause is long-term (e.g. relating to the person's desired state of health) or short-term (e.g. representing an immediate threat to the person's safety) and whether it is controllable by them (see also the discussion on risk perception in chapter 5, pp. 121–30. A more detailed description of Klein's integrated model can be found in Arnold *et al.* (1991).

THE COGNITIVE REVOLUTION: ATTRIBUTION THEORY

The essence of the cognitive approach to behaviour is that individuals are **involved** in understanding and interpreting their environment as essential antecedents (e.g. motivators) to action. Thus, cognitive processes (such as attitudes, motives and beliefs) **mediate** stimuli and responses, that is to say thought influences action and a purely mechanistic or behaviourist approach

---

Summary text 3.6 The power of cognition

A participant in an experiment is occasionally given electric shocks when he makes errors while learning a task. The participant is able to cancel the onset of the shock by quickly pressing a button after making an error – assuming he realizes the error – in which case a shock is no longer given. The behaviourist experimenter disables the shock generating mechanism and then observes behaviour to see how long the participant continues to press the button after making errors. The experimenter is testing how long the now non-functional button pressing behaviour continues to the point of extinction – the point at which the participant realizes that even if he fails to press the button in time, no shock will be delivered. The experimenter records many superfluous button pressings.

The cognitive researcher in the same experiment simply says to the participant, 'please continue with the task, but I'm not going to deliver any more shocks so you don't need to use the escape button any more'. The consequence is that having had the situation **explained** to him, as opposed to leaving him to find out by trial and error, the experimental participant ceases to press the button immediately (assuming he believes that the experimenter is telling the truth, although in any case he is certain to test this hypothesis to confirm that it is true) and gets on with the task.

Thus, if we view human beings as mere recipients of physical stimuli, we cannot advance beyond a behaviourist perspective, whereas if we take account of their complex mental apparatus and explain things to them, then we are dealing with a more complete perspective of what governs or motivates human behaviour.

An analogous situation in the risk management field would be to leave an inexperienced worker to find out for him/herself about the hazards of a job. Eventually, through trial and error this may happen – if the youngster is not killed first. However, if the hazards and necessary precautions are **explained** to the worker, then this constitutes a more immediate and more effective way of getting important safety information across.

---

is inadequate to account for the complexity of human action. An illustration is given in summary text 3.6.

Cognitive approaches to human behaviour straddle the boundaries of the chapters of this book. Thus, cognitive theories which deal with motivation are also likely to cover perception, attitudes and learning for example so that where in this book we describe such theories is to an extent arbitrary. In the remainder of this section, we describe key features of the main 'pure' cognitive theory of motivation – attribution theory.

Attribution theory originated in the study of subjective experience (phenomenology). Stimuli from the environment provide information which is processed to give **meaning** to that environment. Attribution theory is concerned with the way in which individuals **interpret** events which are **caused** in their environment and with **inferential perceptions** of causality. Motives are attributed.

The development of attribution theory was influenced by Gestalt psychology and by field theory (pp. 41–3) – behaviour being a function of person and environment. Early attribution theorists (Festinger, 1957; Osgood *et al.*, 1957; Heider, 1958) all saw disequilibrium as a basic principle of motivation. The individual strives for balance or consonance with the environment and this was considered to be the primary motivating force. However, in modern attribution theory, reducing dissonance (e.g. in the form of conflicts between attitudes and behaviour – chapter 4, pp. 76–84, especially summary text 4.6) or achieving balance is a means to superordinate (i.e. higher order) goals. Thus, attributions are made, first to enable the individual to **predict** events and second, to help them to exert **control** over events. Thus, the need for control is the primary motivation in attribution theory and the prediction of events facilitates this control. The sequence of events in making attributions is shown in figure 3.4.

An important distinction, or attributional bias, is consistently found in attributions made by actors and observers. Because, for the actor the situation is prominent and their behaviour takes place within the situation, the actor tends to attribute cause to factors inherent in a situation. However, for an observer, who sees the behaviour of an actor against the background of the environment, they are more likely to attribute cause to supposed stable dispositions of actors. This attributional bias continues to operate even when situational constraints are made clear to the observer. A good example of this bias in operation is in attributing causes of accidents. Individuals tend to attribute their own accidents to factors in the environment – for example, design faults in apparatus or layout of controls, whereas observers, such as accident investigators or those to whom accidents are reported, such as supervisors, are more likely to attribute cause to imputed individual characteristics such as 'carelessness', 'lack of preparation', 'human error', 'rushing' or 'inexperience'. Given this apparently universal bias, it is little wonder that such a high proportion of accidents are attributed to 'human error', while situational factors such as design or layout or work pressure are much less

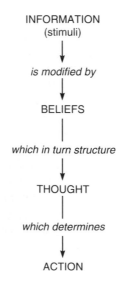

INFORMATION
(stimuli)

↓

is modified by

↓

BELIEFS

|

which in turn structure

↓

THOUGHT

|

which determines

↓

ACTION

Figure 3.4 General attributional sequence.

emphasized. This labelling phenomenon should be recognized for what it is – an attributional bias.

Why should this asymmetry between perceptions of actor and observer exist? The main reason is that the actor is more attuned to the situation and so uses situational factors in making causal attributions. The observer on the other hand, has less information about the situation and thus makes attributions for behaviour which are based more upon the actor. The relative amounts of information available to actor and observer also differ. Thus, the actor has information about his or her own intentions and experience, while the observer must infer information about intentions from the context of behaviour and from general social norms. The importance of this fundamental attributional bias in respect of recommendations for accident prevention is that it devalues the importance of the situation in giving rise to behavioural 'problems'. Recommendations are thus more likely to be aimed at altering the person rather than the setting – hence the frequently seen recommendation for action on accident report forms, 'told him not to do it again'.

This bias towards making attributions in respect of the person rather than the situation extends into the basic motivational tenet of attribution theory – that of the need to control. The sequence is shown in figure 3.5. The notion of controllability in respect of danger is considered as an important dimension of risk perception in chapter 5, pp. 121–30.

As well as this bias in actor/observer attributions, whereby one's own accidents are seen as misfortune or as the confluence of events, while others' accidents are attributed to carelessness or similar personal factors, there are other important biases which can help to explain commonly observed examples of human behaviour. These are described below.

Self-serving bias   This refers to a tendency for a person to take credit for their successes or improvements in their own behaviour but not to take the blame for increasing failure or mistakes – often referred to as 'defensive attribution'.

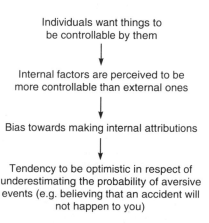

Figure 3.5 Attributional bias sequence.

This bias comes into play when we seek to protect ourselves from blame when things go wrong, for example when accidents happen.

Severity bias   Here, people are held to be more responsible for serious consequences than for minor ones, even if the antecedents are the same. This bias stems from the supposition that serious consequences (such as disasters) should have been foreseen and therefore must have been. Thus, when many people are killed in an accident, an inquiry is almost inevitably held, whereas if few or no people are killed, even if the **potential** for a higher death toll existed then an inquiry is unlikely. Summary text 3.7 illustrates a few contrasting incidents. The literature on making attributions for accidents is reviewed by Hale and Glendon (1987).

False consensus   People tend to think that their own beliefs are universally shared, i.e. that others think the same way as they do. For example, people who believe that most accidents are caused by 'carelessness' might well consider that most other people believe this as well. Children in particular have this bias and need to learn that other people think differently, although some people apparently go through life without making many concessions to others' views!

Situation bias   Here people underestimate the degree to which a person's role situation can modify their behaviour (e.g. in driving). This means that we tend to overestimate the extent to which behaviour seen in one situation (e.g. at home) will be shown in another (e.g. at work). This bias may account for

---

Summary text 3.7 Contrasting incidents

It has often happened that an accident or incident with serious consequences is preceded by a similar occurrence with much less serious outcomes. What is critical is that lessons are learned not from what the outcome was but what it might have been if the environment had been less forgiving. Examples include the Piper Alpha oil rig disaster in which 167 people died (Department of Energy, 1990) which was preceded by an incident with similar antecedents on the rig the Ocean Odyssey in which only one person died and which did not lead to a full scale inquiry. The sinking of the passenger ferry, the *Herald of Free Enterprise* at Zeebrugge (Department of Transport, 1987) in which 188 people lost their lives may be compared with an earlier incident in which a similar ferry, the *European Gateway* left port with her bow doors open, as had the *Herald*. Finally, at Markham Colliery 19 people were killed when winding gear failed (Department of Energy, 1973). A similar incident which did not result in loss of life or extensive damage occurred at Ollerton Pit in 1961.

The chances are you may not even have heard of the second incident in each of these pairs because while the event antecedents were comparable with the first in each case, the loss of life was small or non-existent. The principal lesson to be learned from these examples, which could be multiplied many times over, is the requirement for those concerned with the management of risk to develop effective systems for learning from 'near miss' incidents which could have had more serious outcomes (see for example, van der Schaaf *et al.*, 1991).

the continued popularity of trait theories in personality (chapter 6, pp. 142–9), despite low correlations found between behaviour in different situations. For example, a person who is a very safe worker may engage in what might be regarded as 'risky' behaviour outside work, such as hang-gliding. Explanations for such apparently discrepant behaviour can be found by reference to the voluntariness dimension of risk perception (chapter 5, pp. 119–21 especially figure 5.2) by which people will accept a larger amount of risk which they **choose** to expose themselves to, compared with risks which are imposed on them, as is usually the case at work.

Correlational bias   In this case people underestimate the importance of non-occurrences. We tend to register far more the occasions when X and Y (two events) are found together than when they are not and the causal link – if indeed there is one – is overestimated as a result. This may happen in non-statistical analyses of accidents or diseases when an event – such as working at a visual display terminal is thought to be associated with a variety of conditions, such as migraine or 'flu symptoms. There may or may not be a causal connection and only rigorous research can establish this. Another example is the 'Bermuda Triangle' – an area of the Atlantic Ocean in which a squadron of planes was mysteriously lost and which subsequently acquired mythological status as a place in which ships and planes were prone to disappear. However, no evidence was produced to demonstrate that vessels were more likely to be lost in this area compared with any other part of the world's oceans of comparable size.

Negative weighting   People generally weight negative information more heavily than positive information. This can happen in situations involving personal judgements such as job appraisal, selection interviews or personal relationships (see chapter 5, pp. 114–17), where a single piece of adverse information can outweigh any amount of positive material. In the case of safety, a single accident can blight an extended run of accident-free months and upset large amounts of careful risk planning for safety provision.

Availability bias   People overestimate the probability of events which are easy to imagine or to recall, for example dramatic events like accidents or those within personal experience. Powell *et al.* (1971) found that workers were more likely to think of hazards which resulted in accidents which had happened to them or to their workmates. The literature on risk perception is replete with studies showing that people tend to overestimate dramatic events and to underestimate more common ones (Lichtenstein *et al.*, 1978; Hale and Glendon, 1987). One way of overcoming this bias in considering health and safety is to use a systematic approach to hazard evaluation such as an expert system or safety auditing.

Adjustment bias   In this bias, people estimate the probability of future events by starting from some *a priori* estimate and adjusting this up or down

(Bayesian approach). The probability of conjunctive events, requiring $A + B + C$ is overestimated, while the probability of disjunctive events – requiring A or B or C is underestimated because in each case $p(A)$ is the adjusting factor. For example, for a fire to occur, an ignition source (A), oxygen (B) and fuel (C) are all required. However, we may overestimate the probability of a fire if an ignition source is present because the probability of this $(p(A))$ is known to be 1 and this affects our judgement of the overall likelihood of fire occurring. At the same time, the probability of a fire where there is not an obvious ignition source may be underestimated. An illustration of this is the TV advertisement for the British Gas emergency service in which a couple arrive home and smell gas. Thus, fuel is known to be present (so $p(C)$ is 1 to all intents and purposes as is $p(B)$). One of the couple goes to switch on the light and is stopped just in time by the other with the warning that a spark from the switch mechanism is enough to ignite the gas. In this example, the probability of a 'hidden' ignition source was perceived to be zero – yet it was very nearly equal to 1! Thus, this adjustment bias often means that little realized hazards can be overlooked, particularly when their worst effects operate in conjunction with other events. Careful engineering controls or human reliability analysis (see chapter 9, pp. 275–86) and detailed safety auditing (see chapter 10, pp. 298–312) can help to minimize the probability that human propensity to fall prey to this adjustment bias will not end in disaster.

Representativeness bias   This leads people to ignore the *a priori* probability of an event and be inclined to predict the future as being representative of the past. One result is that we tend to underestimate an important statistical phenomenon – regression to the mean. A good example of this is seen in accident data. When the accident rate rises, we tend to look for causes and when it falls we assume that we must be getting things right. Yet neither of these is necessarily correct. The popular saying 'what goes up must come down' can apply as much to accident rates as it does to share values. The issue is, when is a rise or fall in accident rates a **real** rise/fall and when is it merely random fluctuation about a mean level of accidents? Only proper statistical analysis can reveal this, and to perform it a large enough sample of accidents is required (Petersen, 1978; ReVelle, 1980; Tarrrants, 1980; Krause *et al.*, 1990b). The hours spent by safety committees and other groups trying to find reasons for changes in accident rates which have no explanation outside statistical variability can now be released for positive action on safety and risk management. The need to find meaning for observed events is certainly a powerful motivator!

Small numbers   People tend to treat results from small numbers as being better than they should. An example of this is the gambler's fallacy – a belief in the short-run (it must come up red on the next spin) as opposed to long-run probability consistency. The way to counteract this bias is to collect large enough samples of cases – e.g. accidents, near misses or safety rules breaches, before arriving at a conclusion. Texts can be used to tell you how large a sample should be (e.g. Bensiali and Glendon, 1987; Petersen, 1989).

Anchoring bias   The anchoring effect of predictions and perceptions results in them being very resistant to alteration, once made. Once beliefs have been formed and other cognitions (e.g. perceptions) linked to them, even removing the original data – e.g. that someone has had an incorrect bad credit rating due to mistaken identity – may still not result in them being disconfirmed in the mind of the observer. The expression 'mud sticks' is a popular illustration of this phenomenon and we may continue to believe that someone was responsible for an accident for example, and not trust them again (negative weighting bias) even when they have been proved innocent. This bias may well be compounded by the strong tendency for people to subject evidence in support of a belief to much less scrutiny than evidence against the belief. A safety and risk example of this bias in operation is again the belief that VDU use makes the operator more prone to certain illnesses – a belief that was widely held during the early years of VDU use and which some people may cling to despite a lack of evidence. Professionals such as scientists and police investigators are as much prone to this bias as any other individual.

Overconfidence   People are poor at estimating the odds of something occurring and are overconfident in their judgements about facts, for example typically being wrong 20–30% of the time on general knowledge questions which they were 100% confident in being right about (Kahneman *et al.*, 1982). Thus, when investigating accidents, incidents or patterns of data, it is vital not to jump to conclusions – about which we may be confident, but perhaps incorrect. This effect could also be confounded by the anchoring bias. We need to remind ourselves continually that we could be wrong about something we believe strongly.

Hindsight bias   Reported events are seen as being more likely in hindsight than using *a priori* information. The expression, 'I knew that would happen' illustrates this bias – the point is you **didn't** know it would happen **before** it happened! If we knew **which** 450 or so workers were to be killed next year at work in the UK, we could take them away and give them 12 months' holiday – it would certainly be a lot more cost-effective than killing them! But of course we don't have this information in advance of events and are therefore prey to such beliefs as either 'lightning doesn't strike twice in the same place' and/or 'history repeats itself'. By exaggerating the past, people underestimate what they have to learn from it – this is one of the unfortunate effects of hindsight bias. Anthony Hidden, QC was aware of this bias in investigating the Clapham Junction Railway Accident, when he wrote, 'There is almost no human action or decision that cannot be made to look more flawed and less sensible in the misleading light of hindsight. It is essential that the critic should keep himself constantly aware of that fact' (Department of Transport, 1989, p. 147).

Enough has probably been revealed about this cognitive approach to human motivation to indicate that it can offer important insights to explain much of what is popularly and unhelpfully termed 'human error' (chapter 9, pp. 244–61 explores this fascinating topic further). Human behaviour and motivation is complex and not always easy to take account of in managing risk. However, some understanding of why we behave as we do, for example because of fundamental biases in our view of the world, helps to unravel some of the more intractable issues of risk-related behaviour. Human beings are not logical thinkers (although they have the capacity for logical thought) and are subject to a number of shortcomings in their attempts to exert cognitive control over their environment (after Fischhoff, 1976):

- our everyday learning is not structured to develop cognitive control;
- we use simple (often over-simplified) models of the world;
- our ability to process information is exaggerated;
- we have poor insight into information integration methods;
- we are poor at applying acquired knowledge.

It seems that experts are no less subject to human shortcomings and attributional biases than anyone else. References to such biases in popular sayings are an indication that we have known about such biases in an intuitive sense for a considerable time in some cases. What is new is a theoretical framework ('there is nothing so practical as a good theory' according to Kurt Lewin) for improving our understanding of how these motivational mechanisms operate.

Practical ways of overcoming these adversely operating human factors in managing risk include:

- strategically designed safety training (chapter 2, especially pp. 8–12);
- carefully engineered safety systems;
- detailed planning of safety and risk management (chapter 10);
- expert systems in specific areas of safety and risk control;
- rigorous ways of measuring health and safety performance – such as safety auditing (chapter 10, pp. 298–312).

More ingenious ways of de-biasing people's views are also likely to be required and one recent attempt is described in summary text 3.8. Reber *et al.* (1989) found that employees who saw themselves on video were able to point out their own mistakes and unsafe acts – a form of training which reduced subjectivity and defensive biases. This relates to the important principle of feedback discussed in chapter 2, pp. 15–23 and 25–7.

To complete this section, we review briefly the three main hypotheses on attribution of responsibility (for a more detailed review, see Hale and Glendon, 1987). First, there is what has been called the 'just world hypothesis' (Lerner and Simmons, 1966) which postulates that we need to believe that people get what they deserve and deserve what they get. Thus, if we see a victim of misfortune such as an accident or illness case, we tend either to blame or to derogate the victim(s) because it is psychologically threatening to us as individuals to believe in a world governed by random reinforcements. In this

---

Summary text 3.8 Attempts to de-bias people's attributions

It is a well-known phenomenon that most people (typically 70–80%) consider themselves to be better drivers than their peers (Svensson, 1981; Groeger and Brown, 1989). However, logically this cannot be so because it is only possible for 50% of us to be better than the average for our group. This is an example of an attributional bias in operation – in this case a 'self-serving' bias which leads many of us to believe that we are better than we are (in this case at driving).

To see whether there might be some way to 'de-bias' individuals' perceptions of their own driving abilities, McKenna (1991) undertook a series of experiments. In the first experiment, he asked participants to write a story about a road accident in which they were involved. When the stories were analysed it was found that, as might be predicted, participants mostly wrote about (real or imagined) accidents in which they had been an innocent bystander or in which they had escaped major injury. On testing the participants, no evidence was found that their perceptions of their driving abilities had decreased in any way as a result of writing their stories.

In the second experiment, different participants were asked to write a story about a road accident in which they were seriously injured. It was predicted that having to confront a bad outcome like this might make participants aware of their own vulnerability and hence reduce their overconfidence in their driving ability. However, the effect which was found was only a slight one, and most participants wrote stories in which, although badly injured, they were the victims of misfortune (e.g. as passengers or pedestrians) rather than the perpetrators.

Thus, in the final experiment, a new group of participants was asked to write a story about a road accident which resulted in serious injury and for which they were to blame. Being obliged to write such a story did have a dramatic effect upon the biases of these participants – who, when tested, no longer considered themselves to be such great drivers! In other words, involvement in an imagined accident with serious consequences for which they were to blame was sufficient to de-bias this group of participants – at least in the short-term.

The experiments demonstrated both the relatively enduring nature of the self-serving bias and also the possibility that it can be overcome. Getting people to accept the possibility that they could make an error which has serious consequences has been demonstrated by these experiments to be a potentially powerful component of attributing responsibility for safety.

---

scenario, we like to believe that 'all is for the best in the best of all possible worlds' (Voltaire, *Candide*).

The second main hypothesis is known as 'defensive attribution' (Shaver, 1970) which maintains that causality is assigned in order to maintain or enhance the person's own self-esteem. Again, taking the example of an accident victim, the more that people believe that one day they may find themselves in the victim's position, the more they attribute his or her circumstances to chance. This implies that they will be protected from blame should the same misfortune befall them. Thus, our attributions are motivated by our psychological need to maintain our position at the fourth level of Maslow's hierarchy.

Finally, there is the underlying motivating feature of our desire for control. As the consequences of an unfortunate event, like an accident, become more severe people are increasingly motivated to assign blame to someone who might be responsible for the accident. Assigning blame reassures people that they will be able to avoid similar disasters, for if causality is assigned to unpredictable – and therefore uncontrollable – events then we have to concede that such an event might happen to us. Thus, motivated attributional processes are a means of encouraging and maintaining a person's effective exercise of control in their world in order to maintain the belief in control over their environment. Self beliefs of efficacy – for example believing that you can control a situation, are central to motivation because they influence causal attributions, expectancies (pp. 62–3) and personal goal-setting (Bandura, 1989). This key concept has links with stress and coping efficacy, discussed in chapter 8, pp. 224–32.

MOTIVATION AND WORK

The most heavily researched applied field for motivation theories has been the work environment. A general orientation has been motivational applications used by management to control workers using a variety of financial and psychological incentives or threats to maintain and improve production. Four types of assumptions are represented in approaches to work-based behaviour. These are revealed in different management styles as well as to notions of what motivates people at work. These broadly correspond with the first four levels in Maslow's hierarchy, as shown below:

Management style	Motivation addressed	Level in Maslow's hierarchy
'Scientific'	Economic	1. Physiological needs
Paternalistic	Security	2. Safety and security needs
Human relations	Social	3. Affiliation needs
Participative	Ownership	4. Self-esteem

It is interesting to note that no coherent management style has yet evolved which caters for the final level of Maslow's hierarchy, self-actualization. Given the nature of traditional workplace relations in which one group manages and controls the behaviour of others, this is unsurprising. However, the changing nature of work (Handy, 1984, 1989) does not preclude this as a future possibility. For example, individuals running their own businesses and who are thus effectively 'their own bosses' might well find a route to self-actualization through work activity.

However, leaving aside this possibility, it is worth reviewing briefly the four main management styles. So-called 'scientific management', the brainchild of F.W. Taylor – hence sometimes called 'Taylorism', is the most blatant manifestation of an approach to motivation through managerial control. The basic assumption is that individuals are motivated if rewards and penalties are tied directly to performance. Thus, in practical terms, a scientific management approach to workforce motivation is represented by wage incentives, payment by results and promotion on merit. On the penalty side it is characterized by threats such as of dismissal or 'redeployment'. The philosophy is congruent with McGregor's Theory X, which maintains that people are basically lazy and require external motivation (McGregor, 1960), and with exploitative authoritarian management (also known as Likert's System 1).

Scientific management is workplace behaviourism as it follows principles of reinforcement in that if behaviour is rewarded it tends to be repeated, while behaviour that is punished tends not to be repeated. Taylor's views and work exerted a profound and lasting influence upon management thinking and practices. The aims of scientific management were to eliminate inefficiency, to increase cooperation between management and workers and to reduce conflict and discord at work. Consequences for management are that they should set tasks for workers, plan ahead, regulate work and exert unilateral control. Workers were treated individually – i.e. not in groups or through trade unions. While there is some support for scientific management, for example that it results in increased productivity, it is not without its problems and these are summarized in summary text 3.9.

Assumptions underlying the second approach, paternalistic management, are that people are motivated by the following:

- people work harder if total rewards are increased (but not linked to effort) – e.g. automatic annual pay increases;
- loyalty and gratitude can be expected by satisfying people's needs;
- the organization is the main source of rewards which are important to the individual – e.g. good working conditions, payments and fringe benefits;
- promotion is predictable and based mainly on seniority;
- job security;
- wage levels are high and pay increases are given 'across the board';
- job satisfaction is important.

Thus, under paternalistic management assumptions, it is held that increased

---

Summary text 3.9 Problems with scientific management

There are limitations in any approach which is based upon an external system of rewards and penalties (Gouldner, 1955). This is because not all rewards are under the control of the formal external system; some are under the control of the informal system (see the human relations approach). There may well be conflict between these two. Neither does the approach take account of higher order needs and thus requires a purely instrumental approach to work in which the only satisfaction which may realistically be obtained is the meeting of basic needs through earnings.

Objective measurement of performance in some jobs is impossible and some measures are liable to be subjective and arbitrary. The sheer logistics of a system of information collation and analysis is liable to make a pure scientific management system very difficult to achieve in practice, especially if applied to managerial positions. Thus, it is likely to be difficult to assess the contribution of an individual. In addition, a worker's performance is not the only factor to affect outcomes – external factors such as parts supply or work quality elsewhere in the system will affect output. So, the approach is highly dependent upon control by the individual over work tasks; if this is weak than links between rewards (and punishment) and motivation tend to break down.

rewards lead to increased satisfaction and greater effectiveness. The work contract is that the employer provides good wages and conditions and expects enthusiasm and loyalty from the worker in return. Evidence suggests that management behaviour based on paternalistic assumptions does help to attract and retain employees. However, there is little evidence that such policies have any direct effect on motivation, performance or productivity. The basic problem is that satisfaction with the job (wages, conditions, etc.) is not related to motivation to perform the job effectively.

The third approach, the human relations school of management grew out of the Hawthorne studies (Roethlisberger and Dixon, 1939) and is characterized by:

- taking an interest in employees improves work performance (safety as well as production output);
- social relations in the workplace are important – often more so than physical conditions;
- informal work groups establish their own work patterns and behaviour norms (e.g. for output and safety);
- while each individual (and group) decides how fast s/he/it will work, management can influence this decision – for example in their behaviour towards individual workers and work groups (chapter 7, in particular pp. 170–84).

The first of the above points, that taking an interest in your employees can improve work performance, was termed the 'Hawthorne Effect' from the original studies because of the observation that human behaviour changes when it is studied. A more contemporary example from the field of safety is provided by Della-Giustina and Della-Giustina (1989) who report an improved safety record, as well as better productivity and morale, for an experimental section of a coal mine (Mills, 1976).

The final general approach to workplace motivation to be considered here is that of participative management. This corresponds with Likert's System 4 (Participative) and McGregor's Theory Y, and maintains that basically people want to work and are able to motivate themselves, given the right environment. Assumptions underlying this approach to work motivation are:

- people can derive satisfaction from doing a job as such;
- people are committed to their work and take a pride in it;
- reduce authority as a means of control – assist rather than command;
- managers teach and consult as colleagues;
- use work groups as problem-solving and decision-making units (chapter 7, especially pp. 188–200);
- supervisors meet with work groups;
- participation in decision-making increases involvement and commitment to the organization;
- with greater freedom to do a job, that job becomes more of a challenge – therefore aim to enlarge discretionary job components and reduce programmed components.

The philosophy of the participative approach is that of self-regulation rather than organizational control. Among the main applications of the participative style are management by objectives and some types of performance appraisal. Managers and staff participate in deciding upon their own job objectives but are given discretion in how to reach them. Elements of participative management are also found in:

- job enlargement;
- training/development programmes;
- profit sharing;
- productivity bargaining;
- quality circles;
- some forms of employee involvement.

However, a major problem with this approach to motivation at work is that it is more applicable at higher than at lower levels within an organization. It could be argued that it is seldom properly tried at lower levels. There are also likely to be individual and cultural differences in response to this management style, and it may only be effective in highly developed countries and organizations.

No attempt to motivate employees has met with universal success and most operational systems are a hybrid of two or more of the above types. In general, the more cognitive approach of involving employees has been thought to work best at higher levels, while the behaviourist scientific management approach has been shown to be more appropriate to shop floor employees. However, with work patterns, practices and attitudes likely to continue to undergo radical transformation in future, traditional distinctions between employee categories are likely to continue to erode (Handy, 1989). Thus, the issue of what motivates people to work is likely to become a much more fragmented debate – dealing at the extreme with what motivates any given individual.

A useful basic distinction which arises out of the foregoing discussion is that between intrinsic and extrinsic motivation to undertake a task (Deci, 1975). With intrinsic motivation, the person perceives the task to be interesting or enjoyable in itself. With extrinsic motivation, the person perceives the task as a means of achieving an ulterior goal or reward – for example, a salary or promotion. This is sometimes referred to as an instrumental approach because work is the instrument for achieving some more important goal – for example, status or consumer goods and services. However, extrinsic rewards can dampen enthusiasm for a task which provides intrinsic rewards – for example problem-solving. Extrinsic rewards may be:

(a) contingent on performance of an activity – such as being paid for doing a job (e.g. production manager);
(b) contingent on quality or success of performance – such as being paid a basic salary plus production and safety bonuses.

The former is more likely than the latter to undermine intrinsic interest. However, while rewards may provide valuable feedback about success, knowing that your performance is being evaluated can lead to the perception that it is under extrinsic control. Thus, for positive motivation it is better to tell people that they **are** doing a job well than that they **should** do a job well.

Reber *et al.* (1989) note that setting work safety goals relies upon intrinsic motivation. However, they also observe that employees may also expect extrinsic rewards, for example in the form of an incentive programme, to reinforce this. Kello *et al.* (1988) describe a series of studies involving employee commitment to wearing car seat belts in which rewards were either extrinsic (e.g. entering a raffle for a holiday) or intrinsic, in which on the basis of a group discussion-based awareness session on seat-belt use, participants perceived that they were voluntarily choosing to wear a seat belt rather than being coerced or manipulated. The authors argue that active involvement, in this case via the group discussion, leads to commitment to behaviour change which is both more durable and cost effective than the use of extrinsic rewards. Sundström-Frisk (1989) also used a group-discussion approach to improve safety and found that the most powerful component in motivating workers to use safer methods was the communication of experiences of near accidents and minor injuries.

An extrinsic reinforcement system is analogous with a purely behaviourist approach, and will work as long as it is in force. However, in effect it is the extrinsic reward which is the reinforcer and not the behaviour which is the subject of attempted change. Thus, extrinsic rewards – e.g. for seat-belt or personal protective equipment (PPE) use – may engender overt compliance, but without any change in underlying beliefs and attitudes. This contrasts with a situation in which attitude and behaviour changes are matched – as in an intrinsic reward system – for example, based upon those involved having a real understanding of the reasons for the behaviour change. This issue is explored further in chapter 4, particularly pp. 76–8 and 93–7.

Before leaving the topic of work motivation, we consider two further approaches which have been particularly influential. The first is Herzberg's two-factor theory or motivation-hygiene theory (Herzberg *et al.*, 1959; Herzberg, 1966). This contrasts with single-factor theories which treat motivation as a unitary concept. Herzberg argues that factors which motivate people at work are essentially distinct and separate from those which simply prevent people from becoming dissatisfied with their work – hence 'hygiene' or maintenance factors.

On the basis of his studies, Herzberg distinguished between motivators – factors which relate to what a person does and hence motivate to better performance, and hygiene factors – which relate to the work environment and hence maintain or prevent job dissatisfaction, but which do not motivate as such. These factors are shown in summary text 3.10.

While Herzberg's theory has been influential, as with other approaches to work motivation, it has its criticisms. These are summarized in summary text 3.11.

Hall and Williams (1980) have combined Herzberg's approach with Maslow's more general theory to produce a work motivation inventory which is designed to measure workers' needs at the five levels of Maslow's hierarchy

Summary text 3.10 Factors which motivate and factors which prevent job dissatisfaction (after Herzberg)

Factors which, if adequate prevent job dissatisfaction – hygiene factors	Factors which, if present serve to motivate job performance
Money	Sense of achievement
Status	Recognition
Relationship with boss	Enjoyment of job
Company politics and administration	Possibility of promotion
Work rules	Responsibility
Working conditions	Chance for growth
Supervision	Work itself
Relationship with peers	Advancement

– the first two of which broadly correspond with Herzberg's hygiene factors and the remaining three with Herzberg's motivators. Thus, it is possible to compare the respective needs of different groups of workers as a basis for recommendations for changes in their working conditions. Ratliff (1988) undertook such a study on secondary school teachers and found that, compared with industrial, government and retail workers, teachers were significantly more concerned about the lower order needs (hygiene factors). However, teachers had significantly lower needs for self-esteem and self-actualization because the nature of their job allowed for greater opportunity to satisfy these higher order needs. Ratliff (1988) points to the teachers' conflict of having higher-order needs satisfied to a greater extent than lower-order needs.

Summary text 3.11 Criticisms of Herzberg's two factor theory

From an ideological perspective, the theory assumes a consensus framework, allowing only for managerially defined situations but not allowing for conflicts among goals, motivation or aspirations, and cannot therefore be a universal theory. From a scientific point of view it overlooks contradictions and inconsistencies and is dogmatic over findings. For example, hygiene and motivation factors are not distinct categories but overlap, so that for example some people are genuinely motivated by money and status through their work.

Conceptually, the theory is weak because it assumes that we are all motivated by the same things, and so ignores individual differences. It also ignores external influences such as market changes and the economic climate. Developed in the affluent USA of the 1950s and 1960s it is, like other theories of motivation, culture-bound and period bound, so that it would be unlikely to apply to depressed or developing countries, or indeed to low status jobs.

Methodologically, it may be criticized on the grounds that the researchers defined what motivation was for them and their findings have not been replicated using other methods. While many theories of motivation share some of these criticisms, few share quite so many!

A more sophisticated, and more cognitive approach to work motivation, and one which has also been applied to safety motivation, is that from expectancy theory. The three basic components of expectancy theory (Vroom, 1964) are:

- expectancy – if I tried, would I be able to do what I want to do?
- instrumentality – would doing this lead to identifiable outcomes?
- valence – how much do I value those outcomes?

The basic elements are shown in figure 3.6.
Figure 3.6 is an expansion of the equation:

$$\text{performance (in a job, sport, safety, etc.)} = \text{skill} \times \text{motivation,}$$

and reveals that the skill (or abilities) component comprises both inherent and acquired skills – for example through training (chapter 2). The motivational component is more complex, comprising effort expended and knowing what is expected by those who matter – superordinates and, to a lesser extent peers. The accuracy of these perceptions is important in respect of work performance. The effort component breaks down into two further elements, the first of which is the **value** of a range of rewards from the work – all Herzberg's factors, both hygiene and motivators are included here. Finally, there is the important element of the link between the effort expended by the individual and the rewards – the behaviourist or scientific management component but with cognitive, i.e. thinking and reasoning as part of the analysis.

To illustrate the type of issues underlying this analysis by the individual of the links between effort and reward, we use the example of the line manager who has been informed that there is a safety blitz on within the organization and that line managers' job performance appraisal is going to incorporate elements of safety. The line manager, not accepting this at face value, may well ask the following questions (after Petersen, 1978):

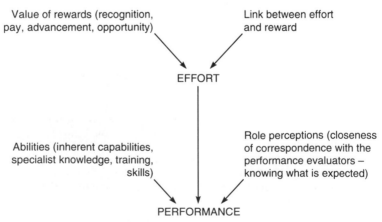

Figure 3.6 Factors affecting work performance.

- will the safety goal actually be rewarded?
- will alternative goals (e.g. output, profitability) be rewarded more?
- does management have other priorities?
- would I get better results in another area (e.g. industrial relations)?
- will my efforts actually bring results, or are many risk factors beyond my control?
- are performance measures effective (e.g. are appraisals fair and objective)?
- will others be rewarded for my efforts (e.g. supervisors, peers)?

Thus, motivation at work – as elsewhere – is complex, comprising many components. There is certainly a reward aspect to motivated behaviour, but a straight behaviourist approach is inadequate to explain all the complexities of human motivation. People give considerable thought to the things which motivate them, to the reasons why they will and will not do things, including putting effort into managing risk and safety. It is vital to understand this if we are to make progress in respect of generating more human activity in favour of risk management. The remainder of this chapter addresses this issue more directly.

MOTIVATING FOR SAFETY

One of the most basic motivators is to induce fear. This addresses one of our real basic instincts – to avoid things that can harm us. Fear may be induced in a variety of ways – for example via films, posters or the written or spoken word. Arousal of fear motivates us to find ways of reducing the arousal (which may take the form of dissonance, discomfort, or stress). One way in which we may act to reduce the negative arousal is to change our behaviour, i.e. to act more safely. However, there are other possibilities, for example that we will change our beliefs rather than change our behaviour (as would be predicted by cognitive dissonance theory – (chapter 4, pp. 76–84), particularly summary text 4.6). For example, if the information is very threatening we may reject it altogether because it is uncomfortable to think about (e.g. the chance that we might be killed or seriously injured or our health severely impaired). We might alternatively consider the information to be inapplicable to our own situation – i.e. that the message is not for us but rather for other people to take note of. Another possibility is that we might seek to justify or rationalize our behaviour in some way – for example, that the rewards we are getting are worth the risks we are taking. Models which seek to explain why we might avoid the most obvious course of action are discussed in chapter 4, pp. 84–8. Finally, we may opt to live with the dissonance of knowing that what we are doing is harmful to our health or threatens our safety – which can be highly stressful.

Evidence from studies of the use of fear suggest that it is only effective as a motivator when individuals feel that they can control the behaviour for which change is sought. Thus, using fear is a good way of strengthening already held attitudes or beliefs, for example on health as it confirms in people's minds that they are already behaving 'sensibly'. For example, Becker and Janz (1987), in a useful review, note that if motivation to improve health is already high then information provision on how to achieve this has positive effects. Otherwise, information provision can have negative effects – inducing fear and rejection of the information. A middle stage is where information provision can induce some motivation and attitude change. In health education, no single intervention strategy can produce long-term changes in important behaviours (Green, 1978).

Thus, by itself fear is not at all effective in changing behaviour. Indeed, it may have the reverse effect – for example, further strengthening an addict's habit – e.g. smoking or other drug use. After all, if anxiety is partly what initially drove a person to the habit, then anything which serves to increase anxiety is likely to drive them back to it. A better approach is to give simple, straightforward information on what the person should do – e.g. 'go for a health check'. There are individual differences (chapter 6, pp. 142–7 and 149–55) in respect of people's susceptibility to anxiety – those who are neurotic (emotionally labile) are more likely to experience anxiety and also be less able to cope successfully with stress (chapter 8, pp. 219–24). For the promoter of a message, the essence of successful communication is to associate the fear appeal with demonstrating that the individual has control over the threat. There are close links here with risk perception, and an example is given in summary text 5.7 in chapter 5. The basic model describing the role of fear in safety motivation and its various possible outcomes, is outlined in figure 3.7.

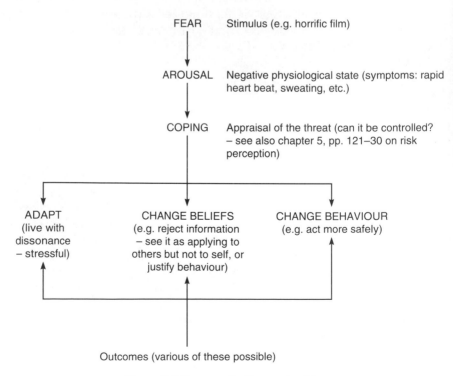

Figure 3.7 Fear, motivation and safety.

Control also relates to a person's self-image. Thus, we tend to reject messages telling us that we are doing something wrong. On the other hand, risk-taking – for which various motivational bases may be discerned – can in some circumstances be interpreted as a demonstration of skill. This may apply to driving as much as to steel-erecting. In some cases, young people's accidents may be due to attempts to emulate behaviour of more experienced (i.e. skilled) drivers or work colleagues, but without the necessary skill to undertake the behaviour successfully on every occasion. To counter the beliefs which underlie a self-image in which an individual equates skilled performance with risk-taking, it is necessary to associate competence with taking precautions – whether this is in the use of motor-cycle helmets, safety helmets or car seat belts – or campaigns such as 'it's fun not to smoke'. These help to overcome the negative image which may attend a safety conscious worker in full safety gear (Pirani and Reynolds, 1976). An interesting example of instilling safety into new workers is given by Kendall (1985) who describes a scheme whereby new site workers wear different coloured helmets for their first 30 days so that experienced workers can ensure that the new employees do their jobs safely. In another construction company all the different trades and professions wear uniquely coloured helmets for ready identification.

Also relevant to the issue of control is the matter of convenience. Thus, good design – of systems as well as equipment, etc. – while it may not have obvious links with motivation, is important from the point of view of how much more trouble it is to take precautions than not to do so (chapter 9, pp. 261–75 for further discussion). It is important to appreciate the relative costs and rewards of different types of behaviour – safe and unsafe. Thus, systems should ideally be designed so that it is at least no more trouble (e.g. awkward, time-consuming) to take precautions than not to do so. It may also be necessary to work hard to change relevant attitudes and behaviour – for example driving at speed in fog or overtaking decisions – because such changes involve changing the perceived relative values of the respective rewards (arriving sooner at your destination, demonstrating skill to self or peers, etc.) and the risks involved (chapter 4, pp. 84–8 considers this issue in more depth). The way to address such risky behaviours is not to attach labels such as 'motorway madness' or allege that drivers are 'careless' or 'stupid' because drivers don't think that these labels apply to them personally – although they may see them as applying to others. Instead, it is necessary to understand the motives underlying fast or 'dangerous' driving and the benefits of so doing and to work on them (see Rolls et al., 1991 for a consideration of this issue).

Allied with considerations in respect of system design are those concerned with the design of payment systems, in particular payment by results systems. Although it is hard to get unequivocal evidence, in their review Hale and Glendon (1987) suggest that there is an association between accidents and financial incentives to take risks. This probably arises from the certainty of a short-term reward (usually payment) set against the uncertainty of a long-term risk – i.e. that some unpleasant consequence may or may not occur. Sulzer-Azaroff (1978) notes that in the workplace, unsafe practices persist because they are 'naturally' reinforced – punishers for unsafe acts may be weak (near misses may actually reinforce perception of skill and ability to avoid an accident), delayed or infrequent. Efforts to improve safety need to overcome these obstacles.

Similar competing values may serve to confound studies of the value of safety incentives (e.g. exchanging goods or services for reduced accident rates) in respect of attempting to change behaviour. Again, individuals will balance the value of rewards with the value for more risky behaviour (e.g. getting the job done more quickly to increase leisure time). Although there are a number of in-house reports on safety incentives, locating published studies which are uncontaminated by confounding factors such as other organizational changes or controls for such matters as reporting (e.g. of accidents) is difficult – although one is described in chapter 2, pp. 25–7. Petersen (1989) points out that incentive programmes don't usually work because incentives are often given for not getting injuries rather than for any specific behaviour – thus rewards are linked to outcomes – which may in turn result from many factors (including chance) and not to specific behaviours. To have a chance of being successful, incentives need to be given at the point when the desired behaviour occurs (to reinforce that behaviour) and this is usually very difficult to arrange.

However, as with learning and training in respect of safety – discussed in chapter 2 – most reported studies of safety motivation are in the behaviourist tradition – linking particular feedback or incentives with a limited range of outcomes (behaviours). Thus, Sulzer-Azaroff (1982) reviews the use of incentives in safety behaviour, and Saari (1990) cites further studies on performance feedback effectiveness. McAfee and Winn (1989) review 24 studies which investigated the use of incentives or feedback to enhance workplace safety. All the studies measured short-term outcome variables, including:

- percent of employees performing the job safely;
- hazard frequencies;
- earplug use;
- number of vehicle accidents.

All the studies found short-term improvements in at least one of the variables measured (although negative findings in any area tend not to be published!). The possibility remains that while the rewarded behaviour improved, other safe behaviours deteriorated and that improvements were not sustained in the longer term. One confounding factor is that most reinforcers are not unitary – for example, praise is both an incentive and provides information (knowledge of results). Some studies reported no improvement effects. However, this is not to detract from the clear evidence that behaviour change is possible by applying behaviourist motivation principles in the workplace. Another problem is that incentives differed considerably, making generalizations difficult. For example, Saarela *et al.* (1989) show the lack of effect of a safety poster campaign upon accident rates. The campaign was well-received but had no measurable effect upon individuals. Petersen (1989) follows Luthans and Kreitner (1975) in charting the historical progress of organizational behaviour modification from motivational origins, and relates reinforcement principles to safety (Petersen, 1989: 73–4).

From the material reviewed in this section, it is clear that motivation in safety is highly situation specific. This means that situation or behaviour-specific campaigns (e.g. 'don't drink and drive') are more likely than general exhortations (e.g. 'be safe') to be successful. However, behaviour change is likely to be short-lived if it is unsupported (for example, by continuing extrinsic motivators such as legislation or company standards) or sustained by intrinsic beliefs. People are motivated to take risks as well as to avoid risk (Glendon, in press) so long as they perceive that they have some control over the risk.

In assessing people's likely behaviour, the respective costs and benefits of both relatively safe and unsafe behaviour need to be taken into account. One problem in motivating for safety is the typical low probability of adverse outcomes (being caught, being involved in an accident, etc.) set against the usually very high probability of benefit (completing a job quickly, getting to your destination sooner, etc.). In general it is better to use less 'powerful' motivators such as praise or feedback of results to achieve positive outcomes (learning as well as motivation) rather than fear or compulsion – e.g. via legislation. The real issue for behaviour modification is, will it be sustained in the long-term? The most likely answer is that behaviour changes will be sustained if they are supported by consistent changes in intrinsic motivation, i.e. if attitudes and behaviour are consistent. If the behaviour is supported only by extrinsic rewards, then once these are removed the behaviour will tend to decline – see also the discussion in chapter 4, pp. 88–90 on compliance, identification and internalization.

Studies which have investigated norms, morale, communication and other organizational factors (chapter 10, pp. 290–1) show positive links between these factors and safe behaviour. However, the direction of cause and effect is hard to establish and is almost certainly complex. Group effects in changing behaviour, for example in the use of participation in decision-making and discussion of change, are also shown to have some effect, for example via group commitment (see chapter 7, pp. 177–80 and 185–8). Examples set by leaders, supervisors and teachers are also important.

CONCLUSIONS

Motivation is a complex concept which can have different meanings involving: movement, energy, self-interest and volition. It is a central concept in psychology, being the crucial link between underlying variables such as personal values, attitudes, personality and behaviour.

There are four main approaches to motivation:

- mechanistic (instinct or inborn urges);
- behaviourist (reinforcement, reward and need satisfaction);
- cognitive (individuals understanding the world so as to predict and control events);
- applied (change and influence – e.g. work, safety).

The various approaches to motivation reflect the complexity of the concept and suggest that no one approach is likely to provide a complete answer in risk and safety applications. It is possible to use something from each of the approaches considered.

Our basic instincts – including avoidance of danger or situations which could cause us harm, are our fundamental survival pack. However, we can learn to override these instincts in order to reward higher goals, for example to experience excitement or to rescue others. Because we have developed ways of overcoming our fears, it is important to ensure that adequate checks exist when people are operating in dangerous environments – such as at heights or in fires.

Maslow postulated a hierarchy of needs as the basis of human behaviour. While safety exists as a second order need in Maslow's hierarchy, this refers to safety in the general sense of a safe, secure home rather than workplace (or road etc.) safety. Thus, while it is of general interest, Maslow's hierarchy does not have anything profound to offer risk management in the pursuit of improved workplace safety.

Motivation is a complex but critical concept in psychology and as such, it is also central to risk management through understanding safe and unsafe behaviour. It has close links with most other behavioural aspects of risk and safety, especially learning, perception and attitudes. However, individuals can differ widely in their motivation to do things, although there are common threads which link us all. No single approach to motivation has a monopoly of being correct or appropriate in all circumstances. Cognitive, behavioural – and even instinctive – approaches have merit. We need to consider all components in order to achieve effective safety and risk management through motivational approaches.

Individuals differ in their need for achievement (NAch). If the safety and risk professional's role is seen as one of implementing engineering solutions to problems, then individuals with low NAch may be considered appropriate. However, if marketing or selling skills – to management and workforce, are considered to be the key component of the safety and risk professional's role, then individuals high in NAch may be more suitable (chapter 6 deals with other personality and selection issues).

In attributing such a large proportion of accident 'causes' to 'human error' or similar personal factors (such as 'carelessness') we are falling prey to the fundamental attributional error – that of ascribing others' accidents to personal factors (and our own mistakes to situational factors such as design or lack of training – or anything but ourselves). One unfortunate consequence of this attitudinal bias is that we underestimate what we have to learn from situational factors (i.e. pertaining to the work environment – chapters 7–10). A classic case is that of the Kegworth air crash in which the principal causal attribution made was that of 'pilot error' (Department of Transport, 1990). The important lesson is that we should first be aware of this bias, and second seek ways to overcome it so as to gain a more enlightened view of the role of the individual in accident causation.

This strong and universal motivator – our desire to protect ourselves from blame (also called the self-serving bias or defensive attribution) can be overcome by getting people to consider their own shortcomings, for example in experiments, watching their own behaviour on video or in group discussions. We all need to be aware of the operation of a range of attributional biases in making judgements about risk and safety issues. Safety and risk professionals need to be aware of the possibilities for reducing these biases and use them whenever possible, for example in accident/incident investigations or in training/briefing sessions.

Various management styles ('scientific', paternalistic, human relations, participative) may be adopted to seek to motivate people at work. None has met with universal success and mostly management is a mixture of styles. It is increasingly likely that effective management will depend upon identifying each individual's unique motivations. This means that management should find out each individual's motivations, in respect of safety, risk-taking and work.

Rewards or reinforcement may be intrinsic (e.g. a job or task is seen as worth doing for its own sake) or extrinsic (e.g. doing a job or task leads to some external reward, such as money or status). In selecting extrinsic safety motivators (e.g. as in incentive schemes), consideration needs to be given as to whether such a behaviour modification approach can be applied consistently in the long term. In promoting safe behaviour, use of intrinsic rewards is more durable and effective than using extrinsic rewards. People need to understand the reasons for engaging in safe behaviour and to be able to participate in decisions which affect them. An optimum strategy would be to combine the best features of both approaches.

Motivation is central to safety and risk-taking and is closely related to a number of topics which are considered in other chapters, particularly learning and training (chapter 2), attitudes and behaviour (chapter 4), perception and risk perception (chapter 5) and human factors (chapter 9).

4 ATTITUDES, BEHAVIOUR AND ATTITUDE CHANGE

❏ This chapter addresses a topic which is generally acknowledged to be central to workplace health and safety – attitudes and their link with behaviour. After evaluating the nature of attitudes, including their components and dimensions, attention turns to theories about links between attitudes and behaviour. Consideration of the functions and levels of attitudes is followed by a review of attitude measurement. The topic of attitude change is next discussed, incorporating a number of case examples of attitude and behaviour change in respect of safety.

INTRODUCTION

> Current studies indicate that the most accurate predictor of actual buying behaviour is consumer attitudes. No other single influence is quite so important to the study of consumer behaviour (Berkman and Gilson, *Consumer Behaviour, Concepts and Strategies*, 3rd edn, 1986).

This observation from a book on consumer behaviour highlights the importance of the study of attitudes in respect of understanding behaviour in this field. This chapter seeks to answer questions relating to the extent to which attitudes on safety and risk issues are critical to safety-related behaviour. The objectives of this chapter are to:

- explain what attitudes are and the functions they serve;
- outline major approaches to attitudes;
- consider the relationship between attitudes and behaviour;
- demonstrate the relevance of attitudes to safety and risk management.

After a review of the relevance of attitudes to safety and risk professionals, various aspects of attitudes are introduced, the important ones being considered in greater detail later in the chapter. Different attitude components are considered – feeling, thinking and tendency to act – as well as a number of different attitude dimensions. Next, given that everyone has a theory about attitude/behaviour links, a series of types of theory about attitudes and behaviour are outlined. Inadequacies of simple theories of attitude–behaviour links are highlighted. It is explained that it is necessary to know about very specific factors in attitude–behaviour links before attitudes can be used as a valid predictor of behaviour. Also discussed are approaches which consider the influence of behaviour upon attitudes, the consistency between attitudes and behaviour and other factors which can affect both attitudes and behaviour.

More complex theories of attitude-behaviour links are next explored and the range of factors which influence behaviour are considered in greater detail. These include beliefs about how others view the behaviour in question, beliefs about the consequences of the behaviour, attitudes towards the behaviour, intentions, perceived risk of outcomes and the degree of control that the individual believes that they have over their behaviour. We next turn to consider the measurement of attitudes, using four different types of scale, each of which is explained with safety examples. The topic of attitude change is next addressed and is considered under the headings: the audience, the persuader, personality factors, presentation of issues, persistence of change. Finally, specific studies on attitude and behaviour change on health and safety, including a number of case studies, are described before the chapter conclusion. Relevant examples and illustrations in respect of health, safety and risk are provided throughout. Practical health and safety applications are derived from the material presented in the chapter both in the case studies and in chapter 11, pp. 331–2.

UNDERSTANDING ATTITUDES

What is the relevance of attitudes to students and practitioners of health, safety and risk management? The answer is that increasingly, safety and risk professionals are becoming aware that there are occasions when people's attitudes and behaviour towards risk and hazards need to be changed. To change attitudes and behaviour requires certain knowledge and skills. Safety and risk professionals know that they require skills which are as much to do with communicating, influencing and negotiating with others as with technical and legal knowledge and expertise in health and safety. They know that having technical expertise is of limited use if that expertise cannot be brought to bear through interacting with other people – both in the workplace and outside. This involves attempts to **influence** significant others (for example, colleagues, managers and other employees) and this in turn can involve attitude **change**.

Thus, like many other groups, safety and risk professionals seek to 'win hearts and minds' in order to be able to carry out their tasks and functions effectively. It is therefore vital that they have a basic understanding of the nature of attitudes and attitude change and how these concepts relate to – and in some cases do not relate to – behaviour. It is necessary to appreciate something of the **complexity** of the relationship between attitudes and behaviour and also to be equipped with theories of this relationship which will be of practical use to them in their work. This chapter makes such tools available and accessible.

'Attitude' is an example of a psychological concept which was long ago incorporated into everyday parlance, so that for example we might comment that someone has 'an attitude' problem (perhaps meaning that we don't agree with their point of view!) or that 'we need to change attitudes in order to improve health and safety' (perhaps meaning that 'we don't know what is wrong or what else to do and thus this must be the solution'!). Thus, 'attitudes' are often ascribed the status of a cognitive (i.e. mental) force which have the potential for either good or evil. Sometimes this force remains within an individual's mind, while at other times it is represented as observable behaviour. In other words, attitudes have the **potential** for influencing behaviour on the assumption that some form of thought process always precedes action.

In this scenario, the task is to discover what attitudes individuals (and groups, e.g. of employees) hold and then to seek to change them in accordance with the agenda of another group (e.g. management) in order to 'improve' their behaviour. This is the simple and original theory behind attitudes and it is one still held by many people, implicitly if not explicitly – namely that if you can change people's attitudes, then you can influence the behaviour which corresponds with those attitudes. Thus, much time and effort has been devoted to attempts to **measure** attitudes and to develop theories that will **explain** how attitudes may be changed and how they can **account for** behaviour.

As we shall see in the course of this chapter, life is rarely so straightforward as would be suggested by this approach to attitudes. However, there obviously **are** links between attitudes and behaviour and a lot of work has been done in seeking to establish the nature of such links. This chapter explains some of the main attempts that have been made to elucidate attitude/behaviour links and review their relevance to psychological components of safety and risk management.

As explained in the introductory chapter, attitudes are one type of individual factor (along with perception and personality – dealt with respectively in chapters 5 and 6) which can influence behaviour via motivation. Thus, some understanding of how attitudes exist and can be changed is important in appraising how such influences may operate.

THE NATURE OF ATTITUDES

Definition

An attitude can be defined as a '**learned tendency to act in a consistent way to a particular object or situation**'. This definition follows the approach to attitudes of a well-known pair of authors in this field – Fishbein and Ajzen (1975). The definition indicates that attitudes:

- are **learned** through social interactions and other influences (i.e. are **not** innate); an example of how such learning might occur in the health and safety field is given in summary text 4.1;
- are a **tendency to act** but are by no means a guarantee that a person with a given attitude will actually act in any particular way; this behavioural component is explored at various places in this chapter;
- have an element of **consistency** about them; we tend to have **clusters** of attitudes which are generally consistent with one another;
- are **specific** to a particular object or situation – i.e. they should not be thought of as being generalizable to **other** objects or situations.

Summary text 4.1 Attitudes in the construction industry: an illustration

Leather and Butler (1983) found that attitudes to safety in the construction industry differed depending upon whether the worker had ever personally experienced an accident injury. Compared with non-victims, victims of accidents considered that construction work was inherently dangerous and that too much familiarity with the job (and reduced danger awareness) was a significant cause of accidents. They also thought that tiredness or fatigue contributed to accident causation and felt that their employers could do more to promote and safeguard their safety.

In contrast, non-victims – unable to rely upon first-hand experience of accidents – tended to stress the importance of their own behaviour in controlling hazards at work in avoiding accidents. They felt positive about the power of their own decisions and behaviour on safety matters – after all, **their** commonsense experience told them that these were reliable. These workers considered individual carelessness to be an important cause of accidents, took a positive view of their employer's concern for safety and were satisfied with the role of the safety officer at their place of work.

Thus, each group's cluster of attitudes appeared to be related to their particular experiences – which influenced the **affective** or feeling, component of their constellation of attitudes towards workplace safety.

The attitudes expressed by the non-accident group may be seen to be subject to the fundamental attributional bias discussed in chapter 3, pp. 46–56, whereby others' accidents are attributed to carelessness. In contrast, the accident victims' attitudes were more likely to be subject to the availability bias as they would recall the circumstances of accidents that were within their personal experiences and the factors which were associated with those accidents.

Thus, attitudes in the safety field need to be seen as specific to particular aspects of health and safety at work. Virtually everyone would say that they are in favour of high standards of workplace safety (i.e. people generally have a 'positive attitude' towards health and safety) but this is not to say anything useful. Thus, we need to specify what **particular** aspects of health and safety people hold attitudes about – for example, using PPE. However, even knowing that workers hold positive attitudes towards using PPE does not mean that we can necessarily predict their behaviour in situations which might require the use of PPE. A number of studies which have focused upon PPE use have shown that both users and non-users feel that using PPE is beneficial – i.e. they hold a positive attitude to using PPE. However, actually being able to **predict** behaviour – i.e. whether they **will** use PPE, does not always match the positive attitude. Why this might be so is dealt with in the course of this chapter when we consider various models of the attitude/behaviour link.

As far as the consistency aspect of our attitude definition is concerned, this affirms that the best predictor of future events is what happened in similar circumstances in the past. Thus the best guide to a person's current attitude to a situation (e.g. as measured on an attitude scale – pp. 90–3) is their past attitude (as measured on the same scale). This obviously has implications for **changing** attitudes – i.e. if we are seeking to change attitudes, for example to using PPE or to some other topic, then it is necessary to pay due regard to principles of attitude change in seeking to achieve this. Attitude change is dealt with on pp. 84–8 and 93–7.

Attitudes may be considered as being located somewhere between deep-seated values and beliefs – which may well remain unchanged over a lifetime – and relatively superficial views and opinions – which may change frequently depending upon what information we have most recently been exposed to (see figure 3.1 in chapter 3). This intermediate position suggests that attitudes **can** be changed, but not too readily – i.e. it is likely to take more than a simple communication such as a poster or a newsletter article.

Attitude components

Attitudes are commonly considered to have three components (Rosenberg and Hovland, 1960):

- Affective – concerned with feelings and emotions. For example, someone who has witnessed a serious accident is likely to feel more strongly about safety than a person who has not learned through such an experience. This is because of the powerful impact of the memory of how they **felt** when seeing the accident. For a personal illustration, see summary text 4.2. However, emphasizing the affective dimension is neither a desirable nor a practical way of teaching people about safety.
- Cognitive – concerned essentially with the **thinking** aspect of an attitude – for example, having an attitude as to whether something is or is not dangerous. This component is subject to influence from a potentially wide variety of influences – e.g. reading an article or seeing a powerful TV documentary on a risk-related topic or an anecdote related by a friend. This is where our risk cognition (see Glendon, 1987b) or risk perception apparatus comes into play – the topic of chapter 5 (pp. 121–30). In its simplest form, we either consider that a particular event is or is not dangerous – e.g. 'scary' fairground rides, bungee jumping or working at heights. We then develop an implicit rank order of different risks (chapter 5, figure 5.5) to which we refer when considering whether the perceived benefits of the activity more than compensate for the perceived risk involved.
- Behavioural intention – is the **tendency to act** component described already, and is the one on which the utility of the concept of attitude stands or falls. If attitudes can predict behaviour, then this **behavioural intention** component has utility value. Behavioural intention is an important component in some models of attitude/behaviour links and relates to specific items, such as intending to acquire further training if you consider that a job or task you are doing is dangerous, or intending to use better PPE the next time you do it, or intending not to do it again at all. The behavioural intention can involve **imagining** yourself engaging in the behaviour which relates to that attitude. While the three attitudinal components can be separately identified, the relationship between them may be problematic, as demonstrated by the experiments described in summary text 4.3.

> **Summary text 4.2** A powerful memory as a safety influencer
>
> One of the authors remembers vividly an occasion as a child of about 4 years old, out walking with his father. A few feet from where we were walking, a child about my own age fell face down from the passenger door of a moving car (this was before the days of seat belts, let alone legislation on such matters). The child's (presumed) father stopped the car, gathered up the child – whose face I remember as being unrecognizable through the mass of blood – to ask my father directions to the nearest hospital. Such an experience – I could take you to the exact place where that event happened well over 40 years ago! – may have something to do with my own obsession with ensuring that my own children (and others who travel with me in a car) have always to wear seat belts on all car journeys (even before there was legislation on this). While I am not continually conscious of the event described above, I acknowledge the impact that it probably had on my subsequent behaviour (early memories for, often violent, impact events can be very powerful in influencing our later behaviour). The feeling (affective) component of an attitude can thus be very potent.

Attitude dimensions

The main characteristics of attitudes, sometimes referred to as attitude dimensions, are:

* valence – the way in which the object of an attitude is evaluated, the degree of positive or negative feeling; this is what attitude scales are often designed to measure (pp. 90–3);
* multiplexity – the degree to which an attitude is differentiated from other attitudes, for example the extent to which attitudes about safety are differentiated from attitudes about health;
* breadth – the number of attributes which characterize the object of the attitude, from very broad (e.g. workplace health and safety) to very narrow (e.g. a particular brand of ear defender);
* intensity – the strength of feeling about an object (e.g. an accident that has been witnessed);
* stability – how resistant to change (pp. 93–7);
* centrality – how much the attitude is part of an individual's self-concept or the extent to which a person feels that it reflects their identity (e.g. a safety and risk professional feeling that holding safe attitudes is part of their self-concept);
* salience – the degree to which an attitude occupies a person's awareness from total preoccupation to complete absence (e.g. a safety and risk professional might be considering safety issues all the time while at work, while most other people would not be);
* interrelatedness – how related the attitude is to other attitudes (e.g. to form a consistent cluster of attitudes towards safety issues);
* behavioural expression – the degree to which an attitude is acted upon (pp. 76–88 on attitude-behaviour links);
* verifiability – the extent to which an attitude can be checked against evidence (e.g. attitudes towards PPE being verified by observing PPE use).

Summary text 4.3 Relationship between attitude components

Kothandpani (1971) studied the interrelationship of the three components of attitudes. However, Breckler (1984) considered that this interrelationship was only of modest proportions. Participants in an experiment were presented with a live snake and their reactions were recorded using verbal measures of the three attitude components. These were compared with their heart rate (affective component) and coping behaviour (behavioural component) – e.g. avoiding the snake.

In another study, participants were put through the same procedure but on this occasion they were merely asked to imagine that a live snake was present. Relying purely on verbal measures, the interrelationships between the affective, cognitive and behavioural components of attitudes towards snakes were found to be higher than in the first study.

The findings can be explained in the following way. When you imagine a live snake in your presence, believed to be harmless (cognitive component), on the basis of verbal statements only, it might be presumed that you would not be afraid of it (fear being the relevant affective component in this case) and that you would be prepared to handle it (behavioural component). However, when actually confronted with a live snake, even a benign one, different reactions may well be seen – i.e. heart rate increases, indicating increased arousal, probably fear or apprehension in this case and avoidance of the snake rather than handling it.

Thus, it may be concluded that merely asking people to imagine what their reactions would be in a situation involving threat, is not a valid predictor of their actual behaviour or of their feelings in respect of the threat. Thus, the power of the actual situation in governing behaviour (and attitudes) is paramount – a point which has been highlighted in a number of controversial psychological experiments in which 'ordinary' people have been persuaded to deliver powerful electric shocks to others (Milgram, 1965) or have behaved brutally when in the role of 'guard' towards fellow citizens playing the role of 'prisoner' (Zimbardo, 1973). Given the powerful influence of a range of situations (e.g. war, opportunities to make money or to exert power over others) it is clear that attitudes are only one source of influence upon behaviour, and perhaps a very weak one.

A parallel divergence between a person's attitude to a particular situation (bungee jumping) and his subsequent exposure to that situation (fear – affective, and withdrawal – behavioural components) was seen in the illustration presented in 3.1 in chapter 3.

ATTITUDES AND BEHAVIOUR: SOME BASIC THEORIES

Everyone has a theory – or a set of theories – about such everyday things as attitudes and behaviour. For the most part, our 'commonsense' theories are not in our conscious minds and therefore generally remain inarticulated. However, it is useful to identify the theory you are using to explain attitudes and behaviour because this then makes explicit the assumptions you are making about other people's attitudes and why you think they behave as they do. Typically, the everyday theories we use take one of the forms described below:

- Attitudes influence behaviour, and thus if we know a person's attitude to something (e.g. using PPE) then we can predict their behaviour towards it.
- Behaviour influences attitudes, and thus if we wish to change someone's

attitude towards something (e.g. using PPE) then we can achieve this by obliging them to behave in a particular way (e.g. by passing legislation or making a rule and enforcing it).

- Attitudes and behaviour mutually reinforce each other and thus if we change either one then this is likely to lead to a change in the other.
- While it is true that attitudes and behaviour are likely to be mutually consistent (see summary text 4.6 for a more detailed explanation of this point), in order to influence them, it is necessary to address both independently – i.e. to influence deliberately attitudes on the one hand and behaviour on the other (in a consistent way).

These four types of theory are considered in greater detail below.

Attitudes influencing behaviour

The first type of theory to be described has already been mentioned in the introductory section, and it is that attitudes influence or predict behaviour. Diagrammatically it can be expressed as in figure 4.1.

Figure 4.1 reflects the view that if we know someone's attitude about something (e.g. using PPE) then we can predict their behaviour in respect of that same thing with a reasonable degree of certainty. Similarly, it also implies that if we are able to change a person's attitude to something then this will also influence – and by implication also change – the relevant behaviour. For example, it is frequently assumed that if people's attitudes towards a particular aspect of workplace health and safety (e.g. using PPE) can be changed then their behaviour will change so as to correspond with that attitude change. However, as has been shown on more than one occasion, merely to express positive attitudes about using PPE is not sufficient to change people's behaviour in respect of actually using PPE – although it is one component of the desired behaviour change.

As another illustration, in 1983 a campaign called **Site Safe '83** was launched in the UK construction industry, one premise of which was that changing attitudes among construction industry workers was the key to achieving behaviour change – and that this would be reflected in a reduction in accidents (for a review of the Site Safe '83 campaign, see Glendon and Hale, 1984). As might have been predicted, such a reduction in accidents did not occur and it could reasonably be surmised that the Site Safe '83 campaign, whatever its other merits, did not effect a detectable change either in attitudes or in behaviour. Thus, the evidence suggests that we should be cautious of any simplistic 'attitudes influence behaviour' type theory as a complete explanation of the attitude–behaviour link.

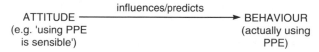

Figure 4.1 A simple theory of the attitude–behaviour link.

What would be valuable would be to specify the conditions under which attitudes are likely to influence behaviour. In a review of over 100 studies of attitude–behaviour links, Ajzen and Fishbein (1977) considered that there were four particularly important factors – action, target, situation and time frame – involved in this relationship. An illustration of the health and safety implications of this review is provided in summary text 4.4. The main conclusion to emerge from the findings of Ajzen and Fishbein's (1977) study is that it is possible to predict behaviour if attitudes are known providing that the attitudes are **highly specific** in respect of that behaviour. By the same token, if we are seeking to change behaviour by the route of attitude change, then we must address those attitudes which are directly and specifically related to that behaviour. An example of the first type of theory is described in summary text 4.5.

Behaviour influencing attitudes

The second type of theory may be represented as shown in figure 4.2.

The type of theory illustrated in figure 4.2 is a straight reversal of that described above. It is this type of theory about the nature of the attitude–behaviour link which can provide the basis for certain types of

---

Summary text 4.4 Important factors in the attitude–behaviour relationship (after Ajzen and Fishbein, 1977)

1. **Action:** The closer is the correspondence between the activity which is the object of the attitude and the behaviour, the greater is the likelihood that the behaviour will be influenced by the attitude. For example, in seeking to predict or to influence behaviour in respect of wearing hearing protection in noisy environments, attitudes towards this specific activity should be addressed (see case study described in summary text 4.15).

2. **Target:** The closer is the target behaviour under scrutiny to the attitude which is being addressed the greater is the likelihood of attitude change. For example, if it is sought to predict or to influence behaviour in respect of using PPE, then it is attitudes towards using PPE which should be addressed. Seeking to change **specific** behaviour by reference to **general** attitudes – e.g. to health and safety – is unlikely to be effective. Thus, campaigns which focus upon the particular attitude–behaviour link (e.g. in respect of a given type of PPE such as eye protection) are more likely to be successful than those which seek to effect behaviour change through generalized attempts to change attitudes.

3. **Situation:** The context within which attitudes and behaviour are linked should be as near identical as possible. Thus, attitudes about using PPE will not necessarily transfer across from one situation to another. This means that if we are seeking to influence behaviour in a particular context – such as a given part of the workplace, then it is attitudes towards using a particular kind of PPE in this part of the workplace which need to be considered.

4. **Time frame:** It is important that the link between the behaviour and the associated attitude is as temporally close as possible for influence to occur. Thus, a past attitude will be less likely to influence a given behaviour than a currently held attitude. For example, a once-held negative attitude towards using PPE will be less influential than a positive one which is held at present – and vice versa.

> **Summary text 4.5** Example of a theory which maintains that attitudes influence behaviour
>
> Fazio (1986) maintains that an attitude influences behaviour by selectively activating various thought processes held in the person's memory. This produces selective perception of the object related to the attitude in question. For example, if you hold a positive attitude towards accident prevention, this could mean that you are more likely to think consciously about positive precautionary measures. Any focus on these measures (e.g. via a safety campaign) will then shape your selective perceptions of what precautionary measures exist to prevent accident occurrences. These processes can then influence a decision to act in the context of accident prevention. According to Fazio, an attitude is anchored in previous positive and negative experiences but it selectively influences the memory of these influences, rather than being influenced by them when deciding on a course of action. Therefore, individuals with different attitudes when confronted by a particular scene or events, are likely to see different aspects of the situation as salient or important.

legislation – in health and safety and in other fields. Thus, it is assumed that if ways can be found to change people's behaviour then their attitudes will change to correspond with that behaviour.

In the case of legislation, an attempt is being made to change behaviour directly – for example by the provision of an agency specifically charged with enforcement and a system of penalties for breaching the legislative requirements which can be imposed through the state legal machinery. Over a period of time, attitudes may change – for example, in respect of workplace health and safety or to seat-belt wearing or to racial or sexual discrimination in employment practices – partly as a result of such legislation. According to cognitive consistency theory (summary text 4.6), if we are obliged (e.g. by law) to behave in a certain way, then whatever our initial attitude towards the topic of the legislation (e.g. seat belt wearing), then to remain consistent we change our attitude so as to correspond with the newly required behaviour. While it is difficult to demonstrate conclusively that any given piece of legislation influenced a person's attitude, it is likely to be among the factors which go to form attitudes. (A comprehensive review of empirical and theoretical work in the attitude–behaviour relationship is given by Kleinke, 1984.)

An alternative interpretation of this type of theory (Bem, 1967) is that we frequently determine what our attitudes are by observing our own behaviour (self-perception). For example, if people repeatedly take various safety precautions at work (safe behaviour or habit) they might conclude that they possess positive safety attitudes. Self-perception theory maintains that a person forms attitudes through observing his or her own behaviour.

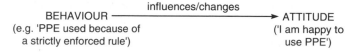

Figure 4.2 An alternative theory of the attitude–behaviour link.

A final example is the link between training as a means to change behaviour (chapter 2, pp. 25–7) and attitudes. For example, the European Commission (1990) emphasize the importance of the link between training and attitudes in the field of safety, maintaining that 'training is the bedrock of an active attitude to prevention' (EC, 1990, p. 75). Their objectives for safety training are stated as being to:

- develop a sense of safety;
- learn how to control the risks;
- promote awareness of the rules of safety.

The first and third of these objectives emphasize the strong attitudinal component of safety training. This is reinforced by the Commission's view that a 'sense of safety' should be developed during basic education – when attitudes are first formed – from the early years at school and followed through during vocational training.

Mutual influence model

A third view of the attitude–behaviour link is represented by figure 4.3 which is an amalgam of figures 4.1 and 4.2, and shows that attitudes influence behaviour and behaviour influences attitudes. Thus, in respect of this type of theory, all that was said in respect of the first two also applies. In effect, this approach reflects one obvious conclusion from the dual premises represented in the two unidirectional theories already described. Therefore, this theory represents an advance on the previous two and is characterized by the notion of consistency between attitudes and behaviour.

The notion of consistency, congruity or balance underlies such theories as those of Festinger (1957) on cognitive dissonance – the basic premise being that people strive to make their attitudes and behaviour consistent. The narrative in summary text 4.6 illustrates the approach to the attitude–behaviour link from the cognitive consistency perspective

Influence of other factors

The fourth type of theory to consider is based upon the premise that while there may be consistency between attitudes and behaviour, this is not

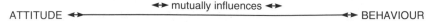

ATTITUDE ◄►━━━━━━━━━━◄► mutually influences ◄►━━━━━━━━━━◄► BEHAVIOUR

In this case, the attitude may be to the effect that 'Because I use PPE (behaviour), then it must be sensible to do so' (attitude) – i.e. attitude is influenced by relevant behaviour.

The behaviour (using PPE) comes about because of the attitude that it is sensible to do so – i.e. behaviour is reinforced by reference to presumed favourable attitude.

Figure 4.3 A combined theory of the attitude–behaviour link.

Summary text 4.6 Cognitive dissonance: a safety example

Cognitive dissonance occurs when our attitudes and behaviour are inconsistent – or dissonant. It is a theory which is based on the assumption that people have a need for consistency in their attitudes and behaviour and that if there is an inconsistency, then they will strive to reduce or eliminate it. For example, if a person smokes (behaviour) and at the same time believes that smoking is harmful (attitude) then they are in a situation of dissonance with respect to smoking.

There are logically only two ways in which they can reduce or eliminate the dissonance; first to change the behaviour and second to change their attitude towards the behaviour. In our example, there is only one way in which they can change their behaviour so that it becomes consonant with their attitude and that of course, is to stop smoking. However there are a number of ways in which they could change their attitude so that it becomes consonant with their smoking behaviour. For example, they could reason that smoking helps them to concentrate at work or that it helps them to feel at ease in social situations or that whatever the possible long-term harm, they still actually enjoy smoking. Alternatively, they might think that they are unlikely to get cancer even if others do, or they might say to themselves that they might die in some other way so why stop smoking or that if they do fall ill they will be looked after, or they might ... and so on. In other words, there are many alternative ways of changing your attitude about something so that it fits with your behaviour, but generally the options for changing behaviour are very few in number.

Thus, when we are seeking to make health and safety improvements which involve human behaviour, it is not enough to change attitudes, as these might simply swing round to remain consonant with risky behaviour in some other way. It is essential to address behaviour directly and also to ensure that attitudes which correspond with that behaviour remain consonant with it. For example, in training people to follow a safe system of work, the behaviour which this involves needs to be reinforced with reminders which will influence attitudes in the same direction – that intelligent people used this method, that it was developed by people experienced in the technique, and so forth. Cognitive dissonance is a theory which has practical application in health and safety.

necessarily a basis for judging one to be a prime causal agent in respect of the other. Thus, while the importance of cognitive consistency is implicitly acknowledged, the possibility of additional factors which could influence both attitudes and behaviour is considered. Figure 4.4 presents a picture of this type of theory – or model – of the nature of the attitude–behaviour link.

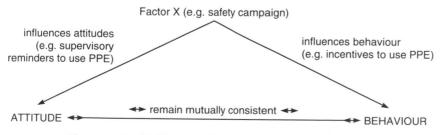

Figure 4.4 A third factor influencing attitudes and behaviour.

Figure 4.4 shows that an underlying factor, for example a safety campaign, might be designed to address both attitudes and behaviour of a section of the workforce. A simple example might be that incentives, perhaps in the form of bonuses, are to be given for achieving a certain safety index score. This might be a combination of: a safety audit score at a specified level (chapter 10, pp. 298–312), a given housekeeping level as revealed by successive workplace inspections and an accident rate target achieved. To reinforce this attempt to influence behaviour, a reminder system is used – for example a combination of: posters showing an appropriate message, toolbox talks with the supervisor and personally addressed letters. Such a campaign would be a variant on the marketing approach to influencing consumer behaviour whereby advertising messages designed to influence attitudes towards a product (but not necessarily to make people buy it) are reinforced by promotional activity such as offers of free flights or price reductions when the consumer enters the store to buy. This approach to health and safety may be represented in a general strategic model, as shown in figure 4.5 – taken from Glendon (1991). It shows that in order to effect change in workplace behaviour in respect of health and safety, it is necessary to address both cognitions (e.g. attitudes, perceptions, motivation) and behaviour directly in order to make progress. This approach to the attitude–behaviour link is a further progression on the first three theories on the nature of this link and is approaching the more sophisticated health belief model (HBM) described on pp. 84–8.

Theory of reasoned action

Before the HBM is considered, one more exposition of the attitude–behaviour link is described – the more complex theory of reasoned action (Fishbein and Ajzen, 1975). This is shown in diagrammatic form in figure 4.6, incorporating a safety example.

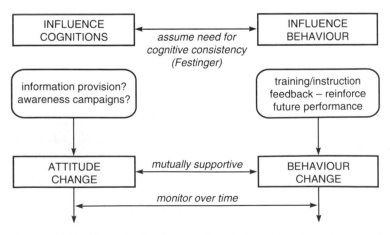

Figure 4.5 Health and safety intervention strategy (after Glendon, 1991).

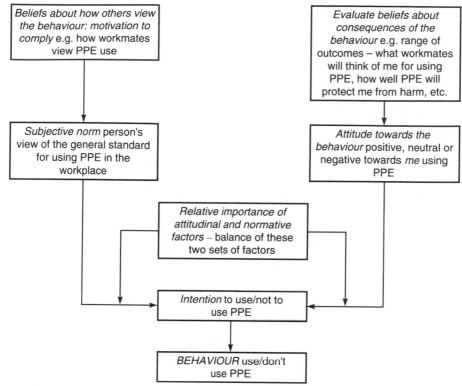

Figure 4.6 The theory of reasoned action (after Fishbein and Ajzen, 1975).

Although in essence, a theory of the first type described above (see figure 4.1) compared with this simple exposition, the theory of reasoned action proposes that more complex processes are involved in the route from attitudes to behaviour. Thus, in this theory it is argued that behaviour can be predicted if we know:

1. the person's **attitude** to the particular behaviour;
2. the person's **intention** to perform that behaviour;
3. what the person **believes** are the **consequences** of performing that behaviour;
4. the **social norms** (socially acceptable behaviour) which govern that behaviour.

However, actually satisfying all the above conditions so as to predict (or to change) behaviour is not easy. For example, workers may be more likely to use PPE in response to pressure from social norms – i.e. colleagues expecting them to behave safely – rather than because they have a positive attitude to using PPE or because they harbour an intention to use PPE. A consideration of attitudes operating at different levels is taken up on pp. 88–90.

Other factors which might serve to promote the continued use of PPE are a desire to obey (safety) rules and the formation of a particular safety habit.

Knapper *et al.* (1976) investigated attitudes towards car safety belts, the results indicating an overwhelming tendency for respondents to express positive attitudes towards the use of seat belts and confidence in their effectiveness. These attitudes existed irrespective of whether the respondents claimed to use their own seat belts. A significant finding was that the main factor responsible for claims by respondents that they were using seat belts was not simply a matter of having a positive or negative attitude, but was predominantly governed by the **habit** of using a seat belt.

Thus, it seems that there is something durable about habits that rest upon previous behaviour, and that changing them could prove to be a greater challenge than seeking to change attitudes and beliefs. For example, health related behaviour – smoking, exercise and diet for example – is frequently at odds with attitudes. Thus, in spite of the assumption of cognitive dissonance, people may continue to engage in behaviour which they know is damaging to their health. One factor is that for some smokers, their behaviour is physically determined (i.e. nicotine addiction) and thus beyond the reach of influence through persuasion, as well as being functional in countering stressful conditions (Eiser and van der Plight, 1988). In addition, while smokers tend to emphasize the short-term benefits of smoking, non-smokers tend to focus upon the long-term consequences of smoking (Eiser and van der Plight, 1982) – an example of the time frame component of the attitude–behaviour link referred to by Ajzen and Fishbein (1977).

Because the theory of reasoned action is a general theory of the relationship between attitude and behaviour, it may be difficult to encompass all instances where the attitude–behaviour link breaks down. It is also a theory which is very much in the cognitive tradition – its very name suggests this. In reality, actions are not always rational because they are subject to emotional factors as well as to cool rational appraisal. Thus, a more specific approach to health attitudes and behaviour which can also take account of emotional factors – the health belief model – is considered next.

THE HEALTH BELIEF MODEL AND OTHER COGNITIVE THEORIES OF ATTITUDE–BEHAVIOUR LINKS

The most widely used model of behaviour change – the health belief model (HBM) (Becker, 1974; Becker and Rosenstock, 1987) – has been used as the basis of many campaigns seeking to change people's behaviour to a healthier way of living. Some of these studies are reviewed by Janz and Becker (1984) while Harrison *et al.* (1992) report on the success of the HBM in predicting health behaviours and outcomes. Summary text 4.7 outlines the essential points of the health belief model while figure 4.7 shows this approach to the (health) attitude–behaviour link in diagrammatic form.

The theory of planned behaviour (Ajzen, 1991) extends the theory of reasoned action, discussed on pp. 82–4, by the addition of an individual **control** component which is influenced by the person's evaluation of factors likely to inhibit or facilitate their performance of the behaviour – analogous to the

Summary text 4.7 The health belief model (after Becker, 1974)

The health belief model offers insight into aspects of human perception and experience which need to be addressed if behaviour is to be changed in the direction of greater health and safety, specifically the likelihood that an individual will take some form of preventive behaviour to improve their health or safety (e.g. use PPE to protect their hearing or reduce/stop smoking to improve their health). Two main factors influence such behaviour; first the individual considers the perceived benefits and disbenefits of taking the action and second the person has a view of the threat which is posed.

An example of taking preventive action to preserve health might be wearing ear defenders. In taking the decision to wear or not to wear, the individual assesses the perceived benefits (e.g. reduced likelihood of long-term hearing loss, less short-term working discomfort from noise) and weighs these against the barriers (e.g. reduced opportunity for social contact at work, physical discomfort from wearing the ear defenders for a whole shift). The benefits and barriers which the individual perceives will be based upon personal experience, education and other factors.

The individual also assesses the threat to their health and in so doing considers their own personal susceptibility to the disease or condition against which they might protect themselves and their perceived severity of the condition should they succumb. This assessment is also influenced by their experience, background and other factors. Finally, the perceived threat of the condition (NIHL) will be influenced by cues to action, for example posters, articles in newspapers, reminders from work colleagues or again, past experience.

In applying the health belief model to any health or safety campaign or attempt to change behaviour so that it reduces the risk to the individual, the following need to be addressed if the campaign is to stand any chance of success.

1. Ensure that the perceived benefits of taking the action are greater than the perceived barriers – e.g. highlight the positive aspects and attend to the disbenefits, for example by providing a choice of ear defenders to improve the likelihood that each person will obtain a pair which is comfortable for them (see for example the case study described in summary text 4.13).
2. Emphasize that the target audience is susceptible and demonstrate this whenever possible. An example is given by Zohar et al. (1980) who used the temporary threshold shift phenomenon to feedback to workers their audiograms after a work shift to show how their hearing had been affected (see the case study described in summary text 4.15). Emphasize also the severity of the long-term condition, for example by playing tapes of how speech and other noises sound to hearing impaired people – not forgetting to explain how the condition can be avoided.
3. Provide appropriate cues for action, for example posters at strategic points, supervisors giving reminders and reinforcing workers when ear defenders are worn. This also serves to demonstrate that individuals have control over the situation and that they can take responsibility for their health and safety.

costs and benefits in the HBM.

Finally, protection motivation theory (Beck, 1984; van der Velde and van der Plight, 1991) considers that health behaviours are affected by:

- perceived severity of outcomes;
- probability of outcomes;
- efficacy of behaviour;
- expectation that the individual will be able to carry out the behaviour.

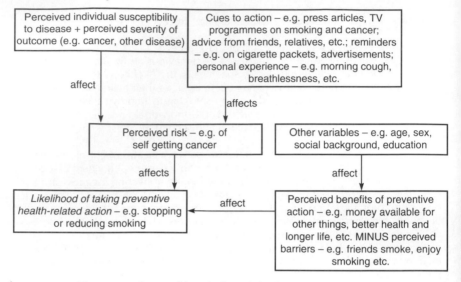

Figure 4.7 The Health Belief Model (after Becker, 1974).

The first two of these factors relate to the individual's perceived risk while the third and fourth factors relate to the likely effectiveness of any individual intervention (akin to perceived control) – the other main dimension of risk or hazard perception (chapter 5, pp. 121–30 for a more detailed exposition). Protection motivation theory introduces the important notion that attitudes and perceptions are linked to behaviour through motivational processes – a theme of this part of the book (for example, figure 3.1 in chapter 3). The four components combine through the notion of protective motivation which arouses, sustains and directs activity to protect the individual from danger. Protection motivation theory is described in figure 4.8, together with safety-related examples.

The complex models described are examples of social cognition models and all emphasize the rationality of human behaviour. They are useful in respect of identifying key variables which link attitudes and behaviour in the health and safety (and other) fields in a coherent and structured way. They have been tested and found to have some validity when they have been used as a basis for interventions (Sheppard *et al.*, 1988; Six and Schmidt, 1992). This is because they help us to identify the relevant factors which need to be addressed – for example in safety or health campaigns.

However, such models tend to ignore the **irrational** – or emotive – aspects of human functioning and also behaviour which is governed more by habit than by reason. External factors also tend to be ignored, such as the social skills required to carry out certain types of behaviour (e.g. using personal protection, stopping smoking) and the complex interactions between individuals in the settings in which the behaviour occurs. Thus, it is assumed in the models that individuals are highly motivated to think about health-related behaviour, whereas in fact there will be competing – and frequently conflicting – attitudes and behaviours to consider.

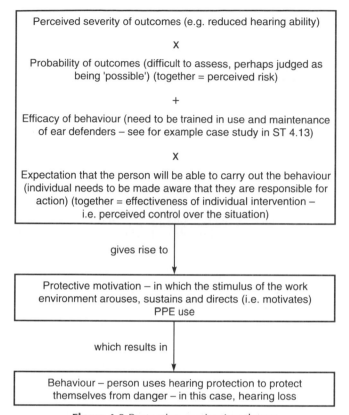

Perceived severity of outcomes (e.g. reduced hearing ability)

X

Probability of outcomes (difficult to assess, perhaps judged as being 'possible') (together = perceived risk)

+

Efficacy of behaviour (need to be trained in use and maintenance of ear defenders – see for example case study in ST 4.13)

X

Expectation that the person will be able to carry out the behaviour (individual needs to be made aware that they are responsible for action) (together = effectiveness of individual intervention – i.e. perceived control over the situation)

gives rise to

Protective motivation – in which the stimulus of the work environment arouses, sustains and directs (i.e. motivates) PPE use

which results in

Behaviour – person uses hearing protection to protect themselves from danger – in this case, hearing loss

Figure 4.8 Protection motivation theory.

Thus, these models can help to unravel some of the main factors which influence behaviour – including attitudes – although they do not yet include all relevant factors. Some authors (e.g. Connor, 1992; Schwarzer, 1992) have produced integrated reviews, from which it is possible to develop a list of the main factors, including those not in the models, which influence behaviour in respect of health, safety and risk. These factors fall under four overlapping headings: attitudes, perceptions, motivation and behaviour, and are outlined in summary text 4.8.

The list in summary text 4.8 can be used as a checklist of items in all circumstances when a change in behaviour is sought. It will be seen that not all influences upon behaviour are attitudinal in nature and that perceptions and motivations as well as past behaviour all play a part.

FUNCTIONS AND LEVELS OF ATTITUDES

Attitude functions

Attitudes are generally considered to perform a number of functions (Katz, 1960). First, they serve an **instrumental** function – serving certain ends and

---

Summary text 4.8 Main factors influencing behaviour in respect of health, safety and risk

Behaviour only
- What is the **social context** (e.g. norms) for the behaviour?
- What are the person's **habits** in respect of the behaviour? (past behaviour is a good guide to future behaviour)

Attitude and behaviour
- What is the nature of any **social pressure** in respect of the behaviour?
- What factors are likely to **inhibit or facilitate** the behaviour?

Attitude only
- What is the person's **attitude towards the behaviour**?

Attitude and perception
- What are the **costs and benefits** of taking a given set of actions?
- What do **relevant others think** about the behaviour?

Perception only
- What are the various **outcomes** possible?
- How **severe** are the respective outcomes?
- How **likely** are various outcomes?
- How much **control** does the individual have?
- How **effective** is the individual's behaviour likely to be?
- What **reminders** are there?

Perception and motivation
- Are there differences between **long term** vs **short term** benefits and costs?

Motivation only
- What is the person's **intention** in respect of the behaviour?
- How **important** is this behaviour to the individual?
- What is the person's **motivation** to comply with **social pressure**?
- What are the **emotional reactions** to the decision and subsequent behaviour?

Behaviour, attitude, perception and motivation
- What are the individual's **personal characteristics** (e.g. age, gender, background, experience)?

---

enabling us to obtain reinforcement for our desires and requirements. Thus, a 'positive attitude' towards people and events is developed with the purpose of satisfying the individual's needs, while 'negative attitudes' are more liable to thwart those needs.

Attitudes are also held to have an **ego defensive** function, whereby they permit the expression of defence mechanisms by an individual. For example, a person may use their attitudes as a means of protecting themselves from certain harsh realities – such as that they are working in a dangerous environment or are pursuing behaviour which presents a risk to their health.

Another function of attitudes is the **value expressive** function whereby attitudes permit a person to express the concept which they have of themselves. Thus, attitudes are part of an individual's self concept, for example considering themselves to be 'safe', or 'normal' or 'independent' partly on the basis of the attitudes which they communicate to themselves and to others.

Finally, attitudes serve a **knowledge** function, being a prime means by which people can order their environment and through which they are able to make sense of and react consistently and meaningfully to the world around them. Without some degree of stability in the way in which we perceive the world, we would encounter many problems in our personal relationships and our interpretation of events.

When a person finds that an attitude, or a set of attitudes, is no longer functional in dealing with the situation in which they find themselves, s/he could well question existing attitudes in the light of new information and, as a result, bring his or her attitudes more in line with 'reality'. Circumstances under which attitude change is most likely are dealt with on pp. 93–7.

Attitude levels

In considering the social influences which impact upon individuals in respect of whether they will adopt particular attitudes and behaviour, it is also useful to consider the **levels** at which attitudes and behaviour are formed. A useful categorization was developed by Kelman (1958). The first level of attitude/behaviour is that of **compliance**. Here a person accepts influence from another party because they hope to achieve a favourable reaction from them – for example, attaining certain rewards or avoiding punishments. In the safety field, an example would be a worker using a particular type of PPE either because s/he wished to please the supervisor or because there were strict rules about wearing it and sanctions, including eventual dismissal, for not using it. However, the attitude–behaviour link in this case is not strong because there is always the possibility that once the reasons for compliance are removed (e.g. a new supervisor arrives who is less readily pleased or the rules are less strictly enforced because of increased production pressure) then the wearing behaviour will tend to lapse because the attitude–behaviour link is basically weak – i.e. the behaviour results from external pressures rather than from internal beliefs.

The second level is **identification** which occurs when an individual adopts behaviour which is derived from another party because of the relationship with that party. A good example would be the operation of group norms, whereby a person uses PPE because others in the group do and the person values their relationship with the group members. Thus, using behaviour is likely to continue as long as the individual remains with that particular group. However, if they transfer to another job and become part of a different group which has different norms (e.g. for non-use or optional usage), then again the behaviour will be susceptible to change in response to changing circumstances (i.e. they now value maintaining their relationship with the new group). Group relationships are considered in greater detail in chapter 7, especially pp. 177–80. Thus, the attitude–behaviour link is again essentially dependent for its continuation upon external factors – in this case social relationships – and is liable to decay if these change.

The final level at which attitudes may be expressed is that of **internalization**.

In this case, a person adopts a particular behaviour because of its functional value (see this section) or because it is in accordance with their existing belief system. At this level, the link between attitude and behaviour is at its strongest because, whatever the external factors operating, an individual engages in the behaviour because they **believe** that it is correct – irrespective of rules or what others choose to do. Thus, in our example a worker would use the protection because they knew it to be the right thing to do – it was in accordance with their own internal belief system about safe behaviour.

There are practical lessons to be drawn from this simple theory about levels of the relationship between attitudes and behaviour and the influences upon them. The critical point about promoting a desired behaviour is that the individual (worker, manager, etc.) must believe that it is correct, in other words should have internalized the attitude–behaviour link. This link should be independent of any external factors. If the whole workforce have developed this belief system, then the group norm for safety will apply throughout and will serve to reinforce the individually held attitude. The existence of rules and sanctions will then serve to reinforce still further the correctness of these attitudes and behaviour. For example, in working with electricity or with other high potential energy sources, trained individuals take all the necessary precautions because they know the danger and behave accordingly. Group norms as well as rules and procedures serve to reinforce and to guide these beliefs. Thus, there is a coherent and consistent system of individual attitudes, group behaviour and a set of rules. Organizations which can successfully achieve the mutual reinforcement and confluence of attitudes and behaviour at these three levels will have taken a vital step along the road towards a positive safety culture (chapter 10, pp. 291–5). However, seeking to change behaviour by the imposition of rules and regulations without changing attitudes, is much less likely to be successful (see the model in figure 4.2).

ATTITUDE MEASUREMENT

There are two main reasons for attempting to measure attitudes. First, we want to know not only whether a person has a positive or negative view of a particular issue or event, but also the strength of that feeling. Second, if we are seeking to change attitudes through some intervention (e.g. a safety campaign), then some objective measure is required to gauge attitudes before and after the intervention. A number of techniques for measuring attitudes have been devised and these can be divided into direct and indirect measures.

An example of an indirect technique is to observe unobtrusively the behaviour of a person, for example by observing and recording their use of a particular type of protective equipment. A measure of their attitude towards that type of equipment may be taken as the amount of time that they use it. The assumption here is that behaviour is consistent with the attitude, although as indicated earlier behaviour may not be a good guide to attitude.

The better known measures of attitudes are the direct measures – usually called attitude scales – which have been developed over many occasions of use and which are considered to be reasonably reliable (being a consistent measure on successive occasions of use) and valid (actually measuring attitude as opposed to something else). The most common types of attitude scale are:

- Thurstone
- Likert
- Semantic Differential
- Visual analogue.

A Thurstone scale is characterized by equal appearing intervals. The procedure for developing such a scale is described in summary text 4.9. The Thurstone scale is among the most time consuming to develop, but gives a more precise measure of attitudes than most other types of scales.

The best-known attitude scale is the Likert scale, the development and nature of which is described in summary text 4.10. It is designed to measure the intensity of an attitude. The Likert scale is relatively easy to construct and administer, but to be used as a valid measure of attitudes, requires attention to development of the scale items so that they represent the best available measure of the attitude.

The Semantic Differential – or Osgood scale after its originator – provides an indication of the strength of an attitude as well as information about its significance to the individual. Scales of this type have nine answer points which are anchored by a pair of polar opposite key words designed to measure aspects of three dimensions of an attitude towards some topic – evaluative, potency and activity. For example, respondents may be asked to rate their attitudes towards a safety film using the bipolar adjectives shown in figure 4.9.

Summary text 4.9 Developing a Thurstone scale to measure workers' attitudes to workplace safety

1. Collect a large number (at least 100) of statements expressing a wide variety of views and feelings about workplace safety – for example by interviewing, holding group discussions or walking around talking to people.

2. A number of workers (similar to those who will be the respondents in the survey) sort the statements into eleven piles on a gradient from very negative to very positive. About a dozen people should be used as judges for this task.

3. The **median** value (mid range point in the 11 piles produced by each of the judges) is found for each item.

4. Inconsistent items are rejected as these are evaluated differently by the judges – and thus would not be reliable attitude measures in the larger respondent group.

5. The resulting scale is tested for item discriminability – the extent to which each item does actually discriminate between attitudes held by different people. Items which have low discriminability are rejected.

6. The final scale should have a relatively small number of items – perhaps less than 20 – which elicit consistent responses and which represent as wide a range of scale values as possible (between 1 and 11).

Summary text 4.10 Developing a Likert scale to measure attitudes towards workplace safety

Statements for inclusion in a Likert scale may be selected in similar ways to that for a Thurstone scale, or may be derived from experts and those knowledgeable in the target area. A reasonable number of items is required to represent the expected range of attitudes on the issue in question – a minimum of 30 may be required in a scale for measuring attitudes to workplace safety. Approximately equal numbers of favourable and unfavourable items on the topic should be included. The following items were included in a study of union and management attitudes to safety (Price and Lueder, 1980).

'Company management plays a crucial role in providing a safe and healthy workplace'
'No monetary value can be placed on human life'
'Unions play a crucial role in providing a safe and healthy workplace'
'There are times when production is at least as important as safety'
'The benefits of safety outweigh its costs'.

Respondents are required to indicate their degree of agreement or disagreement to each statement, usually on a 5-point scale such as: 'strongly agree', 'agree', 'neither agree nor disagree', 'disagree', 'strongly disagree'. Occasionally larger or smaller numbers of categories may be used – for example, a 7-point scale for greater discrimination or a 4-point scale so that respondents cannot opt to be neutral about any item.

In developing the Likert scale, each respondent's scores are totalled and the scores for all respondents on each item are then correlated with the total score – a procedure known as item analysis. The final scale should comprise those items which correlate most highly with the total score – i.e. those which measure most effectively what the whole scale is intended to measure.

To indicate your views of the film which you have just seen, please circle the number which most closely corresponds to your view for each of the pairs of adjectives listed below. There are no right or wrong views – just your views. Go through the list fairly quickly trusting your first impressions. Please ensure that you circle one number for each pair of adjectives.

The film that I have just seen was in my view...

good	1	2	3	4	5	6	7	8	9	bad
credible	1	2	3	4	5	6	7	8	9	not credible
strong	1	2	3	4	5	6	7	8	9	weak
sensational	1	2	3	4	5	6	7	8	9	lacking impact
active	1	2	3	4	5	6	7	8	9	passive
fast	1	2	3	4	5	6	7	8	9	slow

Figure 4.9 Example of items from a Semantic Differential (Osgood) scale to measure attitudes to a safety film.

In the example given in figure 4.9, respondents would be required to rate the safety film on the scale for each of the adjective pairs. In the example given, the evaluative dimension consists of the adjective pairs 'good ... bad' and 'credible ... not credible'. The potency dimension is represented by the adjective pairs 'strong ... weak' and 'sensational ... lacking impact', while the activity dimension adjective pairs are 'active ... passive' and 'fast ... slow'. The evaluative dimension scores provide information on the degree of favourableness of the safety film and the other two dimensions provide information about the significance of the film to each individual respondent. The evaluative dimension is often regarded as the most important of the three dimensions because it measures the strength of an attitude.

The final type of attitude scale described here is the visual analogue scale. This comprises a set of attitude or behaviour statements – obtained in similar fashion to those derived for other types of scales – which describe various examples of the attitude or behaviour being explored, for example road safety. Respondents are required to express their attitude to each illustration of the attitude or behaviour by indicating on a single line of fixed length (usually 100 mm) their view of the attitude item in respect of whether it represents more or less safe or unsafe behaviour. The total score on a number of items – perhaps 20 or more – represents that individual's rating on the scale. An example item is shown in Figure 4.10.

There are other types of attitude scales and those described above require more detailed reading before use can be considered. Therefore, consultation of a textbook on attitudes and attitude measurement (e.g. Oppenheim, 1992) is recommended.

ATTITUDE CHANGE

The title of this chapter, as well as some of the models described on pp. 76–84, indicate that attitudes and behaviour have a cyclical relationship – one follows the other in a developing process. This section considers some of the main factors which affect the attitude change process. Aspects of the attitude change process have already been considered in the form of cognitive consistency theory – the notion that we seek to make our attitudes and our behaviour mutually supportive.

Attitudes can be changed and a number of processes are responsible for bringing about change. A new attitude may be adopted for an ulterior motive such as a desire to make a favourable impression on your boss or a client or to develop a relationship with someone whom you value. These are examples of the **instrumental** function of attitudes. The new attitude may then be embraced as part of your cluster of attitudes towards that party. Membership of a group or organization, whereby the individual is influenced by prevailing practices can also contribute to a change in attitudes, for example when a worker joins a company which has sound and progressive safety practices (see also the discussion on this topic in chapter 7, especially pp. 184–5).

Please mark the scale below at the point which most closely represents your own view of the activity described. For example, if you felt that 'overtaking a vehicle on the inside lane of a dual carriageway if another driver remains in the outside lane' is generally a rather unsafe manoeuvre, then you might mark the scale as indicated below.

Overtaking a vehicle on the inside lane of a dual carriageway if another driver remains in the outside lane is generally . . .

Very safe_____/_____Not at all safe

Figure 4.10 Example of a visual analogue scale item to measure attitudes towards safe driving.

The mass media – press, radio and television – is often held responsible for attitude changes, particularly when recipients of media messages have the opportunity to discuss the issues involved with people whose opinions they have confidence in and who find the message acceptable. Campaigns may be mounted via the media which have a strong safety message – for example, car seat belt wearing ('clunk click every trip'), chip pan fires (brief film sequence showing what to do), looking out for motor cyclists ('think bike') and high-lighting the risks of driving after consuming alcohol. Such campaigns **may** have some influence upon attitudes which begin by being unformulated or are at odds with those implied by the campaign, but are more likely to be effec-tive in **reinforcing** existing attitudes which are consonant with the message. Appealing to the motives and needs of the target group is likely to be the most effective way of promoting attitude change within this group.

A comprehensive set of studies was carried out at Yale University during the 1950s and 1960s and the findings from these have formed a generally accepted set of criteria for effecting attitude change. These will be outlined under five main headings:

- the audience;
- the persuader;
- personality factors;
- presentation of issues;
- persistence of change.

Audience

First, audiences generally self-select, that is they make decisions in respect of what messages they will expose themselves to. This is important for the com-municator of any message to remember – whether in the marketing, safety or whatever fields. It means that to communicate a message aimed at changing attitudes, you need to address this to your audience on their 'home ground'. It is also important to remember that members of an audience will have an existing network of interconnected attitudes and that it is helpful to know what these are – for example, by measuring them (pp. 90–3) – in order to be able to identify those where change is desired and to measure whether any change has taken place. It is also necessary to accept that because there are individual differences, it is unlikely that you will be able to change the attitudes of every person in an audience at the first attempt. There are also important considerations relating to the self-esteem and ego involvement of members of your audience. It is advisable to seek to promote attitude change through addressing needs and motives which are important to the person's self-esteem and in which they are highly involved.

Persuader

As far as the persuader is concerned, it is important that this party should have credibility in the eyes of the audience, for example be seen as an expert in the area and to be trustworthy. The communicator should be seen to derive little personal advantage from influencing others to change their attitudes. A communicator who is attractive to and liked by the audience is more likely to be accepted by an audience and to be able to induce attitude change. They should exhibit characteristics which are similar to, or at least acceptable to, the audience and they should express views which are congruent with those of the audience. For example, in attempting to introduce a new safety rule, it could be pointed out that everyone favours a safer workplace and that the new rule is congruent with this broader attitude. The message should aim to have some immediate impact so that people remember it (salience requirement) and it has been found that if you ask for extreme change in an attitude, then it is more likely that the audience will at least move some way in the direction of change.

Personality factors

A number of personality factors have been found to be associated with the likelihood of attitude change (personality is considered in more detail in chapter 6). It has been suggested that there is a general trait of 'persuasibility', which is another way of saying that individuals differ in their liability to attitude change. It also seems that more intelligent people are more open to attitude change, although individual cognitive needs and styles are also relevant. Some individuals are more defensive than others and those who are very self-defensive may hold attitudes which are very hard to change. Finally, group affiliations are important as people will discuss their views within their peer groups before firming up their own attitudes on a topic (see chapter 7, pp. 168–9 and 171–7).

Presentation of issues

As far as the presentation of issues is concerned, it is usually better to present both sides of an argument rather than one side only as the audience will be wary of a message which presents one side only unless this is one about which there are positive attitudes already – such as workplace safety. There is no particular rule as to where the most important material in a message should be placed, although there are both primacy (first material most likely to be remembered) and recency (last presented material also highly likely to be remembered) effects in any communication. The primacy effect is generally the stronger. When the audience is intelligent and knowledgeable about the topic or where the topic is a fairly straightforward one, they can be left to draw their own conclusions about the topic in question, otherwise it may be helpful to spell out the main findings and issues for the audience. Whether the material should be presented in an emotional or factual way depends upon the nature of the message and the desired change. The most extreme form of emotional appeal for a safety message is usually a fear appeal or threat and this issue is taken up below.

Persistence of change

When it comes to the persistence of any change, this is aided by **active** participation in the delivery of the message. For example, participation through role play has been found to be particularly powerful in changing safety attitudes and behaviour in respect of PPE use (Pirani and Reynolds, 1976). This accords with a training reinforcement principle discussed in chapter 2 (pp. 15–23). Transmitters of messages also rely upon repetition to reinforce a change in attitude and this can be effective if the message is received several times by an audience. Finally, there is the so-called 'sleeper effect' whereby a message is received but the processing takes some time and any change may take time to show.

Studies of attitudes and behaviour change and safety

Safety propaganda campaigns by themselves are likely to have limited success in changing attitudes, particularly where these are not backed up by other measures, such as training. Where the support does not exist, a gradual reversion to previous behaviour is likely (Hale, 1974). In a review of a number of research findings, Sell (1977) set out the conditions necessary for a change in safety behaviour as a result of using safety posters and other propaganda, as well as situations to avoid. Findings from this study are shown in summary text 4.11.

The issue of whether fear arousal should be used in seeking to change attitudes and behaviour has been the subject of much research (e.g. Janis and Feshback, 1963; Higbee, 1969; Rogers and Mewborn, 1976; Sutton, 1982). In general, findings indicate that high levels of fear arousal are counterproductive in changing attitudes and behaviour because the audience erects defensive barriers and tends to reject the information (e.g. that they could be seriously hurt or suffer ill-health). Mildly arousing messages may be more effective, but more important than this is that the audience require the information or perception of control over the threat – whether this is available from the environment (e.g. via some protective barrier) or from their

---

Summary text 4.11 Safety posters and other propaganda (after Sell, 1977)

To be really effective, they should:

- be specific to a particular task or situation;
- back up a training programme;
- give a positive instruction;
- be placed close to where the desired action is to take place;
- build on existing knowledge and attitudes;
- emphasize non-safety aspects;
- be on topics over which the audience has some control.

To be really effective, they should **not**:

- involve horror – this brings defence mechanisms into play;
- be negative as this does not indicate the correct way of doing something;
- be general exhortations as people then think the message applies only to others;
- have a different impact upon different groups – e.g. a positive effect on those already acting safely but a negative effect on those who are not acting safely.

---

personal resources (e.g. in the form of skill or ability). The attitude change models considered on pp. 76–88 are relevant here. In general, considerable caution needs to be exercised in the use of fear in propaganda messages. A more detailed review of studies of the use of fear to change attitudes and behaviour is given by Hale and Glendon (1987).

To conclude the main part of this chapter, a series of four case studies on successful attitude and behaviour change in the workplace are described in summary text 4.12 to 4.15. These are intended to illustrate some of the principles outlined in this chapter and to indicate that quite dramatic changes are possible in respect of safe attitudes and behaviour.

CONCLUSIONS

In this chapter, we have explored the nature of attitudes, focusing upon the vital link between attitudes and behaviour in the context of safety and risk management. The other main focus has been the important topic of attitude change and the strategic approach of ensuring congruence between attitudes and behaviour in effecting change in the workplace.

Workplace attitudes **are** relevant to safety and risk professionals because they are one component of safe behaviour, which in turn is an important feature of the overall safety culture of an organization (chapter 10, pp. 291–5). However, attitudes are only one of the variables which influence a person's behaviour and it is therefore essential that those seeking to effect behaviour changes address a range of issues which also affect behaviour. These include: previous behaviour (e.g. habits), social norms and pressures (chapter 7, especially pp. 177–80), risk perception (chapter 5, pp. 121–30), motivation (chapter 3), individual differences (e.g. personality – chapter 6) and workplace factors which can facilitate or inhibit the desired behaviour – very much under the control of management (chapter 10). Thus, attitudes take their place as

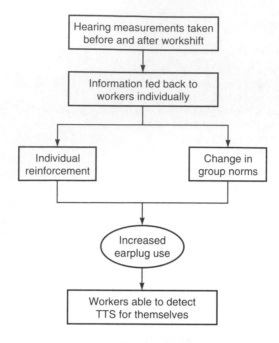

Figure 4.11 Promoting the use of ear protection (after Zohar *et al.*, 1980).

Summary text 4.12 Case study on increasing influence through involvement (after Kjellén and Baneryd, 1983)

In an action research study in three companies in the explosives industry in Sweden, three groups of 8–10 employees were formed to discuss work safety issues and to make decisions on those they considered to be important. Each group, which included the production manager, supervisors, safety representatives and operators was given formal decision-making powers and reported to the safety committee. The groups met regularly for about 3 hours every fourth week and members were paid overtime for their attendance. The production manager chaired the meetings and recorded decisions taken. Workplace briefings for all employees were also held to inform them of progress.

   One aim of the study was to improve the knowledge and attitudes on accident risks and safety activities for the operators by giving them greater influence over these activities. At the end of the experiment, there were indications that worker attitudes to health and safety activities in the departments concerned were more positive than before the experiment. It was felt that the experiment resulted in active efforts to reduce health and safety risks, particularly those relating to explosion. Other benefits to those participating in the study included increased knowledge and broader under-standing of the problems associated with workplace health and safety, and the ready acceptance of remedial action postulated as a result of group decision-making.

Summary text 4.13 Case study of a noisy textile mill (after Hale and Else, 1984)

One hundred and eight people worked in such noise that they should have been wearing hearing protection (HP) for at least some of the time. However, for those who should have been wearing HP:

- 11% said they wore HP all the time;
- 6% said they wore HP some of the time;
- 81% said they did not wear HP.

The main reasons given for not wearing HP were:

- 'irritates ears';
- 'don't like them';
- 'too late/too old (to make any difference)';
- 'confusing'.

A programme to change behaviour was conducted in five stages:

1. An initial course was held on noise control. Among the attenders was the plant manager – it is important to influence top management at an early stage if the programme is to be successful.
2. Seventeen volunteers from a range of affected personnel took part in user trials to reduce the range of theoretically adequate HP. From an initial ten types of HP available, five were rejected at this stage as being too uncomfortable. This should have eliminated one of the main reasons given for non-use of HP.
3. The entire workforce was trained in the use of the five 'acceptable' types of HP and were given a choice as to which type to use for themselves.
4. A retired employee came in on an occasional basis to monitor HP use and to clean and maintain the HP and the machines for dispensing it.
5. An induction package was prepared for new employees.

Eighteen months after the start of the programme, more than 90% of workers aged 40 years and under, and more than 60% of all the workforce, wore HP when necessary. Usage continued to climb as older workers left and younger ones came in. After five years, wearing HP was made a condition of employment.

This is an example of internalization of an attitude (belief that HP is necessary) being reinforced by identification (other group members increasingly wearing HP) and finally by compliance (wearing being made a condition of employment after five years) – see pp. 88–90.

Thus, a combination of approaches for dealing with new and existing employees was adopted. Crucial to the programme was the training and feedback which accompanied it and this was designed broadly along the lines of a structured behavioural model (Hale and Glendon, 1987).

---

one of the factors which influence and are influenced by safety-related behaviour.

Attitudes are complex multidimensional representations of certain aspects of individuals' cognitive functioning. This chapter has illustrated the importance of a thorough and systematic approach to attitude and behaviour change – one which is based upon a sound and relevant theoretical approach to the relation between behaviour and other factors. A considerable volume of evidence has accumulated over the past 40 years in respect of how behaviour

Summary text 4.14 Case study of methods to improve PPE use (after Pirani and Reynolds, 1976)

Five methods of persuading employees to adhere to safety precautions, such as using PPE, were tested. During initial questioning, members of the workforce were asked about their attitudes towards a worker kitted out in full safety gear and the following list emerged: 'good', 'reliable', 'responsible', 'elderly', 'conscientious', 'plodder', 'out of touch', 'rather isolated from the rest of the workforce', 'fastidious', 'compulsive', 'cissy', 'unsociable'. Management attitudes to such a worker were: 'half witted', 'slow', 'reliable', 'gives little trouble', 'could be left safely alone', 'prone to making trivial complaints'. Thus, both management and workforce portrayed such a worker as one reflecting at best neutral, and at worst negative images.

Five methods of attitude change were used in attempts to influence PPE use and the researchers then studied subsequent wearing of safety helmets, gloves, goggles and boots. Management policy during the course of the study provided them with an opportunistic sixth method. The methods, with their corresponding degree of success were:

- **Poster propaganda** produced an immediate effect which was not sustained in the longer term;
- **Film shows** also produced an immediate effect which was not sustained (apart from goggle wearing);
- **Fear techniques** induced fatalism and resignation, indicating a lack of control – i.e. the opposite of what was intended;
- **Group discussions** had very little impact;
- **Role play exercises** in which workers played out roles of manager, safety officer, safety consultants, supervisors and injured workers, resulted in dramatic changes in behaviour which were sustained over time;
- **Enforcement policy** – imposed by management – succeeded in the short term but was counterproductive in the long term. It was seen as confrontational and was not applied consistently – for example, less so when production pressure increased.

The conclusions from this study were that most change methods produced some effect in the short term, perhaps due to a Hawthorne Effect (chapter 7, pp. 171–7). However, only role playing – where workers were actively involved – produced a long-term behaviour change. Using techniques in which fear is aroused and not relieved, means that workers are motivated to ignore the message. Eyes were seen as particularly worth protecting, while a positive overall safety image is required to support PPE usage programmes.

and attitudes may be influenced and changed. It is through the application of structured approaches that we can seriously address human behaviour issues relating to workplace safety and risk.

While the number and variety of theories relating to attitudes and behaviour may at first appear bewildering, most of these share common features and can be encapsulated within a set of generally agreed principles. However, the attitude–behaviour link **is** complex and any theory which failed to reflect this would be neither credible nor useful. One intractable problem in seeking to change attitudes and behaviour is the variability between individuals. This diversity means that some people will change fairly readily, a majority may change after a certain amount of pressure, while a minority may change very

> **Summary text 4.15** Case study of improving the use of ear protectors (Zohar et al., 1980)
>
> These researchers sought to improve the use of ear protectors in noise through information feedback. Workers in a noisy department of a metal fabrication plant took hearing tests before and at the end of their workshifts to ascertain the extent of temporary hearing losses that occurred with and without earplugs being worn. The information was fed back to individual workers to encourage greater use of ear protectors. The programme is illustrated in figure 4.11.
>
> Follow-up observations over a 5-month period showed a steady increase in earplug use, attaining a level of 86%. In a control department, no more than 10% of workers used earplugs after being given a standard lecture on hearing conservation in noise, later augmented by disciplinary threats. The effectiveness of the feedback technique in promoting earplug usage was explained as a two-stage process involving individual reinforcement and subsequent group adoption of new norms for accepted behaviour (internalization of the new attitude plus identification with the new group norm).
>
> The researchers used the temporary threshold shift (TTS) phenomenon and found that feedback of audiometric information to workers on TTS provided a strong incentive to change behaviour towards using ear protection. The results suggested that, without earplugs, there are much larger differences between hearing levels observed before and at the end of the workshift and that these were in a direction indicating noise-induced TTS. Motivation comprised the feedback success for behaviour change (feelings of control over the risk) and the continued use of PPE was reinforced by subsequent noise reduction and associated relief experienced by the users. That users were able to perceive improvements in their hearing was important – they had been made aware of how to detect TTS for themselves. The acceptance of using PPE by a large number of workers in a group creates new norms and a standard for behaviour which becomes self-sustaining after an initial period, meaning that the experiment does not have to be repeated.

reluctantly, if ever. This is a well-accepted phenomenon in the marketing sphere. Thus it may be expedient for a safety and risk professional or other change agent to accept that some individuals will be very resistant to change and that it would be more cost-effective to devote resources elsewhere rather than to put yet more effort into this minority.

Influencing attitudes in the field of safety and risk management has many parallels with analogous efforts in the field of marketing and consumer behaviour. In the latter case, organizations are seeking to increase profits by encouraging the purchase of their products and services, while in the former case they are seeking to improve safety and thereby reduce costs by minimizing loss through accidents and ill-health. Both types of effort therefore make a positive contribution to organizational functioning and business success.

5 PERCEPTION AND RISK PERCEPTION

❏ This chapter first describes the main senses as the bases for human perception of objects, events and other people, before considering the important aspects of the specific issue of risk perception. Included is a discussion of attention mechanisms and warnings as well as other components and biases involved in perceiving risk. A review of risk and society incorporates issues of acceptability, risk preferences and the role of the media.

INTRODUCTION

Perceptions are key cognitions – they are central to our fundamental mental apparatus because they provide the bridge between input from the environment through our senses and also comprise our unique personal appraisal of that environment in conjunction with other cognitions such as memory, learning, decision-making and problem-solving.

The study of risk perception as a particular example of human perception experienced something of a heyday during the 1980s, which appears set to continue through the 1990s as the Royal Society (1992) report extends risk perception into hitherto neglected cultural areas. One reason for this activity is the acknowledgement that perception is a critical behavioural antecedent – the way in which we perceive the world around us is crucial for our behaviour. The objectives of this chapter are to:

• describe and explain basic perceptual processes;
• reveal something of the complexity of human perception;
• explore relevant aspects of risk perception;
• demonstrate parallels between micro and macro aspects of risk perception;
• identify pertinent components for managing risk.

The study of perception focuses on how people discover what is going on around them from data that are registered through the senses (vision, hearing, taste, etc.). A distinctive feature of our central nervous system is its great capacity to store parts of previous perceptual inputs and to interpret new perceptions in some meaningful framework. Cognitive psychology, which embraces the above, treats individuals as active agents trying to make sense of their environment in order to adapt successfully to it and to satisfy personal needs.

Our perceptual system processes and interprets a vast array of stimuli before committing a selection of these to memory. Interpretation and selection of stimuli is influenced both by our genetic inheritance and by our experiences (Held and Hein, 1963). Stimuli perceived by people who need to evaluate risk could include:

- direct experience of accidents;
- reports of accidents from others;
- media accounts.

Perception occurs when such stimuli are evaluated by individuals' unique perceptual structures.

Statistical data on the risk of adverse events are produced by governments and other agencies. Individuals make their own subjective appraisals on the basis of published statistical data in the light of their personal experiences and make-up. For example, some people may neglect certain serious risks because they are relatively indifferent to them (Royal Society, 1983). It has also been shown that the risk of rare adverse events occurring tends to be overestimated, whilst the risk of more common events is likely to be underestimated (Lichtenstein *et al.,* 1978). For example, people in Lichtenstein *et al.*'s study said that murders were more common than strokes, although strokes kill ten times as many people – see figure 5.1. Floods were said to cause more loss of life than asthma, although death from asthma is nine times more likely. Cancer was judged to be about twice as frequent as heart disease, although the reverse was true. The reason that people's judged frequencies of a range of risks differs from their actual frequencies is that our perceptions are subject to a number of biases – described in chapter 3, pp. 48–53. Thus, the availability bias ensures that we are exposed to unusual or bizarre risks through the media – and hence overestimate these, while defensive attribution (chapter 3, pp. 55–6) serves to protect us from acknowledging that we could be struck down by one of a number of common diseases.

Before exploring some facets of risk perception, it is useful to review a few fundamental aspects of human perception. Mowbray and Gebhard (1958) identify five distinguishable 'physical' human senses or sensations. It has been suggested that there are also a number of non-physical or intuitive senses. However, this discussion is restricted to the more commonly known sense modalities.

VISUAL AND AUDITORY SENSES

Our sensory system works through receptors in the body. For example, we receive information from the external environment through receptors in the eyes, ears, nose and mouth as well as via touch receptors in the skin. Information on the body's internal state is received by different types of receptors (proprioceptors), those concerned with motor functions are called kinaesthesis and vestibular. The kinaesthetic sense is located in muscles, tendons and joints and provides information about the activities of these tissues. The vestibular sense, located in the ears, gives information about the position

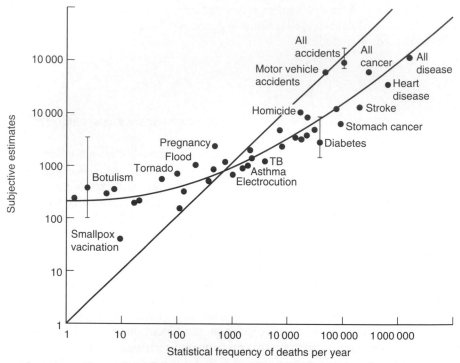

Figure 5.1 Subjective estimates compared with actual frequencies of deaths per year (after Lichtenstein *et al.*, 1978; reproduced with kind permission of the authors).

of the body and its component parts. Sensory organs act as temporary 'reception centres' for energy which is passed to the brain by nerve impulses. This is the **sensation** process.

Nerve impulses entering the brain are interpreted to produce meaningful patterns that we can recognize. For example, we may perceive a quarrelsome situation when we see two people apparently engaged in a hostile exchange. The process of interpretation constitutes **perception**. Perception is highly subjective in nature and is influenced by past experiences, present feelings and intentions about the future. The distinction between sensation and perception is important. Thus, when two people sense the same object, their perceptions always differ, however slightly.

Vision

The visual system comprises our eyes, each connected to the visual cortex of the brain by an optic nerve. Light enters the eye through the pupil. The retina, at the back of the eye, converts light energy into electro-chemical energy. The retina is made up of rods and cones, each performing different functions. The rods are located towards the periphery of the retina, while the cones are found in greater number towards the centre of the retina – the fovea. Rods and cones are sensitive to different wavelengths of light. Rods function better than cones at lower levels of illumination – for example at night. During daylight the cones are more efficient, effectively being used in normal vision. Cones are capable of distinguishing between colours.

Driving illustrates the operation of the visual sense. The driver's eye encodes information received about the road conditions into a form which the nervous system can handle. The resulting impulses which represent this information are conveyed from the retina via the optic nerve to the brain. Then, other nerve impulses travel from the brain to the relevant muscles – these are messages sent to the driver's hands and arms to control the steering wheel and other hand controls and to the feet and legs to control the foot pedals.

It has been known for some time that age can affect visual performance. In one study it was found that 50–60-year-old participants required illumination in the range 100–400 lux to perform as well as younger participants (20–30-year-olds) who functioned with illumination in the range 2–5 lux (Bodman, 1962). Thus, a worker's age may be important when designing visual tasks.

Another problem with increasing age is the reduced ability to focus on objects at different distances. For example, the eyes of an older operator typing text at a computer keyboard move between the written material on the manuscript and the visual display screen. If the respective positions of the screen and manuscript are at different distances from the eye, then the eye needs to accommodate rapidly. With increasing age, the ciliary muscles in the eyes deteriorate, creating a long-sighted effect, whereby the nearest point at which the eye can be sharply focused moves further away. The heavy load on the ciliary muscles accounts for eye strain experienced by VDU operators (Oborne, 1994). To counteract this effect people naturally resort to the use of appropriate spectacles.

Perceptual deterioration is one reason why older people are generally slower than younger people at using software such as word processing (Davies et al., 1991) even where they have comparable typing speeds (Glendon et al., 1994) and at a range of other tasks, for example driving (Davies et al., 1992). A measure of drivers' visual attention and search is the useful field of view (Ball and Owsley, 1991; Owsley et al., 1991). When difficult driving conditions (e.g. heavy traffic or an unusual roundabout layout) are encountered, the amount of visual information to be processed may exceed the capacity of some older drivers, thereby increasing the accident risk (Hancock et al., 1989).

People with normal colour vision are capable of distinguishing between hundreds of different colours – or hues (think of the colour charts which you look through when deciding what colour to paint a room). Colour can therefore be used to help to distinguish between different controls, displays and action signals. The British Standards Institution (BSI), in collaboration with industry, has adopted standards for the best use of colour in coding systems. Colour codes (e.g. in the form of bands) are used to denote different types of fire extinguishers. Colour is also used to distinguish between different conditions, for example industrial and medical gas cylinders, traffic signals and electrical wiring. Colour may be used to denote differences between pipework in work locations or different categories of workers on a construction site may be identified by them wearing different colour helmets. However, beyond about five different colours, confusion may occur, particularly when individuals are under stress (chapter 8, particularly pp. 209–14).

Colour can also be used to help create feelings and moods or to represent a variety of conditions. For example, people are supposed to feel a greater sense of warmth in a situation where red predominates, compared with a situation in which blue prevails. A number of psychological effects are attributed to colour, some of which are shown in summary text 5.1.

In today's world, our eyes have to cope with many coloured charts, diagrams and screen graphics. The cones in the retina respond best to red, green and blue light. The sensation of yellow is created when the cones that capture red and green are equally and simultaneously activated or stimulated. A strong yellow light tends to undermine the strength of the red and green cones, leaving the blue cones with the primary responsibility for controlling vision. As there are fewer blue cones than red or green cones, the response of the blue cones is inferior in controlling vision and thus performance is below optimal. For a more detailed review of vision and performance, see Megaw (1992).

Visual efficiency is much lower when the red, green and blue cones are all fully operational. Significant adaptation by the eyes to the yellow leads to

---

Summary text 5.1 Some psychological attributions of colours

Colour	Positive attributions	Negative attributions
Red	happiness, optimism, strength dynamism, passion, warmth	explosiveness, death, war, debt, anarchy, the devil, blood, anger
Orange	communication, organic, warmth ambition, cheerfulness, richness generosity, receptivity	malevolence
Yellow	cheeriness, enlightenment, youth sunshine, intelligence, action	cowardliness, treachery
Brown	organic, strength, earthiness compactness, health, utility	vulgarity, barrenness, impoverishment
Green	nature, fertility, prosperity, life hope, stability, security, calmness	decay, mould, envy, jealousy, immaturity
Blue	spirituality, devotion, justice, rationality, tranquillity, contentment, hygiene	melancholy, darkness, doubt, discouragement, depression
Purple	royal, loyal, power, truth	lust, decadence, mourning, secrecy
Black	impenetrability, distinction, nobility, elegance, richness	death, sickness, despair, denial, evil, sin
White	purity, refreshment, perfection, infinite wisdom, truth, refined, delicate, peace	blankness, absolute silence, void, ghostliness, surrender
Grey	autonomy, neutrality	indecision, fear, monotony, dirt, coldness, depression, age

Source: Napoles (1988).

changes in the appearance of other colours, so that yellow may be a poor choice in many situations. For example, yellow has a poor contrast on a white visual display screen. Red is a favoured choice for many displays where light-emitting diodes are used, as in electronic calculators, as it appears to be identified more frequently than any other colour of the same brightness.

For those with some defective colour perception, red, orange, green and brown colours generally pose the greatest difficulty, although those affected may remain unaware of their deficiency until an obvious error of judgement is made. Although very few people are completely colour blind (seeing only white, black and shades of grey) Megaw (1992) notes that between 6% and 10% of males and between 0.5% and 1% of females have some colour discrimination deficiency. The most common form of deficiency is confusing red with green and yellow with blue. However, particular colours on certain backgrounds can be a problem for those with normal colour vision. Colour vision defects can be due to genetic factors, although a number of diseases have been associated with such defects. These are summarized in box 5.2. Where effective performance on a job depends upon a certain level of colour discrimination, appropriate tests may be used to diagnose colour abnormalities.

Eyes are particularly vulnerable to material hitting the cornea with force or to splashes from hazardous substances and can suffer damage from excessive light or radiation. Where eye protection is required by the Protective Equipment at Work Regulations 1992, this must conform to BSI specifications. Operatives may remove their goggles because of impaired vision or discomfort, for example if the interior mists up when working in high temperatures. These issues need to be addressed by adequate attention to motivational, attitudinal and behavioural factors, as discussed in chapters 3 and 4, as well as design of the work environment and the equipment used (chapter 9, pp. 266–75) for further discussion.

Summary text 5.2 Diseases which can cause colour vision disturbances

Disease	*Effect upon colour vision*
Addison's disease	Blue-yellow defect
Alcoholism/cirrhosis of the liver	Blue defect
Ataxia (Friedreich's/Spinal cerebellar)	Red-green defect first, then mostly green defect
Brain tumor/trauma/concussion	Red-green or blue-yellow defects
Cerebral cortex disease	Blue defect
Congenital jaundice	Blue and green defects
Cortical lesions	Blue defect
Diabetes mellitus	Blue defects
Malnutrition	All colours
Multiple sclerosis	Red-yellow defects
Pernicious anaemia	Green defect
Syphilis	Red-green defect, blue defect
Vascular accidents/stroke	Various
Vitamin A deficiency	Most colours

Source: Voke (1982).

Hearing and vibration

The ears convert noises received as sound pressure waves into electrical patterns, which as nerve impulses are decoded and measured by the brain's auditory cortex. Sound waves vary in frequency – measured in Hertz (Hz). Sounds sensed by a normal young adult range from a low of 20 Hz to a high of 20000 Hz. Sound below 16 Hz is called infrasound. For maximum effectiveness, auditory warning signals should be designed in accordance with the criteria shown in summary text 5.3.

Different messages can be transmitted by different types of tones – as in the case of a telephone system. The quality of the tone of sound enables people to distinguish between different human voices. Sounds can help airline pilots to steer a steady course. For example, a continuous 1020 Hz tone can be heard when the aircraft is on the planned course, but any deviation is indicated by different sounds. Sounds with little or no quality of tone are called noise – frequently described as unwanted sound. The ear's sensitivity to sound intensity varies with the frequency of the sound. Sound intensity is measured in decibels (dB). The range of audible noise levels is shown in summary text 5.4.

Examples of the use of auditory and visual displays are given in chapter 9 (pp. 266–75). Summary text 5.5 gives examples of adverse and beneficial effects of sound, while summary text 10.17 in chapter 10 gives examples of reducing noise at source as part of a risk management programme.

Hearing loss can result from the combined effects of long-term exposure to noises that people encounter every day, such as those generated by loud vehicles or disco music. Normal ageing also results in hearing loss. Evidence on the role of noise in accident causation is inconclusive and is summarized by Smith and Jones (1992). However, the results from one study indicated that some self-reported everyday errors by people living in a high aircraft noise area were higher than for a comparable group in a quieter area (Smith and Stansfield, 1986).

Summary text 5.3 Recommendations for auditory warning signals

- use sound frequencies between 200 and 5000 Hz – where the human ear is most sensitive
- when sounds must travel long distances (>300 m) use sound frequencies below 1000 Hz – because high frequencies are absorbed in travel
- use frequencies below 500 Hz when signals must bend round obstacles or pass through partitions
- in noise, use signal frequencies different from the most intense noise frequencies to reduce masking of the signal
- use a modulated signal to demand attention – intermittent beeps (1–8 per sec) or warbling sounds that rise and fall in frequency
- use complex tones rather than pure tones to differentiate from other sounds

Sources: Deatherage (1972), Margolis and Kroes (1975), McCormick (1976b).

Summary text 5.4 Noise levels and environmental conditions

dB	Example of noise
140	Pain threshold
130	Pneumatic chipper
120	Loud automobile horn
110	
100	Inside underground train
90	
80	Average traffic on street corner
70	Conversational speech
60	Typical business office
50	Living room
40	Library
30	Bedroom at night
20	Broadcasting studio
10	
0	Threshold of hearing

(dB stands for decibels, a logarithmic measure of sound intensity)
Source: Oborne (1994).

While noise is sound transmitted through the air and detected by the ear, when transmitted through a solid and detected by the body, it is vibration. Sound at the low end of the range is felt as vibration. Levels of vibration experienced by vehicle drivers who drive on rough ground can cause structural damage to the body. In a study of 371 tractor drivers who frequently drove over rough ground, those who operated for long periods reported stomach complaints and spinal disorders, particularly in the lumbar and thoracic

---

Summary text 5.5 Examples of adverse and beneficial effects of sound upon human performance

Both intermittent and continuous noise can have detrimental effects on behaviour. For example, Crook and Langdon (1974) found that aircraft noise impacted on a group of school children thus:

• increased fidgeting, irritability, tiredness and headaches among pupils;
• disruption of lessons;
• reduced teacher satisfaction and increased irritability and tiredness.

   Nemecek and Grandjean (1973) found that percentages of employees in a landscaped office reported that they were distracted by noises from conversations (46%), office machinery (25%) and telephones (19%). Similar problems were revealed in a study by Waller (1969). Noise in the environment interferes with sound reception and decoding because of masking – which weakens the perception of a signal in the form of speech or sound from an auditory system.

   Some sound may have positive effects. For example, Fox (1983) found beneficial effects of background music in the work environment, such as reduced absenteeism and turnover, improved timekeeping and productivity.

regions (Rosegger and Rosegger, 1960). Prolonged exposure to high frequency vibration is also likely to cause injuries. This is common among workers who use hand-held powered equipment such as road drills, stone breakers and chain saws. Intense vibration can be transmitted to the operator's fingers, hands and arms, producing effects such as intermittent numbness or clumsiness and perhaps damage to bones, joints or muscles as well as restriction of the blood supply (as in vibration induced white finger). Prolonged rest is the only cure for all or some of these symptoms, although they can reappear if the worker is again exposed to the vibrating stimulus. Vibrating structures can also produce motion sickness and headaches – as on board a ship. A vibrating source can also provide useful information. For example, a particular combination of noise and vibration from a car engine can inform the driver that something is amiss. Effects of vibration on human performance are complex – for details, see for example McLeod and Griffin (1989) and Griffin (1992).

OTHER SENSES

Smell and taste

Olfactory (smell) and taste sense rest on chemical processes. The taste receptors are cells in the taste buds of the tongue, cheeks and throat. The smell receptors are located on the roofs of the nasal passages. When certain chemicals come into contact with these cells, nerve impulses are triggered and directed to the brain. The sense of smell can have particular relevance as a warning device in the context of some hazards. For example, inhalation of vapour from chlorinated solvents in degreasing agents has a potent anaesthetic effect.

Skin

Receptors for four different senses are found in the skin: touch, pain, warmth and cold. The skin can be vulnerable to hazards. Industrial dermatitis has become more prevalent with greater application of chemical-based products (e.g. organic solvents, tar, paints, thinners). When the outer layers of skin are damaged, the skin is vulnerable to contamination by particles and bacteria. The skin's natural protection is reduced further by cuts, scratches and blisters resulting from handling rough substances and objects. Irritant dermatitis usually attacks areas of the skin in direct contact with the harmful substance.

Kinaesthetic sense

This is one of the two proprioceptive senses concerned with perceiving the body's own movement. The kinaesthetic (feeling of motion) system consists of sensors in the muscles, tendons and joints. These sensors inform us of the relative positions and movements of different parts of our body. Thus, a normal person can climb stairs efficiently because of kinaesthetic feedback from muscles, tendons and joints in motion. When walking or climbing we do not always have to look at our feet to know where to place the next step. Kinaesthetic sensory receptors in hand, arm and shoulder muscles allow the worker to use the hands efficiently above the head or out of sight.

A proprioceptive sense (e.g. kinaesthetic), unlike other senses (e.g. vision) does not have a visible organ. However, kinaesthesis does underpin a visible sensory organ (eyes). The position of the eyes is maintained by muscles which attach the eye within the socket. Kinaesthetic receptors in these muscles provide information about the degree and direction of the eye's movement.

The kinaesthetic system is of crucial importance in training and utilization of motor skills (e.g. manual dexterity, finger dexterity, wrist and finger movement and reaction time). Feedback from kinaesthetic receptors in fingers, arms, shoulder muscles and joints provides essential information which allows a typist to sense where the fingers ought to be placed without recourse to a series of conscious acts. Lifting activity uses the kinaesthetic sense and if not done properly, may result in discomfort or back pain, and in extreme cases permanent disability. Nurses are a high-risk group, in particular student nurses and auxiliaries (Stubbs *et al.*, 1983),

Vestibular sense

The vestibular sense (the other proprioceptive sense) is located in the ear and is primarily concerned with maintaining the body's posture and equilibrium. The vestibular receptors enable a person to maintain an upright posture and to control the body's position. These receptors also provide information about the speed and direction of the body, the head's rotation and its position when static. The vestibular system triggers the sensations associated with motion sickness. Damage to the system – as in cases of severe head injury – can affect the balance organs, producing symptoms of dizziness, nausea and disorientation.

While walking, slips can occur when turning and matters can be made worse if the worker is carrying a load. Slipping is a common cause of accidents on the job, and it is estimated that injuries resulting from slipping, tripping and falling can account for up to 40% of time lost due to accidents (Davies, 1983). People may adapt to conditions such as slippery conditions on a greasy factory floor, for example by shortening the stride. However, if the muscles are used too often to overcome the tendency to slip they will quickly become fatigued. Design features of floor and shoe materials can help to reduce these problems.

Ideally, a person's sensory and physical characteristics would match their job requirements. However, if a person's sensory or physical characteristics are deficient then extra time and precautions are required for safe performance. This is referred to as compensatory behaviour. In one study of disabled people it was found that disabled workers generally had a lower accident rate than did able-bodied workers (Kettle, 1984).

ABSOLUTE AND DIFFERENTIAL THRESHOLDS

A stimulus or level of energy must be of a certain strength before perception can be organized. An absolute threshold is the minimum level below which stimuli cannot be perceived. The absolute threshold for light is a candle flame at 50 km on a dark clear night; for sound it is the tick of a watch under quiet conditions at 7 metres; for taste it is one gram of sugar in 10 litres of water; and for smell it is one drop of perfume diffused into the entire volume of a three-room apartment. Perception which occurs below the threshold is often referred to as **subliminal** perception. A differential threshold arises when a perceiver can see differences between two stimuli which others fail to see. For example, a professional wine taster can frequently **see** a difference between two wines that an amateur cannot differentiate.

Absolute and differential thresholds are known to fluctuate – this fluctuation being referred to as sensory adaptation, for example visual adaptation. When dusk descends, the rods take over from the cones in the retina. The reverse happens when light reappears. We generally encounter no difficulties when adapting to different illumination levels, but temporary blindness can appear with rapid changes in illumination. For example, a rapid change from darkness to light increases the level of illumination falling on the retina. In such circumstances, the rods no longer function and the cones require two minutes to adapt to the new conditions.

As we move from light to darkness, the rods take about half an hour to react fully. It is for this reason that coloured goggles (e.g. red) are worn by workers having to work in a dark environment, as in the photographic industry. They would normally wear the goggles for some time before entering the dark room. Red is an appropriate colour for the goggles because it has little effect on the visual pigment in the rods (Cushman, 1980).

Colour adaptation can be illustrated by the example of a person viewing a bright red stimulus for a few minutes and then focusing on a yellow stimulus – which then appears to be green. Gradually the eyes will adapt and recover to normal colour perception. However, such processes may have important implications for operators who spend lengthy periods viewing different colours on screens or other displays.

PERCEPTUAL ORGANIZATION AND INTERPRETATION

Organization

After concentrating on the relevant stimuli, we proceed to organize the incoming information. When people watch a safety film, the soundtrack and visual images are complementary and help the audience to organize the messages. Repetition of a message – as in advertising or a safety campaign – also contributes to perceptual organization. However, this can be difficult in circumstances where the stimuli are ambiguous or difficult to grasp. Thus, people tend to make their world more understandable by emphasizing stability and constancy.

Constancy is illustrated in situations where objects are perceived as stable (e.g. in size) despite significant changes in the stimuli reaching our senses. Thus, a person who is close to us rather than distant produces a larger image on the retina, but we make allowances for the differences and we still see a normal sized adult. Likewise, we make adjustments for variations in the effects produced by light on different surfaces, seeing colour as we expect it to be, rather than how it is. For example, sunlight coming into a room with a white ceiling and a blue carpet may make the ceiling appear blue from the reflected light. However, because of the constancy effect we still see the ceiling as white.

Under certain circumstances constancy does not hold good, so that what we see appears to be quite different from what we know to be true. In such circumstances illusions occur as errors of perception. For example, when we see the moon near the horizon, it looks larger than when we see it high in the sky, even though the moon produces the same sized retinal image in both cases. One explanation for this illusion is that the perceived distance to the horizon is judged to be greater than that to the zenith and it is this greater perceived distance that leads us to see the moon as larger at the horizon (Holway and Boring, 1941). Illusions of movement arising from stationary stimuli are not uncommon. For example, an isolated stationary light in an otherwise dark visual field appears to wander after observing it for a while. This is called autokinesis and is often encountered in flying (Hawkins, 1987). There are numerous reported cases of mistaken identity of lights, such as a pilot circling round the wing tip light of the aircraft to identify it.

There are also examples of illusions arising from moving stimuli. For example, a person on a stationary train looks out of the carriage window and sees another train moving out from the adjacent platform. The illusion is that the person's own train is moving – the illusion of induced movement. Another common illusory problem experienced in visual flights relates to the evaluation of the relative altitude of approaching aircraft and the subsequent assessment of collision risk. At a distance, an aircraft appears initially to be at a higher level but may eventually pass below the level of the observer. Mountains at a distance appear to be above the aircraft, but are eventually seen well below it. Two aircraft separated by 1000 feet may appear to be approaching each other's altitude, and both pilots have been known to take unnecessary evasive action, possible increasing the risk of a collision with another aircraft (Hawkins, 1987).

Interpretation

Interpretation of information or stimuli of interest to us follows the organization of our perception. This is aided by our cognitive processes, i.e. the way we think and feel about things, and we are highly selective in the way we attend to stimuli. This is unsurprising, given our different needs, values, objectives, education, training and experiences.

Information is filtered through a person's frame of reference – or personal model of the world. Information which challenges cherished positions may be rejected unless it is accommodated in some way within the individual's belief system (chapter 4, especially pp. 93–7). Information may have to be fed to the individual on a piecemeal basis if a behaviour or attitude change is sought. Information which is absorbed into the person's belief system is afforded some form of protection (Ross *et al.,* 1975). As discussed in chapter 4 (pp. 80–2) people strive for consistency in their mental models and can unconsciously modify their existing belief systems by appealing to hindsight (Fischhoff, 1975). With the benefit of hindsight, an unexpected outcome, such as an accident can be seen to have some purpose and can to some extent compensate for poor prediction. This means that the individual does not have to overhaul their ideas completely.

If we are concerned with communicating safety messages which are designed to challenge people's frames of reference, it is important to consider strategies for effecting such change. One approach is to challenge current frames of reference dramatically. An example would be a person who is involved in an accident or hears about a friend who has been involved in an accident. Such an event can pose a substantial challenge to a prevailing negative perspective about the need for cautionary measures. However, because accidents remain relatively rare events, this option cannot be relied upon.

An alternative is to use a training programme to change the foundation underpinning the frame for reference. For example, organizations may use case studies of major accidents in other organizations in training sessions. The case studies are used on the grounds that the training organization could, given similar circumstances, find themselves in the same position as the organizations in the cases. Thus, the use of such case studies can help to promote a profound learning experience, leading to changes in management, working practices, training, design and other components of risk management.

PERSON PERCEPTION

We are constantly perceiving the personality characteristics of people with whom we come into contact, and we normally note a number of conspicuous features – facial expressions, gestures, tone of voice, posture, etc. The signals we pick up in social encounters are used in the interpretations we place on other people's behaviour. However, making accurate interpretations of the behaviour of others is fraught with difficulties, and it is not surprising that misinterpretations arise. Thus, an opinion of another person may be compiled from incomplete information. For example, somebody who was held responsible for an accident might be deemed to be careless on the basis of this one piece of information. This is similar to the 'horns' effect in which an individual who is perceived to be bad in one respect is viewed negatively by the perceiver in all other respects. The 'halo effect' is the same phenomenon except that a perceived 'good quality' – e.g. physical attractiveness – is generalized to all characteristics of another person. A common social situation in which these biases can operate is the selection interview – see chapter 6, pp. 149–55 for a review of personality and selection issues. Misperception of other people is also prone to many attributional biases and heuristics, such as those discussed in chapter 3, pp. 48–56 – see also Hinton (1993) for a review.

Hinton (1993) notes that person perception depends not only upon information from the person being perceived (dress, hair style, accent, etc.), but also upon:

- the perceiver – whether they pay attention to the information, their expectations (e.g. held as stereotypes – see below) and past experiences (used as frames of reference for judging others);
- the relationship between the parties (e.g. whether they are friends, strangers, or in a professional relationship);
- the social context (e.g. public or private);
- the cultural setting (e.g. in different cultures, individuals have different preferences for how close they stand when talking – for example, Hall (1966) noted that Arabs stand closer in conversation than Americans do, and Argyle (1988) reports on cultural differences in patterns of gazing).

As well as halo effects which operate when individuals make judgements about other people, other biasing effects include assuming that certain characteristics go together – for example, that intelligence is always associated with honesty. A leniency effect may also be exhibited by people who are generally optimistic and tend to rate others positively on a number of characteristics. Bruner and Tagiuri (1954) concluded that:

- people are better at judging others who are similar to themselves;
- people are better at judging others on traits that can be observed through a person's behaviour (e.g. politeness);
- people who can emotionally detach themselves from their judgements are better at judging others;
- being able to empathize – to see things from the other's point of view, increases the accuracy of person perception.

Individual differences exist in people's ability to perceive others accurately. For example, because their social competence and standing depend more upon accurately judging others, introverts may be more astute than extraverts at perceiving others (chapter 6, pp. 144–7 discusses these terms). Factors that determine whether an individual (A) will like another individual (B), include: B's physical attractiveness as perceived by A, the perceived similarity (e.g. in attitudes), the amount of time two individuals spend in each other's company and the extent to which B likes A (reciprocity) (Byrne, 1971). Self-disclosure – at an appropriate level of intimacy, also increases liking (Duck, 1988).

All 'normal' individuals engage in impression management to some extent (Leary and Kowalski, 1990), whereby they portray a particular image to others, even if this is unconscious (Tetlock and Manstead, 1985). However, there are individual differences (Snyder, 1979) so that high self-monitors adapt themselves more to their surroundings – like a chameleon – some politicians may be good examples of such individuals. One problem in judging others is the difficulty of defining a criterion adequately. For example, if individual A rates individual B as 'friendly', what does this mean? Is A's perception of 'friendliness' the same as that of person C or D? To attempt to overcome this type of problem, psychologists have developed personality tests to seek to produce more 'objective' measures of personality. Some of the main approaches to personality are described in chapter 6.

Stereotyping

Misperception can also occur when we rely upon stereotyping – popularized by Lippmann (1922). Stereotyping is an attempt to force people into certain categories or 'pigeon holes' without accommodating personality traits that a person actually possesses. Stereotypes persist because they help to simplify the very complex task of perceiving others and predicting their behaviour. However, they are distortions of reality and result in bias and prejudice. Stereotyping involves three stages (Secord and Backman, 1974):

1. identifying a set of people as a specific category on the basis of defining characteristics – e.g. skin colour, age, sex, height, hair colour, religion, nationality, occupation, etc.;
2. assigning a range of characteristics to that category of people (e.g. lazy, intelligent);
3. attributing these characteristics to every member of that category (i.e. in the form 'all X are Y').

One problem with stereotyping is that it can lead to self-confirming predictions in respect of how members of that category are treated (Snyder *et al.*, 1977). Thus, members of a group may end up behaving more like the stereotyped views held about them than they otherwise would have done (e.g. Christensen and Rosenthal, 1982). In accordance with attributional biases (e.g. illusory correlation, see chapter 3, pp. 49–51) we tend to look for confirmation for our views rather than to seek disconfirming evidence. A conclusion based on empirical evidence suggests that we process information supportive of a stereotype more intensively than information inconsistent with it (Bodenhausen, 1988). It seems that our desire to stereotype others is associated with our need to paint a picture of our social world in which the person's identity of others finds expression in membership of groups. This view is contained in social identity theory, which has been applied to group interactions within organizations (Ashforth and Mael, 1989).

Stereotyped images emerged from a study of managers' and workers' perceptions of workers who wore PPE (Pirani and Reynolds, 1976). Workers perceived such individuals to be: good, reliable, responsible, elderly, conscientious plodder, out of touch, isolated, fastidious and compulsive. Managers' descriptions included: reliable, slow, gives little trouble, half-witted, can leave safely alone, makes trivial complaints. Many of the attributed generalized characteristics of PPE wearers had negative connotations, suggesting that major problems could be encountered in overcoming social barriers to wearing PPE in these workplaces.

Funder (1987) argues that the 'errors' made by people in perceiving others are a necessary part of our learning about others – as such, our biases and stereotyping in such situations may therefore be analogous with errors made in other situations – see chapter 9 (pp. 244–61) for a consideration of human error as it is more usually understood.

ATTENTION MECHANISMS AND WARNINGS

We live in a world where a wide variety of stimuli compete for our attention. Physical stimuli likely to attract our attention include large objects, loud sounds, strong colours, repeated occurrences, a moving object in a stationary setting, and an event which contrasts sharply with its surroundings (e.g. an accident or, to an astute observer, a near miss). Since we cannot attend to all stimuli coming our way we are obliged to select those which we consider to be most relevant to our needs. A real challenge for safety and risk professionals is how to influence people's perceptions so that they are motivated to select safety relevant information at appropriate times.

Apart from the effects of physical stimuli attracting our attention, our mental condition is also important. This is affected by our personality (chapter 6), motivation (chapter 3), learning ability (chapter 2), etc. and we are inclined to attend to signals or cues which are of interest to us. For example, a safety and risk professional may take a keen interest in the safety aspects of a media report of a major disaster. Likewise, a safety and risk professional's motives in respect of his or her professional activities will alert that person to see things in a safety or risk context. Thus, perceptions can be selectively biased by motivations.

Where stimuli are related to a need awaiting gratification (e.g. hunger), perception of those stimuli can be pronounced. For example, a hungry person pays selective attention to images of goods on display posters because of the association between food and gratification of the hunger need. This is called **selective perception**. In coping with a threatening situation, selective perception can come to our assistance. This manifests itself when a person ignores stimuli considered to be mildly threatening but attends to stimuli posing greater threats. Apart from the person's specific motives, the person's experience of the stimulus can aid perception. This can be seen when an audible sound signifying a hazard is isolated as being more important than a number of other sounds that are heard at the same time.

Attention mechanisms

Because humans attend **selectively** to phenomena, in order for a message to be successfully delivered it must be presaged by some mechanism which alerts the receiver. It is like tuning in a radio to a particular frequency so that a specific channel may be picked up. This 'tuning in', which applies to all the senses, is akin to another important aspect of perceptual and attention mechanisms and that is expectation. What we perceive (using data from eyes, ears, nose, etc.) is governed very much by what we **expect** to perceive. This in turn is largely determined by our previous experience. The expectation of perceiving a particular set of circumstances – often known as 'perceptual set' can be a powerful determinant of whether we are able to take in and act upon new information.

For safety and risk professionals, breaking a perceptual set – for example in a group of employees – can be a real problem. Human beings, unlike computers, are not very good at picking up minor deviations from sequences or small changes in routine. It is essential to use machines or computers for the task which they perform best – an issue considered in greater detail in chapter 9, especially summary text 9.8 and 9.9.

Effectiveness of warnings

Warnings can take many forms – verbal, written, pictorial – as appealing to human cognitions; or they may appeal directly to the senses – as in the case of alarms, bells or other noises, smells or sights. Like any message to be communicated, if a warning is to be effective, then certain conditions must be fulfilled. These are shown in summary text 5.6.

From the information contained in summary text 5.6, it should be clear that the presentation of warnings is no simple matter. The most important things for warnings to be effective are:

- timing – the warning has to be given at exactly the right moment;
- audience – the warning has to reach all those for whom it is intended, and should not be wasted upon those for whom it has no use or meaning;
- explicitness – the warning must tell those for whom it is relevant **exactly** what they should do, i.e. general exhortations are no good.

An example of a warning which meets these requirements well is given in summary text 5.7.

The style and format of an effective warning will be dictated very much by the nature of the danger and those who might be affected by it. Thus, in the example given in summary text 5.7, a combination of written and pictorial warning messages was effective. There are criteria available for deciding when to use auditory or visual presentation of warnings, and these are shown in

---

Summary text 5.6 Conditions required for effective communication

Sender should be	Message should be	Channel should be	Receiver should be
Active	Accurate	Open	Present
Aware	Adequate	Capacious	Attentive
Sensitive	Addressed correctly	Economical	Literate
Selective	Economical	Low noise	Perceptive
Sympathetic	Direct	Secure	
	Timely	Swift	
	Reliable		
	Up-to-date		
	Actually sent!		

Summary text 5.7 A case study in communication (after Piccolino, 1966)

An airline was becoming increasingly embarrassed by accidents to passengers falling down the steps to the tarmac after alighting from its aircraft. It had tried various means of reducing the passenger accident toll, including in-flight warnings and cabin crew members instructing passengers to 'mind how you go' as they left the aircraft, but none had any noticeable effect.

The airline's management then called in a research team to see whether they could provide a solution. The researchers tried a number of alternative solutions before coming up with one which seemed to work. The method was as simple as it was elegant. As passengers left the aircraft and walked onto the platform at the top of the steps they were confronted with a poster on the side panel of the platform. The poster displayed the words HOLD THE RAIL, underneath which was a picture of someone lying on the tarmac at the foot of the steps. Following the introduction of the poster on all its airport steps, the airline found that a significant reduction in passenger falls resulted.

The poster which was used in this case fulfilled the essential criteria for effective communication in safety. It was given at exactly the right moment – when passengers were about to descend the steps; it was available only to those for whom the message was intended and not 'wasted' on anyone else; and it gave an explicit instruction as to what to do. The written message was backed up by a picture of what could happen if you didn't follow the instruction. As a general principle, if fear or threat is used in safety propaganda then this must be accompanied by explicit instruction on how to avoid the threat.

---

summary text 5.8. Less predictable or immediate dangers will require different approaches. The different dimensions which are available for the perception of risk or danger have been identified by Pérusse (1980) and are shown in figure 5.2. The crucial dimensions used are those shown at the top of figure 5.2, namely scope for human intervention (i.e. what could I do about this risk?) and dangerousness (what is the worst thing that could happen as a result of this risk?). The components of each of these major dimensions are discussed in various publications, for example HSC (1993a).

Summary text 5.8 Guidelines on the use of auditory or visual information (after Deatherage, 1972)

Use auditory presentation if:	*Use visual presentation if:*
Message is simple	Message is complex
Message is short	Message is long
Message will not be referred to later	Message will be referred to later
Message deals with events in time	Message deals with location in space
Message calls for immediate action	Message doesn't require immediate action
Visual system is over burdened	Auditory system is over burdened
Receiving location is too bright or dark adaptation is required	Receiving location is noisy
Job requires continually moving about	Person's job is in one position

---

People may adapt to repeated stimuli by developing reduced awareness. For example, a worker may become oblivious to the dangers of operating certain types of machinery and consequently the risk of having an accident is increased. Accounting for this phenomenon, it could be argued that a repeated stimulus contains no new information. This is analogous to people living near to a nuclear power station adapting to this situation in the absence of an accident. Anxieties subside with the accompanying cognitive reassessment of the probability of an accident. However, those living at a slightly greater distance may experience greater anxiety of dissonance (chapter 4, summary text 4.6 discusses this term) as they are still close enough to perceive the risk but not sufficiently close to reduce the dissonance, for example by gaining benefits such as employment or obtaining support from others in the community.

There are occasions when some workers take short cuts, acting in a 'cool' way, and as a consequence send out the wrong signals as they act as unacceptable role models for other workers. To counteract portrayal of the wrong stimuli, in the form of unsafe behaviour, safety campaigns should be designed to link competence and safe behaviour as natural allies in people's minds. In this way, safe practices are seen as the outcome of competence in the

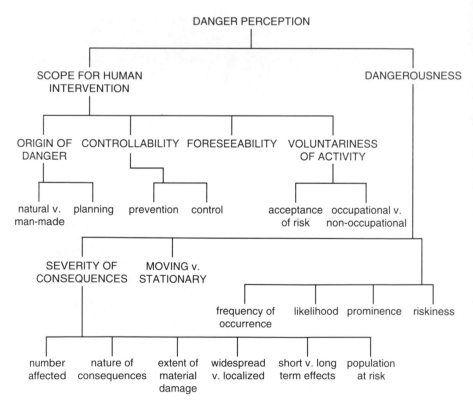

Figure 5.2 Dimensions in the perception of danger and risk (after Pérusse, 1980; reproduced with kind permission of the author).

performance of a task. For example, much of industry has been successful in promoting safety gear such as hard hats, boots and safety harnesses as symbols of the true professional. Helmets used by motorcyclists have been upgraded in image, design and styling. For the male motorcyclist the helmet has become a symbol of masculinity (a form of competence), and the motorcyclist of the 1930s speeding along country roads with the wind blowing through his hair has been replaced by the rider suitably clad with helmet and other protective gear. A similar transformation is the linking of safety helmets and competence in pedal cyclists.

PERCEIVED RISK

Reactions to perceived risk

People differ in their reactions to perceived risk so it should not be expected that different categories of people will react in the same way. An example of what this might mean in practice – which is also relevant to warnings – is given in summary text 5.9.

The example in summary text 5.9 indicates that we need to consider the strong possibility that people will be motivated (chapter 3 discusses motivation) to act differently in response to the same hazard. Thus, some people will accept that the hazard represents a real risk to them and react in an aversive manner. Others, however, will acknowledge the risk, but perceive it as a challenge – to their skill for example. For these people, perceived risk could serve as a source of stimulation. Chapter 6 examines personality differences which might underlie some of these different approaches to risk perception and subsequent action.

In other cases, a warning about a risk can produce a rejecting reaction. This means that the person reacts against the information given or the warning provided and rejects the information. Every time a smoker opens a packet of cigarettes and smokes one, he or she is effectively ignoring the warning message on the packet. The reason that people do this is because the risk presents too much of a threat to the person. In order to control this threat, they adopt the simplest option – they reject the information which reminds them of the threat, in this case to their health.

Factors which affect individuals' reactions to perceived risk in general include:

- individual differences – e.g. age, sex, personality factors (chapter 6);
- perceived control by the person over the risk;
- the person's existing behaviour – specifically, does it contradict the perceived risk? (cf. cognitive dissonance – summary text 4.6 in chapter 4) – if so changing the behaviour will be made particularly difficult;
- the individual's 'set' or state of alertness – the extent to which they are 'tuned in' to receiving information about the risk.

This last point is interesting from the point of view that there are often

Summary text 5.9 Are warning signs in swimming pools effective?

Goldhaber and deTurck (1988) carried out an interesting study on the effectiveness of a warning sign put up in a college swimming pool over a 4-week period. The NO DIVING sign contained four essential elements of a warning:

- an appropriate signal word – DANGER;
- a statement of the hazard – shallow water;
- the effects of the hazard – paralysis or other injury;
- how to avoid the hazard – no diving.

The warning which they used for the study is shown below.

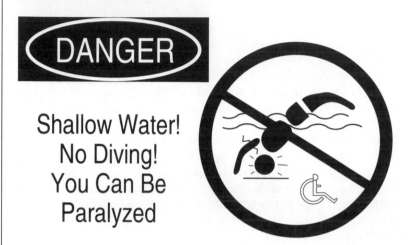

Reprinted form Goldhaber and deTurck (1988), with kind permission of Elsevier Science, Kidlington.

One-hundred-and-eighty male and 148 female (students) took part in the study. It was found that:

- despite the fact that swimmers were exposed to the sign for a month, the majority either did not recall seeing it or were uncertain that it was there;
- males were almost 3 times as likely to report accurately that they saw a sign (unprompted);
- a large majority of respondents understood that by diving into shallow water they risked paralysis – males were more aware;
- but, males were more likely than females to dive into the shallow end of the pool – this effect being more pronounced in the college with the NO DIVING sign!
- thus, the NO DIVING sign had a 'boomerang' effect – increasing the likelihood that males would dive into the shallow end;
- those with a history of diving into the shallow end and students who had a history of diving into other pools and students who were in the swimming team: perceived less danger from diving into the shallow end and were more likely to dive into their pool's shallow end.

In seeking to explain and draw lessons from their findings, the researchers make a number of points. The relative ineffectiveness of the NO DIVING sign supports other research. As only a fraction of the swimmers recalled seeing the sign, this could explain the lack of effect upon swimmers' perceived danger and lack of intention to comply.

Summary text 5.9 (continued)

When a message is difficult to understand and contains many facts, written warnings are more effective than other media. When messages are short and easy to understand, audio and audiovisual messages are better. The effects of a warning are maximized when communicated face-to-face as:

- the source can target the message directly to those needing the information, thereby increasing awareness;
- there is the maximum feedback possibility from the recipient so that the source can determine whether the message was understood and the likely extent of the receiver's compliance with the warning.

Thus, swimming pool owners and attendants should be responsible for giving oral warnings and making sure that they are understood and complied with. The boomerang effect for males may be due to:

- the NO DIVING sign being seen as restricting their freedom so that they responded in a manner contrary to the message;
- males are motivated more by internal cues (e.g. attitudes and beliefs), are more competitive than females, and so saw the NO DIVING sign as a challenge and responded accordingly.

Final points of relevance to this study:

- males tend to process fewer pieces of information from a persuasive message than females do before formulating an opinion;
- females tend to process all or most of a persuasive message before deciding on an appropriate response;
- if a user has some experience of a hazardous product without checking a safety warning and has experienced no personal injury from it, then they are likely to feel confident about using the product.

windows of opportunity for presenting risk information so that it is likely to have maximum effectiveness. These windows of opportunity are most likely to occur when someone has experienced a recent event which has alerted them to a particular risk. For example, if a relative or well-known personality (e.g. a film star) has recently died of cancer as a result of smoking or from AIDS, then an individual who smokes or who indulges in sexually risky behaviour may be sensitized to the possibility that they could die in this way too. However, for behaviour to change there has to be relevant information provision and, most important of all, the person has to perceive that they have the ability to change their behaviour – i.e. that they are in apparent control of the situation. This is often the single most important aspect of individual behaviour change.

Näätänen and Summala (1976) note a number factors which decrease the subjective danger of traffic for road users, and hence increase the likelihood of risk taking:

- deluding perceptual/cognitive processes – e.g. adaptation to speed, underestimation of speed or physical forces in an accident, not learning from others' accidents;
- learning inappropriately from the consequences of 'near misses' – the illusion that one can control such situations;

- subjective feelings about driving – e.g. that it is an easy task;
- feelings of control of driving situations;
- expectancy – generally poor at estimating accident likelihoods;
- little traffic supervision – low likelihood of being caught for violations;
- norms and rules seen as applying to others not to oneself – can lead to perception of low vulnerability.

Responses to risk

A central human factors problem for those working in the area of safety engineering or risk management is that of ensuring that individuals affected by danger or responsible for it are alerted to it at the right time but not at other times. To take a simple example; designers of fire alarm systems need to ensure that the systems work as they are supposed to when required – i.e. when there is a fire. However, everyone knows that fire alarm systems are tested from time to time and that there are also fire drills when the fire alarms also sound. We also know that there are false alarms – when the fire alarm (or a burglar alarm on a house or car) goes off and that no action is necessary. One problem is that most of the alarms we hear are false alarms and thus there is a very real problem for the individual in sorting out which are false alarms and which are real alarms.

A comparable problem arises in many jobs – how does a control room operator or train driver, etc. learn which alarms should be taken note of and which should be ignored or even cancelled? The answer is that we learn by experience – thus, what guides our behaviour is based upon what has happened in the past – we use our statistical repertoire of events to guide our current behaviour. Thus, if our experience has told us that most fire alarms do not really mean that there is a fire or that control panel annunciators or alarms can usually be ignored or that red signals can be passed without undue consequences even if they are supposed to mean 'danger', where does this leave the status of alarms? For an example of how the misperception of an alarm had tragic consequence, see summary text 5.10.

The answer is that alarms may alert us to the **possibility** of danger but that we require some additional evidence to confirm this possibility. Thus, for the individual in an office building, either physical (smell of burning or sight of smoke or flames) or social (others taking action) evidence is required before the possibility is registered as a real probability of danger. In the control room, an unusual combination of alarms or a slight change in the plant monitoring print-out pattern may convert a routine event into a potentially dangerous happening in the operator's mind. A train driver may be alerted to a real probability of danger only when another train is seen on the line ahead – by which time it may be too late to take effective avoiding action.

Thus, as these examples show, designers of safe systems have a real problem in overcoming people's everyday experience that most of the time there is no real danger to them – even when things intended to act as warnings are present. An alternative scenario of continually contemplating danger is not a

---

Summary text 5.10 An accident resulting from misperception of an alarm state

In the public inquiry into the circumstances surrounding the collision of two British Rail trains at Colwich Junction in 1986, there was evidence to indicate that the driver of the northbound train had difficulty in perceiving the significance of the red lights. The northbound train passed through the red lights before stopping, resulting in the death of the driver of the southbound train and injury to 52 passengers. The driver of the northbound train, who jumped clear just before the crash, in his evidence to the inquiry stated:

As a railwayman with 42 years service, I saw a double flashing yellow light which means 'caution', followed by a red signal. I was surprised, as I expected the red signal to change to green, but it stayed at red. I am familiar with the use of flashing lights, but I never had formal training or seen training videos about the lights.

The signalman, in his evidence, said that he had given clear signals for the northbound train to stop as the southbound train was coming from the tunnel. A point worth noting in connection with this incident is that the driver of the northbound train was accompanied in the cab by an off-duty trainee driver. Could an animated exchange between the two at the critical moment have led to the delayed response to the stimuli in the form of the lights?

Sources: Department of Transport (1986), reports in the *Sunday Times* (21.9.86), the *Guardian* (24.10.86).

---

viable option as we would be incapable of performing any other useful tasks. Thus, the intractable problem is: 'when does an alarm really mean danger?'

One approach to this problem is via systematic study of operations (e.g. using task analysis) and to use an appropriate model as a basis for operator behaviours. In a comprehensive study of human factors aspects of alarms, Stanton (1992) and Stanton *et al.* (1992) propose a 6-stage iterative model of alarm initiated activities, comprising the following stages:

- observe
- accept
- analyse
- correct
- investigate
- monitor.

These can be applied to alarm handling activity in a wide range of circumstances.

Because there may be large differences between individuals in their propensity to report hazards (Powell *et al.*, 1971; Pérusse, 1978), any approach to this problem should take account of these differences by providing a general model which can cope with all variants of behaviour. In their model of behaviour in the face of danger (shown in its complete form in figure 5.3), Hale and Glendon (1987) divide the hazard detection process into four main stages:

1. is there an obvious warning? (such as an alarm);
2. is hazard seeking initiated? (i.e. an active search for evidence);

3. are tests for danger known?(to [dis]confirm danger);
4. are tests for danger carried out? (by individual operator, driver etc.).

If the answer to all these questions is 'yes' then it may confidently be expected that the person involved will avoid the danger. However, if any of these questions is answered in the negative then the danger will remain unaffected by the actions of the individual (other events may of course progress or reduce the danger). Thus a 100% correct response is required for detection of danger and subsequent correct action. It follows from these steps in the hazard detection process that system designers should ensure that:

1. warnings of danger are obvious;
2. there are prompts to individuals to search for danger;
3. relevant individuals are aware of what to do;
4. they carry out the required actions.

The task for designers and managers is then to translate these principles into specific components of a system which is 'tuned in' to danger but which otherwise operates in a normal state. For example by:

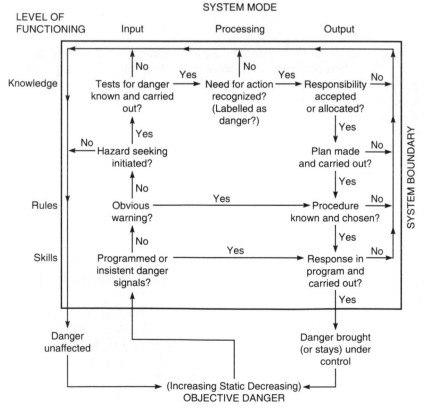

Figure 5.3 Individual behaviour in the face of danger model
(after Hale and Glendon, 1987).

1. minimizing the use of alarms which do not actually mean 'danger';
2. backing up all genuine alarms – e.g. by a voice prompt 'this is a real fire!';
3. training personnel appropriately;
4. refreshing them in the sequence of events to be followed.

Individuals' ability to estimate risk

In general, we are rather poor at estimating the degree of risk to ourselves. As described in figure 5.2 a personal risk calculation involves at least two major components (and possibly more, taking economic, social and political considerations into account). One important distinction to make is that between objective risk and subjective (perceived) risk. Rothschild (1978) maintained that people were poor at estimating objective risks and were therefore illogical in their behaviour (e.g. they could not accept that nuclear power was safe because it presented less of a risk than say traffic). However, such arguments have at least two problems.

1. **Measurement** – 'objective risks' are usually calculated on the basis of accident rates (frequency or incidence usually) – often fatal accident rates. It is therefore assumed that these represent a good measure of the risk. However, there are many difficulties associated with using accidents as a measure of risk – these are reviewed in chapter 10, summary text 10.6.
2. **Populations versus individuals** – measures of objective risk apply to populations and not to individuals – it is effectively impossible to calculate an objective risk for any given individual if objective risks are defined in terms of aggregates and averages. Therefore, exhortations by proponents of objective risk cannot logically be made to individuals but only to populations. Because populations cannot take collective decisions spontaneously – they elect representatives (in democracies) to take such decisions, this means that there may be no mechanism by which the arguments of objective risk proponents can be taken by individuals as such. To take a simple example – car seat belts; it is statistically uncontentious that if all drivers and passengers wear seat belts then the risk of serious injury is reduced for the population of drivers and passengers. However, for any individual driver or passenger, the likelihood that **they** will be killed or seriously injured as a result of not wearing a seat belt on any particular journey is very small (too small for the individual to calculate). Thus, for any given journey, it is immaterial in the total context of 'objective risk' whether that individual wears or does not wear a seat belt.

A second important factor to consider is that, because we are poor at estimating risk, we tend to use heuristics (Kahneman *et al.*, 1982). A number of these were described as motivational biases in chapter 3 and some of the most relevant to risk estimation are considered in summary text 5.11.

The sort of biases outlined in summary text 5.11 make it essential that we understand the nature of subjective or perceived risk in making decisions about safe systems (Hale, 1987; Hale and Glendon, 1987). DeJoy (1990)

Summary text 5.11 Biases in estimating risk

Availability – the tendency for us to judge an event as frequent or likely if instances of it are easy to imagine or to recall. Thus, dramatic causes of death – or those recently encountered (e.g. among family or friends) tend to be overestimated. More common, yet less dramatic events involving only one person at a time, such as diabetes or bronchitis, tend to be underestimated (figure 5.1).

Overconfidence – this tendency often compounds the availability bias, because typically people do not realize how little they know about a given risk. Experts as well as lay people are prone to this particular bias. Thus, potential risks, such as might be created by human error or deliberate violations of safety rules, tend to be overlooked, for example in the design of systems or in risk calculations.

Desire for certainty – because we get anxious when we are unsure about something and as this anxiety is uncomfortable we tend to seek certainty. However, this desire for certainty can result in risks being played down because their frequency of occurrence is not known (e.g. the *Challenger* shuttle disaster). It is important to note that individuals differ in their propensity to accept uncertainty or ambiguity and thus, one antidote to this particular bias is to ensure that in any system in which safety features are important a team of people, each from a different background, is involved. With a heterogeneous group, it is more likely that at least one individual will be able to cope with high uncertainty and that this particular bias is then less likely to affect decision making (see also chapter 7 on group roles, especially pp. 188–200).

Anchoring bias – partly because of our general desire for certainty, we tend to anchor our beliefs and attitudes as a result of information which may be quite inaccurate – e.g. an article about contact lenses becoming fused with the cornea as a result of welding flash or a newspaper report about radiation from visual display screens. The problem with anchoring biases is that they can be remarkably resistant to extinction – even in the face of new and more convincing contradictory evidence.

---

stresses the importance of subjective appraisal of risk in respect of protective behaviour.

Economic and other factors affecting acceptance of risk

We accept risks all the time for all sorts of reasons. Some risks we are totally unaware of and therefore the issue of 'acceptance' is theoretical. Other risks we might know about but still be unaware of the real impact upon us – for example, our chances of succumbing to heart disease or schizophrenia are influenced by genetic factors, but we may still not know whether we personally will be affected.

However, other risks we apparently take in full knowledge of the potential consequences. There are a number of reasons why this might occur. The first reason is economic necessity – applying particularly to workplace risks. In the early days of the industrial revolution or when countries are in economic recession or when unemployment is high and there are few jobs available, people are often obliged to work in jobs with high physical risk. However, given that all jobs carry some degree of risk to a person's health and safety, the decision has to be made (explicitly or implicitly) by each worker as to whether to accept the risk and how much to seek to increase or decrease the risks associated with a particular job. An illustration of this – from a paper prepared for the Robens Commission in 1970 – is given in figure 5.4.

Eldridge and Kaye's occupational stress model (figure 5.4) shows that economic and other circumstances may lead to a worker becoming stressed at work. This stress may give rise to a number of outcomes, one of which is accidents. All the outcomes identified in figure 5.4 have some evidence for a link with stress (this theme is taken up in greater detail in chapter 8). However, workers may be prepared to 'accept' a degree of risk which they would refuse if given a genuinely free choice – i.e. if the economic and other pressures did not exist. If we do not have a free choice when it comes to risk acceptance then this term is problematic.

Linked with the issue of choice in respect to risk is the point that people are more likely to accept risks which they regard as voluntary. Thus, we may regard our mode of travel to work – whether this is by car, motorcycle, pedal cycle or public transport – as being determined voluntarily by us and therefore accepted because of this. However, risks which we perceive as being 'imposed' upon us by others or simply because they are part of the job that we do, may be accepted only in the sense that they are tolerated (see the debate on the distinction between acceptance and tolerability – HSE, 1988 reviewed in the next section). Voluntariness of risk acceptance is now considered to be less clear-cut than it used to be, but perceived voluntariness remains a factor in risk acceptance or tolerance.

Of greater importance in risk acceptability is the issue of control. If people feel that they have control over a risk source, then it is more likely to be accepted by them. This issue was at the root of much of the public debate on nuclear power – where the risk issue (economic and political factors apart) was one not so much of the 'actual' (or objective) risk (notwithstanding the

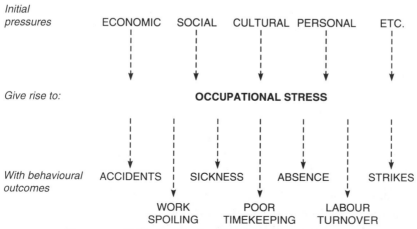

Figure 5.4 Risk-taking: antecedents, stress and outcomes
(after Eldridge and Kaye, 1970).

already noted comment that it is impossible to determine this for an individual) of a nuclear accident say, but of the degree of control, or lack of it, which individuals feel that they have over such an energy source. This is associated with the extent to which individuals have faith in the political system in meeting their needs and in the scientific experts in providing unbiased information.

RISK AND SOCIETY

Risk acceptability

The issue of 'acceptable risk' has been debated at some length (e.g. Fischhoff *et al.,* 1981; Royal Society, 1983; Perrow, 1984; HSE, 1988) and an important question to ask is 'acceptable according to what criteria?' Different acceptability criteria which might be applied include:

- legal – does it conform with legal and enforcement standards?
- managerial – is it consistent with organizational standards?
- cultural – how does our society view this risk?
- market – will our competitiveness be compromised by the cost of reducing/eliminating this risk?
- political – will there be a political price to pay for not/reducing this risk?
- public – how influential are media and pressure groups on this issue?

Decisions on risk control are not limited to technical or scientific considerations. Acceptability of risk often involves complex social processes in which scientific and legal requirements are juxtaposed with broader social notions of acceptability which are influenced by media and political statements. This makes knowledge of how to reduce risks to acceptable levels problematic because of the range of acceptability criteria. For example, does one seek to meet legal requirements on risk or is there another 'lower' level of acceptability which can be used as a reference point? The answer to this problem cannot be found by reference to technical scientific literature because it is not an empirical question. Ultimately, issues of risk acceptability involve social and political value judgements and a trade-off between risk and costs of reducing or otherwise avoiding the risk. These judgements are part of managerial decision-making on risk.

Perceived risk and acceptability

The problematic nature of risk acceptability has already been discussed. In an attempt to address this problem, the HSE (1988) suggest the following definitions:

- **acceptable risk** – 'the risk, although present, is generally regarded by those who are exposed to it as not worth worrying about';
- **tolerable risk** – 'a risk that society is prepared to live with in order to have certain benefits and in the confidence that the risk is being properly controlled'.

The HSE note that a risk greater than the tolerable risk cannot be justified on any grounds. However, both definitions beg further questions. For example, do those who are exposed to an 'acceptable risk' have comprehensive knowledge about it in order to make their decisions? and do they genuinely have a choice to 'accept' the risk? The HSE definition of tolerable risk encounters the problem of the heterogeneity of society – the fact that some groups will be exposed more than others to any given risk and that attributions made in respect of society conveniently labels the problem of tolerability but does not resolve it.

Nevertheless, the distinction between 'acceptable risk' and 'tolerable risk' is useful in principle because the latter involves the benefits side of the equation – the notion that risks are only ever accepted or tolerated because they are associated with some benefits. A major problem for policy makers is that parties who are obliged to accept or tolerate the risks are often not the same as those who reap the benefits.

For example:

- those living near chemical or nuclear plants are exposed to higher risk than the rest of the community, yet the wider community shares any benefits from these plants;
- road systems and vehicles designed to reduce risks of accident and injury to motorized vehicle users may increase risks to cyclists and pedestrians (Adams, 1990);
- workers are exposed to risks at work to produce goods and profits which benefit customers and shareholders (while workers do derive benefits from work, the other parties are not exposed to the workplace risks).

These examples indicate that issues of risk acceptability are political questions and that the way in which risk is perceived is also at least partly a political issue. This is because different interests are involved and, in a pluralist society, there is the potential for conflict between parties. For further debate on these issues, see for example: Fischhoff *et al.* (1981), Perrow (1984), Glendon (1987b), HSE (1988), Booth (1990).

Revealed and expressed preferences

Among the ways in which decision-makers and policy-makers have sought to measure risk acceptability when considering the introduction of products or processes which involve new risks are those known as revealed preference and expressed preference.

Revealed preference refers to the amount of risk 'accepted' – or, more accurately, tolerated – by people at present – for example, the number of road deaths per annum. This might be used as a basis for the introduction of some activity which has a risk attendant upon it, the criterion being that if people 'accept' a risk of (say) 1 in 10000 of being killed on the roads each year, then they would be willing to accept a new activity which incurs a risk of death which is no more than this figure. However, this approach to risk assessment is flawed for two main reasons.

First, just because a certain risk may be measured 'objectively' (pp. 127–30 discuss problems relating to objective risk), does not mean that people accept the risk willingly – i.e. given a real choice they may actually prefer a lower level of risk. Because most people need to work to live and in order to do their work in most cases they have to travel to get there and be exposed to risks once they are there, this degree of choice does not exist in reality. Thus, the revealed preference approach presumes that people do actually choose their current level of risk in an absolute sense – which is not usually the case. Second, the same problems arise here as for 'objective' measurement of risk – i.e. while it may be possible to assess risk for an aggregate or population, this is not the same as being able to calculate a level of risk for an individual. Therefore, trying to apply a risk acceptability formula upon individuals is not valid using this approach.

Expressed preference is essentially the questionnaire approach to measuring risk. For example, respondents may be presented with pairs of risks and asked which of each pair they would prefer. This is a notional exercise as it cannot be based upon people's real options or experiences and thus falls under the heading of hypothetical questioning – to be avoided in question- naires or interviews as producing unreliable results. For example, if someone is asked 'would you rather have a nuclear power station sited 5 kilometres from your home or smoke 20 cigarettes a day?' the question may have no meaning if the person does not smoke and doesn't want the nuclear power sta- tion either! This extreme example reveals that getting people to express gen- uine preferences in this way is problematic and respondents are understandably cynical about the motives of those asking the questions – thinking perhaps that the real decisions have already been taken.

Another approach which has been used is to ask people to state how much they would be willing to pay in order not to experience a particular risk. For example, people may be asked to indicate how much additional income tax (or some other tax) they would be prepared to pay to reduce, say, a risk to their local environment or to improve health service provision or to reduce road accidents. This approach suffers from the same difficulty as that described above in that these are hypothetical questions – anyone can say that they would be prepared to pay a certain amount in the full knowledge that this amount would not actually be added to their tax bill. In fact, it is possible to get some people to agree to 'donate' more than their total income in order to reduce many of the risks which they might face! Clearly, this method of measuring risk is invalid – indicating once again the com- plexity of this concept.

Reaction of society to risk

In effect, 'society' does not have a single reaction to risk because society com- prises numerous different groups, each with their own interests and objectives (pluralism). Thus, to talk about society's reaction to risk is to oversimplify the issue. However, policy-makers and decision-makers do seek to measure the reactions of different groups within society to risk and in general parlance, we do refer to 'the public interest' or to effects of risk upon local communities. Nevertheless, it is important to disaggregate our approach to society to see what features lie underneath.

There are various ways in which risks may be expressed, for example:

* frequency of deaths per year (absolute numbers);
* fatal accident rate (e.g. a rate per 1000 exposed);
* probability of death per annum (a ratio – e.g. 1 in 10 000);
* loss of life expectancy (in days, years, etc.);
* dreadfulness of outcomes (e.g. injury severities).

When it comes to ranking or estimating different types of risk, people are generally poor at these tasks, being subject to the types of biases discussed earlier. For example, when asked to estimate the numbers of people killed annually from 40 main causes, people's estimates are on average fairly accurate around the middle of the scale. For example, many people know the numbers killed on the road each year (around 4000 in the UK) or the numbers killed as a result of accidents at work. However, numbers dying of the most common diseases – stroke, cancer or heart disease – are typically **underestimated** by a factor of 10 (Lichtenstein *et al.*, 1978 – see figure 5.1).

At the other end of the scale, unusual or 'dramatic' ways of dying   such as botulism – which rarely claim any lives in any given year, may be **overestimated** by a factor of 100. The general picture of subjective estimates is therefore one of a truncated scale in which frequencies which in fact cover six orders of magnitude (1 to 10^6) are perceived to be over only 4 orders of magnitude (10 to 10^5) (Lichtenstein *et al.*, 1978).

This finding, that generally people are unable to differentiate between risks which have large numbers attached is a common one and relates to our limited cognitive processing capacity. Thus, while we have created mathematical representations of large numbers, our own ability to comprehend such numbers and relate them to our everyday lives is limited. However, this does not mean that groups in society are unwilling or unable to express preferences in relation to risk (despite the flawed methodology discussed above). For example, Slovic *et al.* (1979) obtained rankings for 30 risks from four different groups and found that while there were positive correlations between all the rankings, there were some interesting differences. Thus, students and women voters ranked nuclear power as their number one risk, while experts ranked this number 20. However, experts ranked x-rays as number 7 while all other groups ranked this risk around 20 on the list. The full lists are shown in figure 5.5.

The risk ranking example highlights the important point that when it comes to measuring 'society's' reaction to risks of various types there will be differences of opinion between groups about the relative importance of different risks.

	League of Women voters	College students	Active club members	Experts
Nuclear power	1	1	8	20
Motor vehicles	2	5	3	1
Handguns	3	2	1	4
Smoking	4	3	4	2
Motorcycles	5	6	2	6
Alcoholic drinks	6	7	5	3
Private aviation	7	15	11	12
Police work	8	8	7	17
Pesticides	9	4	15	8
Surgery	10	11	9	5
Firefighting	11	10	6	18
Large construction	12	14	13	13
Hunting	13	18	10	23
Spray cans	14	13	23	26
Mountain climbing	15	22	12	29
Bicycles	16	24	14	15
Commercial aviation	17	16	18	16
Electric power (non-nuclear)	18	19	19	9
Swimming	19	30	17	10
Contraceptives	20	9	22	11
Skiing	21	25	16	30
X-rays	22	17	24	7
High school and college football	23	26	21	27
Railroads	24	23	20	19
Food preservatives	25	12	28	14
Food colouring	26	20	30	21
Power mowers	27	28	25	28
Prescription antibiotics	28	21	26	24
Home appliances	29	27	27	22
Vaccinations	30	29	29	25

Figure 5.5 Ranking of risks by four different groups (after Slovic *et al.*, 1979; reproduced with the kind permission of the authors).

Summary text 5.12 The King's horse

Centuries ago, a man was condemned to death. His appeal was turned down and in a final bid for life he made a plea to the King. He asked the King for a year, during which time he said that he would make the King's horse talk. Intrigued by this possibility, the King agreed and gave the man a year to make his horse talk. The man's friends were scornful, saying 'you know very well that you can never make the King's horse talk – it's impossible'.

'Aha but', the man replied, 'I now have a year of life which I would not otherwise have had and therefore this was a good ploy'.

'Yet', replied his friends, 'at the end of that year you will be no better off because you will simply be condemned to death again'.

'That may be so', replied the man, 'but consider, during that year the horse, which is no youngster, might die and then I could be freed or at least be allowed to work on another horse and have another year's freedom. Then again', he added, 'during the year I might die of some disease or other and I will then still have had those extra months of life. Or, he went on, the King might die – he does after all have a risky lifestyle. Or', he added after a pause', 'the horse **might** talk!'

Risk of catastrophic events and long-term health risks

Catastrophic events include that class of accidents which involve sudden failure to danger of a system which usually results in substantial loss of life in the short-term. Examples include: releases of toxic agents, fires and explosions, building or other structural collapse, sinkings, earthquakes, flash flood, volcano. Usually excluded from these 'natural' or technological disasters are acts of war, although large-scale terrorist attacks would be a marginal event which might be included on the grounds that breaches of security – and therefore safety – could be involved.

Attitudes to risk such as these are frequently determined as much by personal experience as by any other factor. For example, Green (1990) reviews a number of studies of flood risk and found that people at risk do not worry enough about the risk of flooding, that they tend to discount the risk and to underestimate the potential severity of flooding to them personally. These features may well be characteristic of people's attitudes to other major risks and present an obvious problem when it comes to the provision of effective warnings.

When it comes to attitudes towards long-term health risks as opposed to risks of sudden death, the health belief model (summary text 4.7 in chapter 4) is a useful reference point. Generally, people are willing to accept a higher risk for delayed death than they are for sudden death because of the discounting factor. As we all have to die eventually, the risk of future death from a particular event or agent is set against all other risks which could be encountered in that time. It is like the story of the condemned man who offers to make the King's horse talk (summary text 5.12).

In statistical terms, death from all causes is about 10 times more likely at age 60 than it is at age 40. Booth (1990) argues that the maximum tolerable risk for death arising from risks with delayed effects should be greater – by up to 10 times – than the risk of immediate death to take account of the increased likelihood of the risk of death from other causes. Kinchin (1982) argues for a figure which is 30 times greater. Whatever figure is taken, there is the problem of difficulty for people in estimating the extent of the risk because of cognitive limitations referred to earlier. However, it also means that programmes to reduce the risk can be planned over a longer period of time. For example, Marks (1990) describes a successful 6-day programme – spread over a period of time – for stopping people smoking whose positive effects could be detected (50% success rate) four months later.

Media, government, communities and risk

Saarinen (1990 p. 279) records that:

> People have difficulty grasping the significance of predicted rare events and relating them to their own location and circumstances. Efforts must be made to establish the credibility of the risk, to communicate the warning message in a form in which it can be understood, and the consequences of

the forecasted events need to be made tangible. Information on what to do to reduce the risk is also needed.

This is a useful summary of the requirements of a successful warning campaign which might be organized by government using various media.

Winchester (1990) draws attention to the basic social and economic differentiation within societies and the widely different perceptions of risk and responses to warnings which are essentially based upon differential access to resources. His case study of reactions to a flood warning in India revealed that most of the rich households left their houses and went to high ground before the warnings of a severe cyclone and storm surge were given. The poor households stayed behind, not because they had not received the warnings but because they could not afford to leave the area or take the risk of leaving – and losing – their few possessions.

Problems from the villagers' perspective were:

- **costs** – the costs of moving were high – prohibitive to most households;
- **erosion of traditional coping methods** – the commercialization of agriculture, along with other factors, had impoverished the majority of the population, who now lived in areas stripped of their natural vegetation;
- **coercion by the government** – positive inducements to leave included the prospect of a family receiving a concrete house or access to bank loans; negative inducements included the possibility of a household or village being struck off the hand-outs register after a cyclone for refusing to obey orders to leave; both types of inducement led to ...
- **over-dependence and rising expectations** – a large government public works programme after the 1977 cyclone created over-dependence and expectations that more would be done; however, villagers who rejected the offer of concrete houses in the hope of getting better ones ended up without even these after the government withdrew the offer.

The government's perspective in this situation was:

- **penalties and rewards** – there are high potential costs for failing to warn exposed populations as well as cost penalties in warning and evacuating areas when nothing then happens (a comparable dilemma faces a railway management when a station bomb threat is received);
- **costs and risks** – there are difficulties in predicting a cyclone risk and differing perceptions of the risk; relief costs are high – 10 times that of warning and evacuation; compensation costs are also very high; a difficult equation has to be worked out.

This case study illustrates well some of the main problems and criteria used by governments and communities in evaluating risk and what to do about it. Different criteria are used by each party according to their own circumstances. Neither is 'correct' in any absolute sense because each is driven by different needs.

In general, the media can play an important role in the public's risk perception, for example:

- providing information about consequences or risk (as in government or other health warnings which receive media coverage);
- translating expert views about the probability of risks (as in articles written by scientific correspondents);
- giving details of case histories of victims ('human interest' stories);
- informing the public of their own perceptions (as in opinion polls);
- acting as a medium of debate about risks (as in editorials and correspondence columns);
- giving warnings of impending disasters and what to do (e.g. of storms at sea or potential flooding);
- drawing differential attention to risks (e.g. in articles about safety).

For a review of media coverage of disasters and hazards, see Wilkins and Patterson (1990).

CONCLUSIONS

Perception is a complex process, whether it relates to objects, people, or to abstract concepts with important consequences – such as risk. Humans develop strategies to simplify perceptual processes. Thus, people attend selectively to physical or social phenomena in order to reduce the amount of information to be processed, for example by stereotyping other people. Complex concepts like risk are made more manageable by using a few of many possible dimensions. More cognitively complex individuals, though still prone to these strategies, are able to embrace a wider domain and to use more dimensions in their perceptions. However, all individuals use simplified models of the world as a basis for their perceptions.

Perceptions are also subject to distortion. In perceiving things, the visual sense in particular may be subject to various illusions. In perceiving people, a first impression, based upon small amounts of information, may be wildly inaccurate. Perception of a particular risk may be adrift by orders of magnitude. Even awareness of these biases and distortions may not protect us from them.

Objective risk is problematic – thus it is essential that the bases and biases of subjective (perceived) risk are understood. The Royal Society (1992) considers subjective risk to be as valid as objective risk – experts' views are just another type of subjectivity. Therefore, managing risk involves not only managing the objective risk, but also managing subjective aspects of risk. The latter is the result of individual perceptions of risk – which are the outcome of continuing experiences, influenced by knowledge from the environment and underlying cognitive biases, about which people may be able to do little, even if they are aware of them.

Risk acceptability is also problematic as people may in reality have little or no genuine choice about accepting a range of risks and this forced choice is likely to influence their perception of risk. Risks over which the individual has no control may be perceived as acceptable only in the sense that this lack of control is acknowledged and as a way of reducing cognitive dissonance.

Risk in the general sense, the product of likelihood, outcome severity and exposure of individuals over a given time, has a corresponding pattern in individual perceptions of risk – essentially the product of scope for intervention (how likely is it that I could affect this risk?) and dangerousness or severity of outcome. Thus, managing risk is an issue for individuals as much as it is for organizations.

Interaction of individuals with risk processes is complex, both because of the complexities of risk perception and the range of possible behaviours in response to risk. However, it is clear that adequate models of risk and individuals' reactions to it are needed if there is to be any realistic expectation of addressing the human risk interface as part of attempts to reduce risk exposure for workpeople and others.

Ultimately risk is a political issue, and as such may be part of managerial decision making on risk control. Different parties or groups will perceive risk differently, based for example upon their status or class group in society, the degree of expertise which they possess, their position of responsibility and the criteria which apply to them personally. Society cannot therefore have a single perception of risk and it is as complex a problem for societies as for individuals.

6 PERSONALITY, WORK AND ACCIDENTS

❏ This chapter completes the part of the book which deals with individual factors – those characteristics which make us both unique and which we share to some extent with other people. After reviewing some of the main approaches to personality, the discussion turns to personality in the work environment and a consideration of accident proneness.

INTRODUCTION

> A person is like some other people, all other people and no other people
> (after Kluckholn and Murray, 1953).

Why should safety and risk professionals wish to know about personality? In psychology, the individual is the prime focus of attention – the ways in which we are similar to and different from other people and what makes each of us unique – is the particular blend of measurable individual characteristics. If we can better understand the nature of these characteristics – or traits or dimensions – and link them with particular job requirements, then first we should be better able to **predict** job performance – including safety requirements, and second we should be better able to **select** for those individual characteristics. Thus, understanding relevant aspects of personality should help the safety and risk professional to manage this particular aspect of human resources.

Personality can be defined as those relatively stable and enduring features of an individual which distinguishes each of us from other people, and which forms the basis of our predictions of other people's future behaviour (Pervin, 1993). This approach to personality follows from the discussion of person perception in chapter 5 (pp. 114–17). For example, having consistently observed a person as being a safe driver, we may conclude that they have a personal **trait** which encapsulates that quality. Each of us possesses a unique combination of traits (e.g. honesty, perseverance, assertiveness) which we share with others to a greater or lesser extent.

This chapter considers some of the main approaches to the study of personality, including the current dominant view of the major dimensions of an individual's personality. Discussion in the first part of the chapter focuses upon the main personality dimensions – especially extraversion – introversion and neuroticism. The chapter also considers personality in the work environment with particular reference to personnel selection. A final section before the conclusion deals with the interesting but problematic topic of accident proneness.

The objectives of this chapter are to:

- review the origins and main types of personality theory;
- provide a contemporary view of the trait approach to personality;
- examine relevant aspects of personality in the workplace;
- consider the evidence for accident proneness;
- determine which, if any, aspects of personality may be identified in applications and interventions when managing risks arising from human behaviour.

THE PSYCHOANALYTIC TRADITION

Freud's approach to motivation was briefly reviewed in chapter 3. His allied theory of personality, which began the psychoanalytic tradition, has been very influential. However, his analysis of factors which shape individuals' personalities from early childhood has also been very controversial. Freud (1938) developed a comprehensive theory of personality, with primary emphasis on the role of unconscious forces. Central to his approach is that the ultimate objective of human behaviour is the pursuit of pleasure (although he also postulated a 'death instinct').

For Freud, personality comprised three main components – id, super-ego and ego – interactions between these components producing behaviour. The id, anchored in our biological inheritance, subscribes to the pleasure principal and is intent on immediate and total satisfaction of instinctual urges regardless of other considerations. The super-ego internalizes parental and societal values, often unconsciously, and is the conscience, being preoccupied with controlling behaviour in accordance with its strict view of morality. The ego takes a balanced view in the face of pressures from the id and the super-ego. It conforms to the reality principle and attempts to control the id as well as trying to neutralize unrealistic demands from the super-ego.

Conflicts between the three components can generate undesirable side-effects, which in severe cases can result in abnormal behaviour such as obsessions and neuroses. According to Freud, a number of mechanisms to cope with these conflicts are available to the individual. These are called defence mechanisms and the more important ones are reviewed in summary text 6.1.

While some early attempts were made to explain accidents in the light of Freud's theory of personality – that accidents are caused by unconscious desires within us – these have not been demonstrated to have any validity. However, some observable aspects of behaviour might be attributable to conflicts which arise between different components of personality as conceived by Freud.

Other theorists of the psychoanalytic school proffered alternative views of personality, mainly centred upon components of neuroticism – which may be

Summary text 6.1 Defence mechanisms arising from conflicts between personality components (after Freud)

1. **Repression** is where an individual is motivated to forget an unpleasant event. For example, involvement in a serious accident is likely to be a traumatic event which might lead to some memory loss (amnesia). In this case, the memory is tucked away in the sub-conscious mind (i.e. is repressed), but many find expression through dreams or in psychotherapy.

2. **Projection** occurs when for example a worker feels anxious about not taking adequate safety precautions and, rather than accept personal responsibility for this, projects the problem onto others. For example, a supervisor or colleagues may be blamed for being lax in monitoring safety procedures.

3. **Reaction formation** – here behaviour is exhibited that is the inverse of the person's previous disposition, perhaps as a result of some 'conversion' (akin to a religious conversion). For example, a worker with a previous track record of carelessness and disinterest in safety matters develops a pattern of behaviour which indicates exaggerated attachment to safe systems of work.

4. **Denial** – the person appears not to notice something which, for example poses a threat to his or her self-esteem. A worker is aware of the supervisor's growing dissatisfaction with the quality of his work, and denies having heard a recent verbal criticism made by the supervisor.

5. **Regression** – occurs when a person slides into an earlier pattern of behaviour when trying to cope with an incident similar in some respects to an earlier experience. For example, a supervisor reprimands a worker for removing a guard from dangerous machinery. The worker responds by silence and withdrawing from the situation in a similar way to behaviour earlier in life when reprimanded by a parent or other authority figure.

6. **Displacement** helps the individual not to react in a predictable way to a particular stimulus; instead he or she reacts in a different setting. For example, if in the above case, the supervisor reprimands in a harsh or unjust manner, the displacement response of the subordinate is to feel angry but to contain the anger and to release it later in the family setting, perhaps in response to mild provocation. The family situation response appears totally unjustified, but is understandable in the light of the earlier incident.

described as emotional instability, often associated with feelings of anxiety. These included: Adler (inferiority feelings, superiority striving and compensation striving), Horney (basic anxiety leading to: moving towards others, moving against others or moving away from others) and Sullivan (emphasizing personal and social influences). The best known of those who broke with Freud was Jung. A central feature of Jung's approach was how people struggle with internal opposing forces, for example masculine versus feminine or the face (or mask) we present to others (persona) and the private self. Jung also developed the concepts of introversion (inner orientation) and extraversion (outer orientation). In Jung's theory, our lives are a continuing struggle to harmonize the conflicting components of our being.

TRAITS AND TYPES

Traits are dimensions of personality along which each individual has a position. For example, we might describe one person as very outgoing, another as very reserved and a third as somewhere in between. An individual's personality comprises the aggregate of their scores on each trait. A trait summarizes past behaviours and predicts future behaviours (Cook, 1993). The first major attempt to identify the main personality traits was that of Cattell (1965) who found 16 such traits or personality factors – hence his well known 16PF. Cattell's 16 personality factors are shown in summary text 6.2.

Cattell calls the 16 primary factors the source traits, which form the underlying personality structure. He felt that, once a person was positioned on the 16 dimensions of personality, much of that person's behaviour could be predicted, although he recognized that many variables other than the source traits also determined behaviour. For example, people's motives need to be considered (chapter 3), along with their mood states (e.g. depression, anxiety) and the particular roles and settings in which people behave. Thus, aggressive behaviour may manifest itself when a person is driving but not at other times. The 16PF questionnaire has been used extensively in occupational settings to match 'ideal' personality profiles for managers and around 50 other occupations (Cattell *et al.*, 1970). Higher order factors which emerge from the 16PF are extraversion/introversion (labelled exvia–invia by Cattell) and anxiety (akin to neuroticism).

While Cattell's work focuses upon traits, Eysenck's work is mainly concerned with personality **types**, although their methods are similar. Although Eysenck is strongly antagonistic in respect of the methodology of the psychoanalytic tradition, his theory of personality uses some of its terminology and broad descriptions – for example as used by Jung and Horney. Eysenck's classification identifies three major dimensions of personality – extraversion/introversion, neuroticism and a less commonly used psychoticism dimension. His descriptions of typical extraverts and introverts (e.g. Eysenck, 1965) are shown in summary text 6.3.

Most people fit somewhere in between the extreme positions of extravert and introvert (i.e. are ambiverts), although their positions can vary from day-to-day according to their mood changes and life experiences. The personality types made up of a collection of traits used by Eysenck appear in figure 6.1. The four temperaments of Galen* – Sanguine (hopeful, confident, optimistic); Melancholic (depressed, pessimistic); Choleric (active, irritable, aggressive); and Phlegmatic (sluggish, apathetic) – are displayed in each of the four cells representing the personality types from Eysenck's two main dimensions. The lists of characteristics in each cell are derived from factor analysis – a statistical technique which can be used to interpret personality traits – also used by Cattell. For a review of this method as used in personality testing, see for example Cronbach (1984).

*Galen of Pergamum, the second century Greek physician and founder of experimental physiology, who was the dominant influence in medicine in Europe during the Middle Ages and Renaissance.

Summary text 6.2 Cattell's sixteen personality factors

High-score description	Factor	Low-score description
Outgoing, warm-hearted, easy-going, participating	A	**Reserved**, detached, critical, cool
More intelligent, abstract thinking, bright (higher scholastic mental capacity)	B	**Less intelligent**, concrete thinking (lower scholastic mental capacity)
Emotionally stable, faces reality, calm (higher ego strength)	C	**Affected by feelings**, emotionally less stable, easily upset (lower ego strength)
Assertive, independent, aggressive, stubborn (dominance)	E	**Humble**, mild, obedient, conforming (submissiveness)
Happy go lucky, heedless, gay, enthusiastic	F	**Sober**, prudent, serious, taciturn
Conscientious, persevering, staid, rule-bound (stronger super-ego strength)	G	**Expedient**, a law to himself, by-passes obligations (weaker super-ego strength)
Venturesome, socially bold, uninhibited, spontaneous	H	**Shy**, restrained diffident, timid
Tender-minded, dependent, over-protected, sensitive	I	**Tough-minded**, self-reliant, realistic, no-nonsense
Suspicious, self-opinionated, hard to fool	L	**Trusting**, adaptable, free of jealousy, easy to get on with
Imaginative, wrapped up in inner urgencies, careless of practical matters, bohemian	M	**Practical**, careful, conventional, regulated by external realities, proper
Shrewd, calculating, worldly, penetrating	N	**Forthright**, natural, artless, sentimental
Apprehensive, worrying, depressive, troubled (guilt proneness)	O	**Placid**, self-assured, confident, serene (untroubled adequacy)
Experimenting, critical, liberal analytical, free-thinking (radicalism)	Q1	**Conservative**, respecting established ideas, tolerant of traditional difficulties
Self-sufficient, prefers own decisions, resourceful (self-sufficiency)	Q2	**Group-dependent**, a 'joiner' and sound follower
Controlled, socially precise, self-disciplined, compulsive	Q3	**Casual**, careless of protocol, untidy, follows own urges (low integration)
Tense, driven, overwrought, fretful	Q4	**Relaxed**, tranquil, torpid, unfrustrated

Source: Cattell (1965).

Eysenck's approach to personality types is loosely based upon Jung's typology. Jung (1953) revealed that neurotics will display different symptoms depending upon whether they tend to introversion or extraversion. Eysenck maintained that introverts suffering from neurotic disorders develop anxiety states, depressions, phobic fears and obsessive compulsive habits. Extravert neurotics developed personality disorders, histrionic behaviour, memory lapses, paralysis and physical disorders with no apparent physiological cause. In extreme cases, a psychotic personality could be revealed, with characteristics shown in summary text 6.4.

Summary text 6.3 Descriptions of typical extraverts and introverts (after Eysenck, 1965)

Extraverts
Typical extraverts are sociable, like parties, have many friends, need to have people to talk to, and do not like reading or studying by themselves. They crave excitement, take chances, often stick their necks out, act on the spur of the moment, and are generally impulsive. They are fond of practical jokes, always have a ready answer, and generally like change; they are carefree, optimistic, and like to 'laugh and be merry'. They prefer to keep moving and doing things, tend to be aggressive, and lose their tempers quickly. Altogether, their feelings are not kept under tight control and they are not always reliable.

Introverts
Typical introverts, on the other hand, are quiet retiring sorts of people, introspective, fond of books rather than people; they are reserved and distant except with intimate friends. They tend to plan ahead, 'look before they leap' and distrust the impulse of the moment. They do not like excitement, take matters of everyday life with proper seriousness, and like a well-ordered mode of life. They keep their feelings under close control, seldom behave in an aggressive manner, and do not lose their temper easily. They are reliable, somewhat pessimistic, and place great value on ethical standards.

	Stable	*Unstable*
Introverted	Phlegmatic	Melancholic
	passive	moody
	careful	anxious
	thoughtful	rigid
	peaceful	sober
	controlled	pessimistic
	reliable	reserved
	even-tempered	unsociable
	calm	quiet
Extraverted	Sanguine	Choleric
	sociable	touchy
	outgoing	restless
	talkative	aggressive
	responsive	excitable
	easygoing	changeable
	lively	impulsive
	carefree	optimistic
	leadership	active

Figure 6.1 Galen's four 'temperaments' compared with modern personality characteristics (after Eysenck, 1965).

Summary text 6.4 Characteristics of the psychotic personality (after Eysenck, 1977)

- sensation-seeking – emphasis upon immediate goals rather than remote or deferred ones;
- impulsive behaviour or apparent incongruity between stimulus strength and behavioural response to it;
- inability to form deep or persistent attachments to others;
- poor judgement and planning in attaining defined goals;
- apparent lack of anxiety and distress over social maladjustment and unwillingness or inability to consider maladjustment as such;
- tendency to project blame onto others and to take no responsibility for failures;
- meaningless prevarication, often about trivial matters where detection is inevitable;
- almost complete lack of dependability and of willingness to assume responsibility;
- emotional poverty and lack of empathy towards others.

Individuals who are high on neuroticism tend to be very excitable and respond quickly to stimuli. Neurotics also tire more quickly, suffer from strain and often have impaired psycho-motor control (Eysenck, 1964). It may be difficult to separate out neuroticism from traits such as anxiety, depression or impulsiveness (Eysenck and Eysenck, 1977; Gray, 1981; Revelle, 1987; Deary and Matthews, 1993). However, while neuroticism is virtually identical to trait anxiety, it is only weakly related to impulsiveness. Mueller (1992) considers two components of anxiety – (1) arousal and (2) worry – the latter being the main predictor of performance impairment. Some anxiety improves performance (facilitative anxiety) but beyond a certain point, performance declines with increasing anxiety (debilitative anxiety). A vital distinction is between **trait** anxiety – a relatively enduring (i.e. personality) disposition to anxiety, and **state** anxiety – a transitory experience triggered by some current outside stimulus (see for example, Cattell and Scheier, 1961; Spielberger, 1966; Spielberger *et al.*, 1980; Spielberger, 1983). However, these two types of anxiety are positively correlated, particularly when people are subjected to evaluation or exposed to some form of threat.

Tests (particularly the Eysenck Personality Inventory or EPI) have been developed to measure personality on the dimensions of extraversion–introversion and neuroticism (Eysenck and Eysenck, 1968). Psychoticism can be measured on a scale along with other dimensions of personality described by Eysenck as part of the Eysenck Personality Questionnaire (EPQ). Whereas neurotic disorders involve emotional disturbance while cognitive processes remain normal, psychotic disorders also involve abnormal cognitive processes. The psychotic dimension of personality is strongly associated with masculinity – males scoring higher than females. Different crimes correlate with different personality types, although criminals in general have higher than average scores on psychoticism, extraversion and neuroticism (Eysenck, 1977).

A range of functions have been found to be related to extraversion, including perception (chapter 5), attention, memory and other cognitive processes (Eysenck and Eysenck, 1985). Many individual differences emerge between extraverts and introverts, this being the most studied dimension of personality, and some of these are shown in summary text 6.5.

In seeking to explain some of the differences outlined in summary text 6.5, Matthews *et al.* (1990a, b) postulate that extraverts have greater processing

---

Summary text 6.5 Differences between extraverts and introverts

Conditioning
- extraverts are more difficult than introverts to condition (Eysenck, 1977);
- effects of conditioning wear off more quickly in extraverts (Eysenck, 1977);
- extraverts are harder to condition to socially acceptable behaviour and are more likely to break moral codes and behave anti-socially (Eysenck, 1977);
- extraverts condition more readily to rewards, introverts to punishments (Gray, 1981).

Perceptual tasks
- compared with introverts, extraverts detect a lower proportion of visual (in particular) and auditory signals in vigilance tasks (Davies and Parasuraman, 1982);
- in tasks demanding attention, introverts are superior at vigilance and it seems that extraverts have poorer visual perception – e.g. poorer perception of flicker (Davies and Parasuraman, 1982);
- extraverts' attention is poorer when driving for long spells, but their driving is improved by playing the car radio (Fagerstrom and Lisper, 1977);
- extraverts recover less quickly from glare and cannot maintain concentrated effort without repeated involuntary rest pauses (Eysenck and Eysenck, 1985).

Other cognitive tasks
- extraverts are superior on more demanding tasks such as those requiring two tasks to be done simultaneously and are also more resistant to distraction (Matthews, 1992a);
- extraverts perform better than introverts on more difficult tasks and worse than introverts on easier tasks (Eysenck and Eysenck, 1985; M W Eysenck, 1981; Matthews *et al.*, 1990a);
- while extraverts tend to do better on demanding, but relatively straightforward information processing tasks, introverts may do better at problem solving tasks that are complex as well as difficult (Matthews, 1993);
- extraverts have better short-term retention and recall than introverts do (Eysenck, 1982; Dickman and Meyer, 1988);
- introverts have better long-term retention (Matthews, 1992a).

Arousal and stress
- extraverts perform better than introverts in highly arousing conditions (e.g. noise) but worse than introverts in de-arousing conditions – e.g. a quiet room (Eysenck and Eysenck, 1985);
- extraverts' performance is facilitated by caffeine, while introverts' performance is impaired by caffeine (Lieberman, 1992);
- introverts perform better in de-arousing conditions such as sleep deprivation (Corcoran, 1972) and alcohol ingestion (Jones, 1974);
- extraverts perform better than introverts under high stress conditions while introverts perform more efficiently at low levels of stress, this finding being consistent for different sources of stress – for example, noise, caffeine, anxiety and incentives for performance (Eysenck and Eysenck, 1985).

Further discussion of stress and its effects is given in chapter 8.

resource availability, being generally faster. However, extraverts seem to deal with complexity by adopting somewhat counter-productive impulsive strategies (Matthews, 1993). Extraversion is also associated with sensitivity to signals of reward and punishment (Gray, 1981) suggesting that extraverts pay greater heed than introverts do to these forms of social cues. A greater availability of resources for verbal processing might account for extraverts' greater social interests and skills (Wickens, 1984; Matthews, 1992a).

It has been suggested (Humphreys and Revelle, 1984) that it is impulsiveness rather than extraversion which affects performance (impulsive individuals tend to rush in to situations rather than giving a considered response), and some evidence for this is outlined in summary text 6.6.

EMERGENCE OF THE 'BIG FIVE'

While debate continues on the number of essential personality traits (e.g. Hough, 1992), many psychologists now accept that there are strong grounds for accepting five basic personality dimensions – sometimes adding a sixth individual difference, intelligence.

The idea that there are five main personality dimensions is not new (Fiske, 1949; Tupes and Christal, 1961), but the labelling of these as the 'big five' by McCrae and Costa (1985, 1987) spawned great interest and continuing debate, not least because of the considerable overlap of these with other studies and approaches. The big five personality factors, as described by a number of writers (e.g. Brand and Egan, 1989; McCrae and Costa, 1989; Barrick and Mount, 1991; Costa, McCrae and Dye, 1991; Deary and Matthews, 1993) are:

1. extraversion (vs introversion)
2. neuroticism/emotionally (vs stability/equanimity)
3. openness/tender-minded (vs tough-minded/practical)
4. agreeableness (vs autonomy)
5. conscientiousness (vs impulsiveness/casualness).

While there is some modest overlap between the five main dimensions, they are generally held to be distinct. More detailed lists of characteristics which have come from a number of studies are shown in summary text 6.7.

Summary text 6.6 Effects of impulsiveness

- caffeine can facilitate the performance of impulsive individuals (measured on the impulsiveness scale of the EPI) and impair the performance of non-impulsives taking complex cognitive tests in the morning – the effect is the opposite way round in the evening (Revelle et al., 1980, 1987);
- high impulsives seem to be lower in arousal in the morning and higher in arousal in the evening (Revelle et al., 1987);
- in carrying out tasks, high impulsives respond faster and less accurately than do low impulsives – i.e. they trade speed for accuracy (e.g. Edman et al., 1983);
- high impulsives respond more slowly than low impulsives when extensive processing is required – i.e. when task requirements are complex (Barrett, 1987).

Summary text 6.7 Detailed descriptions of the 'big five' personality dimensions (after Brand and Egan, 1989; McCrae and Costa, 1989)

1. **Extraversion** (vs **introversion**)
venturesome, assertive, energetic, spontaneous, talkative, frank, enthusiastic, uninhibited, sociable, outgoing, affiliative, socially confident, controlling (others), lacking emotional control, persuasive, warm, gregarious, active, excitement seeking, positive emotions.

2. **Neuroticism** (vs **emotional stability/adjustment**)
neurotic, tense, apprehensive, defensive, highly strung, strong moods, vulnerable, over-sensitive, labile, worrying, anxious, emotional, hostile, depressed, self-conscious, impulsive.

3. **Tender-minded** (vs **tough-minded**)
affectionate, trusting, understanding, aesthetic, sensitive, feminine, imaginative, unusual, intellectual, tolerant, culture-oriented, responsible, open, conceptual, innovative, change-oriented, independent, behavioural, fantasy, feelings, actions, ideas, values.

4. **Autonomy** (vs **agreeability/sociability**)
self-sufficiency, dominance, radicalism, will, independence, bohemianism, imagination, experimenting, rebelliousness, assertive, quarrelsome, detached, non-trusting, selfish, non-compliant, devious, immodest.

5. **Conscientiousness** (vs **impulsive**)
conforming, general inhibition, conventional, careful, self-controlled, orderly, compulsive, obsessive, productive, cognitively structured, striving to achieve, responsible, superego strength, plans ahead, persevering, disciplined, precise, industrious, detail conscious, competent, dutiful, self-disciplined, deliberate.

Note that opposite lists would be applied to the other end of each of the five dimensions (in parentheses).

Conscientiousness has been found to be closely aligned with motivation (chapter 3) and is related to performance (Barrick and Mount, 1991) and intelligence (Goff and Ackerman, 1992). This factor has also been called dependability – including planning, responsibility and carefulness (Hough *et al.*, 1990). Openness to experience is related to learning capacity and other abilities (McCrae and Costa, 1985) and to training proficiency (Barrick and Mount, 1991; see also chapter 2).

More enduring personality traits should be distinguished from **mood** states, although there are correlations between mood and some personality traits – e.g. extraversion and neuroticism (Matthews, 1992b). Matthews *et al.*'s 1990c model of mood has three components:

1. hedonic tone (pleasure vs displeasure dimension);
2. energetic arousal (energy, activation, positive effect);
3. tense arousal (tension, stress, negative effect).

Further work is required to establish the validity of the 'big five' personality factors and their associated behaviour patterns, although their rediscovery has given a new lease of life to personality trait theory and has in effect brought together much previous work on personality – including that of Eysenck and Cattell as well as elements of the psychoanalytic tradition. However, it appears that there are cultural differences in the way in which personality dimensions are perceived. Thus, Bond and Forgas (1984) found that conscientiousness was more important to a Hong Kong Chinese sample, while extraversion was more important to a sample of Australians. Yang and Bond (1990) found a 'big five' for Taiwanese, but not one-to-one correspondence with the US/UK dimensions.

The trait approach has been criticized by authors such as Mischel (1968) on the grounds that correlations between personality traits and behaviour are very modest and that much of our behaviour is socially shaped. However, studies indicate that in the region of 50 percent of the variance in the major personality dimensions (extraversion, neuroticism) is inherited, which indicates some degree of stability (Deary and Matthews, 1993). These authors argue that although the expression of personality traits is filtered by the environment – e.g. social situations, the reasonable degree of consistency for behaviour across situations shown by a number of studies argues for the relative durability of personality traits.

The 'truth' as usual lies between extremes, so that social situations shape a person's behaviour to an extent, but are also partly determined by the individual seeking out or exploiting certain social factors. For example, aggressive children **expect** others to be hostile, which may elicit the (expected) hostile behaviours (Dodge, 1986) and we may all be prone to self-fulfilling expectations (pp. 49–53 on attribution in chapter 3 and pp. 114–17 on person perception in chapter 5). The midway interactionist view of personality maintains that to some extent situations determine how people behave, but at the same time, people have some influence over events in their environment and they also help to create the situations that surround them. Thus, personality and environmental influences interact to produce observed behaviour.

There are a number of other approaches to personality; summaries of five of the main ones are shown in summary text 6.8. Relevant aspects of some of these for safety and risk management are considered in other chapters – e.g. chapter 2 on learning, chapter 3 on motivation and chapter 4 on attitudes. Further details of these and other theories are given in numerous textbooks on personality (e.g. Pervin, 1993).

PERSONALITY AT WORK

Personality has been used as a variable in occupational settings for some time. For example, Anderson's (1929) survey of staff at Macy's department store in New York found that 20% of employees fell into the 'problem' category – can't learn, suffer chronic ill-health, in constant trouble with fellow employees and can't adjust satisfactorily to their work. Culpin and Smith (1930) surveyed over 1000 British workers and found 20–30% suffering some level of neurosis (around 1 in 5 maladjusted people in a heterogeneous population is typical).

Summary text 6.8 A summary of other personality theories

1. **Person-centred** (e.g. Carl Rogers) – concerned with how the individual **perceives** and **experiences** the self and the world (phenomenological approach). Part of the humanistic, human potential movement, emphasizing self-actualization and the fulfilment of growth potential.

2. **Cognitive theory** (e.g. George Kelly – Personal Construct Theory) – concerned with how the individual perceives, interprets and conceptualizes events and the environment. The individual is a scientist who develops a unique set of theories (constructs) to predict events (Fransella and Bannister, 1977).

3. **Behavioural approaches** (e.g. J. B. Watson, B. F. Skinner) – are based upon principles of learning (see also chapter 2) – conditioning and stimulus-response learning. Recognizes the role of situational and environmental variables in determining behaviour – being concerned with what is observable (contrasts with phenomenological, humanistic and trait approaches to personality).

4. **Social-cognitive theories** (e.g. Albert Bandura, Walter Mischel) – emphasize **social** origins of behaviour and the importance of cognitive processes. Particular attention paid to how people learn complex patterns of behaviour, how individuals achieve goals (self-efficacy) and sees people as **active** agents in influencing events in their lives (contrasts with being the passive 'victim' of possessing certain personality traits).

5. **Psychographic ('lifestyle') approaches** – psychographics is used to segment consumer markets and provides marketers with general consumer profiles, analogous with personality types. Probably the best-known exposition of consumer psychographics is the values and lifestyle (VALS) typology. The original typology portrayed nine consumer groups (market segments) within four main categories (need-driven, outer-directed, inner-directed, integrated) to reflect their consumer orientation (Mitchell, 1983; Holman, 1984). The revised VALS typology portrays three general consumer groups divided into eight segments (Graham, 1989, Schiffman and Kanuk, 1991). Consumers are characterized on two main dimensions (analogous with trait or type theories in personality) – available resources (abundant-minimal) and primary orientation (principle – guided by beliefs; status – guided by social approval; action – guided by activity, variety and risk taking). The VALS hierarchies are modelled along similar lines to Maslow's hierarchy (chapter 3, summary text 3.4).

US nuclear power industry officials listed over 150 cases of distracting behaviour in nuclear power plant operations – argumentative hostility and impulsive action were considered to be particularly risky (Cook, 1993). Psychologists advised testing and periodic retesting (Dunnette *et al.*, 1981). Other studies have found that extraverts tend to leave jobs sooner (Cooper and Payne, 1967), are less satisfied than introverts with clerical jobs (Sterns *et al.*, 1983) and that stable extraverts were generally better in flying training (Bartram and Dale, 1982). Matthews *et al.* (1992) found that extraverts were better at mail sorting.

Hough *et al.* (1990) found that personality traits similar to the big five could be used to predict some job-related criteria. For example, extraversion predicts effort and leadership in military personnel, while dependability (conscientiousness) predicts personal discipline. However, Hough (1992) reviews a number of studies which indicate that further personality dimensions may be required to predict job related criteria. Hough points out that if the relatively poor predictive validity of personality tests for job performance is to be improved, then further work is required. Schmitt *et al.* (1984) found small correlations between personality traits and job performance.

Personality tests

In order to improve the ability of personality tests to be used as valid predictors of work activity, attempts have been made to develop personality tests which are specifically occupationally oriented. A prime example is the Occupational Personality Questionnaire (OPQ) (Saville and Holdsworth, 1984, 1985). The OPQ was developed as a means of measuring personality factors which were deemed to be particularly relevant to occupational environments. There are several forms of the OPQ; summary text 6.9 describes the three main domains – relationships with people, thinking style and feelings and emotions, as well as the traits and descriptions within each domain.

Matthews *et al.* (1990d) and Stanton *et al.* (1991) factor analysed the OPQ and found a factor structure which corresponded with the big five. Thus, some underlying common features do emerge in many personality tests, although some researchers consider that even the best personality tests do not predict job performance (Blinkhorn and Johnson, 1990). One problem is that many jobs involve a wide variety of activities (e.g. the job of a safety and risk professional) and thus it would be difficult to find a single test which could predict for all aspects of such jobs. As Deary and Matthews (1993) point out, in many jobs, where a variety of types of processing (i.e. mental/physical activity) are required, stress, motivation (and other factors) vary over time so that (personality) trait effects are swamped by overall performance measures (and external demands). Robertson and Kinder (1992) found that OPQ personality variables were associated with job competencies such as creativity, analysis and judgement. Hesketh and Robertson (1993) explain the necessity of examining the relative contributions of personality and situation in job performance as a basis for measurement. Thus, personality tests may most appropriately be used to predict relatively homogeneous aspects of job performance or those aspects which are critical – for example to safety systems.

While the OPQ is frequently used as part of a battery of occupational selection predictors, another test which has been in occupational use since the 1950s is primarily designed for use as a tool for counselling, personal development and team-building (chapter 7). This is the Myers-Briggs Type Indicator (MBTI), derived from Jung's theory of personality types and based upon individual differences in perception and judgement and their relation to motivation, interests and values. Four dimensions, which in Jung's theory structure an individual's personality, are ascribed:

1. extraversion (relating best to people and things) vs introversion (relating best to inner ideas).

Summary text 6.9 Domains, traits and descriptions of the dimensions of the Occupational Personality Questionnaire

1. **Relationships with people**
   (a) Assertive
      • Persuasive (enjoys selling, changes opinions of others, convincing with arguments, negotiates);
      • Controlling (takes charge, directs, manages, organizes, supervises others);
      • Independent (has strong views on things, difficult to manage, speaks up, argues, dislikes ties).
   (b) Gregarious
      • Outgoing (fun loving, humorous, sociable, vibrant, talkative, jovial);
      • Affiliative (has many friends, enjoys being in groups, likes companionship, shares things with friends);
      • Socially confident (puts people at ease, knows what to say, good with words).
   (c) Empathy
      • Modest (reserved about achievements, avoids talking about self, accepts others, avoids trappings of status);
      • Democratic (encourages others to contribute, consults, listens and refers to others);
      • Caring (considerate to others, helps those in need, sympathetic, tolerant).

2. **Thinking style**
   (a) Fields of use
      • Practical (down-to-earth, likes repairing and mending things, better with the concrete);
      • Data rational (good with data, operates on facts, enjoys assessing and measuring);
      • Artistic (appreciates culture, shows artistic flair, sensitive to visual arts and music);
      • Behavioural (analyses thoughts and behaviour, psychologically minded, likes to understand people).
   (b) Abstract
      • Traditional (preserves well-proven methods, prefers the orthodox, disciplined, conventional);
      • Change-oriented (enjoys doing new things, seeks variety, prefers novelty to routine, accepts changes);
      • Conceptual (theoretical, intellectually curious, enjoys the complex and abstract);
      • Innovative (generates ideas, shows ingenuity, thinks up solutions).
   (c) Structure
      • Forward planning (prepares well in advance, enjoys target setting, forecasts trends, plans projects);
      • Detail-conscious (methodical, keeps things neat and tidy, precise, accurate);
      • Conscientious (sticks to deadlines, completes jobs, perseveres with routine, likes fixed schedules).

3. **Feelings and emotions**
   (a) Anxieties
      • Relaxed (calm, relaxed, cool under pressure, free from anxiety, can switch off);
      • Worrying (worry when things go wrong, keyed-up before important events, anxious to do well).

Summary text 6.9 (continued)

(b) Controls
  - Tough-minded (difficult to hurt or upset, can brush off insults, unaffected by unfair remarks);
  - Emotional control (restrained in showing emotions, keeps feelings back, avoids outbursts);
  - Optimistic (cheerful, happy, keeps spirits up despite setbacks);
  - Critical (good at probing the facts, sees the disadvantages, challenges assumptions).
(c) Energies
  - Active (has energy, moves quickly, enjoys physical exercise, doesn't sit still);
  - Competitive (plays to win, determined to beat others, poor loser);
  - Achieving (ambitious, sets sights high, career centred, results orientated);
  - Decisive (quick at conclusions, weighs things up rapidly, may be hasty, takes risks.

Source: Saville and Holdsworth Ltd (1987) and is reproduced with their kind permission.

---

2. sensing (preferring known facts) vs intuition (preferring to search for possibilities and relationships);
3. thinking (judgements based more on impersonal analysis and logic) vs feeling (judgements based more on personal values);
4. judgement (preferring a planned orderly way of life) vs perception (preferring a flexible spontaneous way of life).

The four dimensions of the MBTI result in 16 personality types – each with a characteristic description. These descriptions can be used for a variety of purposes, including: providing individual feedback, as a basis for group discussion or for career counselling. Those completing the MBTI may also be counselled in respect of ways to develop their weaker aspects of the four dimensions which comprise their personality profile with the aim of helping them to achieve greater harmony and balance between the various contrasting elements of these dimensions. More detailed description of the MBTI and its underlying rationale, as well as further explorations of its uses may be found for example in: Briggs Myers and Briggs Myers (1980), Kroeger and Theusen (1988, 1992) and Bayne (1994). Bridges (1992) has expanded the MBTI notion to organizational 'characters'.

Using personality tests in selection

Various authors provide advice and guidance on a variety of selection procedures (e.g. Lewis, 1985; Herriot, 1989; Shackleton, 1989; Smith and Robertson, 1989). Testing is basically of two types – aptitude (e.g. intelligence or various types of ability – spatial, speed, accuracy, programming ability, etc.) and personality (e.g. using 16PF, OPQ, etc.). Dorcus and Jones (1950) note that in the US, use of psychological testing grew rapidly between 1910 and

1948, while in the UK and the rest of Europe it remained at a relatively low level. There is a very large number of personality measures available (Buros, 1970; Conoley and Kramer, 1989), many of them quite dated. During the 1980s, personality testing increased in UK organizations' selection procedures (Robertson and Smith, 1989), although this may have levelled off by the 1990s (Williams, 1994).

Although there has been criticism of the validity of personality tests in job selection (e.g. Blinkhorn and Johnson, 1990), there has been strong support for personality testing (e.g. Day and Silverman, 1989; Gellatly *et al.,* 1991; Tett *et al.,* 1991) providing that:

- relevant personal qualities are identified;
- personality measures used are rationally selected and are valid;
- personality-oriented job analysis is used as a basis for test selection.

Jackson and Rothstein (1993) conclude that personality testing can be a useful component of personnel selection, if:

1. well constructed and validated personality measures are used;
2. the choice of personality measure is guided by job analysis and prediction;
3. appropriate statistical analyses are used to validate the measure;
4. economic benefits are evaluated in respect of improving job performance.

To this list, one could add that personality tests should be used in conjunction with one or more other selection techniques, for example those listed in summary text 6.10, and it should be ensured that the personalities of those selected are consistent with the culture of the organization (chapter 10, pp. 291–5).

When considering personnel selection in a strategic context, such as one provided by human resource management, the contribution of personnel selection to the organization's corporate objectives needs to be considered as an investment in human resources. Cook (1993) argues for a systematic approach to selection as a means of improving productivity, and it is increasingly recognized that poor selection decisions can be very costly for an organization. One principle of human resource planning is to use selection procedures systematically. Part of this process is the use of job analysis, often

---

Summary text 6.10 Selection techniques to complement the use of personality tests

Interviews – should be structured and interviewers properly trained
Biographical data (biodata) – to indicate relevant aspects of experience, qualifications and background
Ability tests – to assess relevant cognitive or behavioural components of job performance
Work sample/simulation tests – to replicate the type of work environment to be encountered for assessing a sample of performance
Assessment centres – to collect data from a range of different tests and exercises which focus upon job (particularly managerial) performance.

done by observation of those doing the job and by interviewing present incumbents. The job description drawn up should show:
- responsibilities involved in the job;
- skills and knowledge required;
- authority level and position in organization;
- how the job is to be performed;
- personal factors required – e.g. age range, qualifications, experience, abilities and personality factors – required, desirable and undesired.

From a detailed job analysis, including the safety and risk aspects of the job, an appropriate personality measure may be a useful component of the selection process. For more detailed information on the role of personality differences in the work environment, see Furnham (1992).

ACCIDENT PRONENESS

There is some evidence that extraverts have more accidents (Fine, 1963; Craske, 1968), although this may partly be due to a reporting effect – i.e. extraverts also report more of their accidents (Powell *et al.*, 1971). Sutherland and Cooper (1991), in a study of offshore oil and gas industry workers, found that while extraverts reported having more accidents than introverts did, the difference was not significant. However, they found that workers who scored highly on the EPI neuroticism scale did report significantly more accidents than more stable individuals, and suggest that both the neuroticism and the extraversion–introversion dimensions need to be considered in respect of accident involvement. This also has implications for attending to human resource management issues such as selection (pp. 149–55) and training (chapter 2).

The search for personality characteristics which might affect accident involvement has a long history. Shaw and Sichel (1971) used Eysenck's personality model as a basis for relating personality characteristics to accident liability and found some relationship – see figure 6.2.

Shaw and Sichel (1971) built up more complete personality profiles of the different categories of accident risk, their work being part of the accident proneness tradition – which in its extreme form maintains that enduring personality factors exert a detectable influence upon accidents. Of all the presumed personality 'traits', accident proneness is the one likely to be of greatest interest to the safety and risk professional. However, the fact that accident proneness has never emerged as a personality trait or type in any general study of personality should be sufficient to ring alarm bells in respect of whether this is a genuine personality trait.

Intuitively we may feel that there is such a trait as accident proneness and many of us have stories to support such a feeling. One of the authors was told of an apprentice fitter in a large transport company who kept on having accidents until one day he had a fatal accident, and of the guilt of his colleagues in not taking action before this happened. A factory manager, faced with a high incidence of lifting and handling accidents is reported as saying

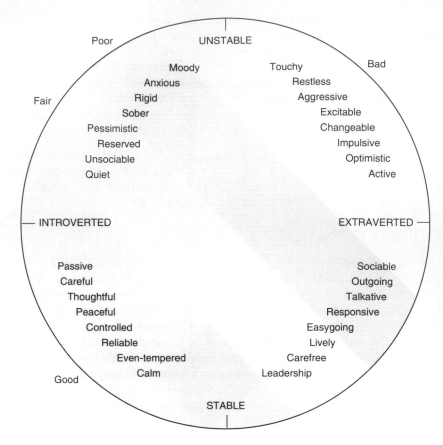

Figure 6.2 Personality characteristics and accident risk (after Shaw and Sichel, 1971 and Eysenck, 1964).

'unfortunately, the majority of our people are accident prone' (Lindsay, 1980). Wong and Hobbs (1949) described accident prone workers as:

individuals who showed most frequent errors in their work, had the poorest attendance, and were vocational misfits given to inattention and worry and demonstrating unwillingness to accept supervision. In addition, they tend to be foolhardy, foolish in the sense of being impulsive and not stopping to think, easily distracted, likely to hurry a job, and to display anger and annoyance.

The concept of accident proneness developed from work by Greenwood and Woods (1919) in UK munitions factories during the First World War. They found that some workers had more than their fair share of accidents, but drew no firm conclusions about personality. Accident proneness has two central tenets: (1) people exposed to equivalent hazards do not have equal numbers of accidents; (2) observed differences in personal accident numbers result from enduring individual differences.

Farmer and Chambers (1926) examined the accident record of a large group of drivers, and found that a few had more than their fair share of accidents. They administered psychological tests, including personality tests, to both accident-free and accident-repeater groups. The outcome of the tests was not clear-cut in distinguishing between the two groups, but nevertheless they confidently announced that, 'Accident proneness is no longer a theory but an established fact'.

As a result, the term 'accident prone' entered the vocabulary, and was defined by Farmer and Chambers as 'a personal idiosyncrasy of relative permanence predisposing the individual who possesses it to a marked degree to a relatively high accident rate'. What this means is that certain durable personality characteristics associated with accident prone individuals cause them to have mishaps or accidents, regardless of environmental circumstances. Effectively, it is an admission that the seeds of our own misfortune as accident victims lie exclusively within. The term 'accident repeater' has been suggested as a recommended alternative to being 'accident prone' because it removes something of the notion of an attribution being made in respect of an individual's personal characteristics. While accident proneness relates to supposed personal characteristics, the term 'accident repeater' refers to an observed behavioural outcome, both of being accident prone and of having many accidents (i.e. a purely statistical phenomenon).

By accepting that some people are endowed with an 'accident prone personality', the next step would be to create a personality profile of accident repeaters, and establish trait(s) which are common to all of them. Personality tests would then be used to screen out job applicants whose personality profile matches that of the typical accident prone person. However, in practice this approach proved to be elusive and even if researchers had been successful in their endeavours, the incentive to falsify personality tests would be overwhelming – who would wish to project the image of an accident prone person? While faking can be a problem in using personality tests, there are ways of dealing with this – see for example Cook (1993), who also describes a number of personality inventories and their application in work settings.

A major problem is that many characteristics (e.g. aggression, hostility, overactivity) have been associated with accident repeaters. Where one encounters many and varied characteristics, it is difficult to graft them into one type of personality. Being unable to produce any overall stable profile of the accident prone person, it is obviously not possible to use a reliable yardstick in establishing whether someone has an accident prone personality. Reflecting on the relationship between personality and accidents, Hale and Glendon (1987) point out that in a limited number of studies personality factors are related to accidents, but correlations are often very low and non-existent in some specific tasks.

The evidence is more substantial for driving tasks than it is for industrial tasks. Perhaps personality has a freer hand when people are behind the wheel of a car than when they are performing most industrial tasks. Thus, it is not so much that an individual's personality changes but rather that its 'darker' sides are more able to exhibit themselves. Willett (1964) notes that once behind the wheel of a car, people are able to let all of their unfavourable and anti-social traits show, with little fear of popular disapproval. Signori and Bowman (1974) claim that both accidents and driver behaviour are dependent not only on driver skill and the driving environment but also on the driver's personality.

While driving offences are not homogeneous – for example in their severity – they may be separated in the public mind from other criminal offences, for example being perceived as 'bad luck' or accidents. However, in a study of 653 driving offenders, Willett (1964) found that 151 had criminal records for non-motoring offences, 60 more were known to the police for other reasons and 157 had previous motoring offences. Thus, over half the offenders had previously exhibited some form of criminal or anti-social behaviour. The personalities of accident repeating drivers have been studied by a number of authors and have been found to include larger than expected proportions of aggressive, ruthless, psychopathic, impulsive and neurotic individuals – see for example, Tillman and Hobbs (1949), McGuire (1976).

Personality dimensions have been correlated with driving offences and accidents, specifically:

- driver inconsistency has been associated with neuroticism and extremes of extraversion and introversion (Venables, 1956; Singh, 1978);
- extraverts have significantly more traffic accidents and violations than introverts do (Fine, 1963; Craske, 1968; Smith and Kirkham, 1981);
- multiple accident drivers are less likely than single accident or accident free drivers to be extraverts (Pestonjee and Singh, 1980).

Quenault (1966, 1967a, 1967b, 1968) developed a typology of drivers and the propensity of each of four types to have accidents. These he labelled 'safe', 'dissociative active' (aggressive drivers who ignored other road users' rights), 'dissociative passive' (unaware of what was going on around them) and 'injudicious' (poor at monitoring their own behaviour and prone to making faulty judgements in manoeuvres such as overtaking). Such an approach, which focuses upon individual (personality type) differences in respect of a specific task, may be a promising route for safety interventions. The Driving Behaviour Inventory, used to measure driver stress (Gulian et al., 1989; Glendon et al., 1993), has been shown to be a strong predictor of mood and performance in simulated driving (Matthews et al., 1991; Matthews et al., 1994).

In the aviation field, researchers have also sought relationships between personality and accident involvement. In a review of studies, Farmer (1984) found some evidence that extraversion and neuroticism traits were involved in accidents, although the data were not clear cut, while Sanders and Hoffman (1975) and Sanders et al. (1976) also had difficulty in obtaining stable correlations between personality traits and accidents.

In a study of 149 RAF accidents, Chappelow (1989) designated 23% at least in part due to 'personality factors'. In these 34 cases, the personality of a crew member or other relevant person was considered to be a possible contributory factor. Terms used to describe these individuals in their personal records included: 'underconfident', 'nervous', and 'prone to over-react' – although it appears that these were only revealed in a trawl of accident-involved crew members' records. Other descriptions included: 'over confident', 'reckless', 'disregards rules', and 'deliberate excitement seeking'. However, it is unclear as to whether this analysis was based upon a systematic appraisal of the personalities of accident-involved aircrew and there is no indication as to whether this group was compared with a matched group of non-accident involved crew. It is interesting that personality factors were considered to be important in such a large number of cases.

Another category of accident caused cited by Chappelow (1989) was 'over-arousal' (e.g. being overloaded through having to cope with a large number of stimuli at once) and in 12 of these cases, a crew member's personality was also considered to be a contributory factor, particularly a 'lower than average tolerance for stress'.

'Predisposition to anxiety' was also judged to have contributed to other accidents. These findings are suggestive of a high neuroticism score, but no evidence is presented to confirm or refute this supposition. However, the author tentatively concludes that, 'it seems likely that both unstable introverts and unstable extraverts have their own idiosyncratic risks', also drawing attention to the difficulty of demonstrating a simple relationship between the extraversion/introversion dimension and 'accident proneness'. Chappelow also notes that, 'there seems little prospect of identifying the high risk personalities … at the second stage', although suggests that personality test results might be used for individual counselling and supervisor guidance.

Chappelow (1989) concludes that two distinct classes of personality problem are discernible from the data, 'one involves overarousal in response to emergencies or other demanding circumstances, and appears to be the province of unstable introverts. The other involves excitement seeking and disregard of risks by unstable extraverts'.

It can readily be acknowledged that certain people are more liable than others to have accidents. For example, Mayer *et al.* (1987), in a study of over 7000 accidents, found that 3.4% of the employees in an oil manufacturing plant had 21.5% of the minor accidents and that many more employees suffered repeat minor accident injuries than would have been predicted by chance. The differences for major accidents (i.e. injuries) were less striking, but still significant. However, the authors note that this is a statistical phenomenon which describes the 'problem' but does not explain it. We are therefore extremely cautious when it comes to attributing specific personality characteristics to those with high accident repetition rates. Of accident repeaters, Reason (1974) states:

> Examination of accident repeaters over a lengthy period indicates that they are members of a club which is continuously changing its membership. New people are added, while long-standing members cease to qualify. It is possible that in some people accident proneness is a passing phase, while in others it is more enduring.

In her review of over 80 studies of accident proneness, Porter (1988) points to the difficulty of using a statistical approach to study human characteristics which cause accidents and reinforces Reason's contention that the accident prone group is a shifting one. This suggests that accident proneness is not an enduring trait which attaches to an individual. If it does exist, accident proneness is unlikely to be a single trait, more a combination of factors and circumstances.

In an attempt to identify individual accident prone characteristics, over the years various tests have been administered, including those to measure:

- psychomotor skills
- visual skills
- perception and attention
- intelligence
- life events and specific types of stresses (chapter 8)
- personality factors (e.g. extraversion).

While major life events seem to be associated with accidents (e.g. Selzer and Vinokur, 1974), these are likely to be temporary and therefore hard to develop preventive measures for. Those who are most vulnerable to stressors are most likely to be the accident prone group. The underlying personality factor is likely to be to do with 'attitude to life' – described as a person's 'underlying cognitive architecture' – basically the way in which s/he sees the world and adjusts in the light of life experiences. Approaches to the accident problem which are exclusively concerned with personality tend to ignore underlying cognitive processes – for example, to do with coping, although neurotics are more liable to the adverse impact of stress. This theme is revisited in chapter 8, especially pp. 219–24.

Reviewing the effects of personality factors through motivational influences, Hale and Glendon (1987) note that the following personality factors have been linked with accidents (Surry, 1969; Hale and Hale, 1972);

- aggression predisposes people to be unwilling to endure inconvenience and frustration – e.g. from safety precautions;
- anxiety can result in more obsessive checking of actions and a lower tolerance for danger – this could be positive in increasing caution but negative in interrupting the smooth flow of routine actions;
- extraversion leads individuals to seek out sensations, including risk, and because of their lower response to feedback, they learn caution more slowly (Eysenck, 1964).

Of the other factors listed above which have been examined, many have been found to be associated with accidents. The best predictors of accident liability (a tendency to have accidents – independently of any personal ascription, such as 'accident proneness') according to Porter's (1988) exhaustive study, appear to be poor attention and experience of recent major life events. This raises the issue of whether the concept of accident proneness is required at all, for if accidents can be explained by reference to such factors as attention and life events, then accident proneness as a hypothetical psychological construct is redundant and only has descriptive statistical value.

In conclusion, it is almost certain that a combination of factors is responsible for the phenomenon that has been labelled as 'accident proneness' and that different clusters of factors attach to each individual. No personality trait for accident proneness has ever been isolated and it is unlikely to be worth looking for. Porter (1988) considers that to unravel some of the confusion surrounding the accident proneness concept, it is necessary to identify two distinct types:

1. a reasonably stable characteristic, for which individuals cannot identify the cause (but which is likely to be associated with a combination of factors such as poor attention and possibly a variety of personality factors);
2. a temporary state, due to an obvious stress, which the individual can easily identify.

While it is very difficult to intervene to prevent accidents to those in the second of these categories – apart from counselling for example, solutions to the first category may lie in attending to a combination of workplace and human resource management factors – including ergonomic design, training and refreshing, safety procedures, adequate supervision, job transfer and monitoring systems, selection and appraisal. In other words, it is one more facet of managing the risks and the human beings which are exposed to those risks – the theme of this book.

CONCLUSIONS

On the face of the evidence reviewed in this chapter, personality theory as it has been developed to date, has still to realize its undoubted potential in managing individual risk in the workplace. A major problem with an approach through accident proneness is that accidents are 'caused' by many factors and trying to isolate one which itself is a collection of different components is unlikely to be worth the effort involved. However, for safety and risk professionals, it is useful to know where to look for solutions to health, safety and risk problems. For example, for any given type of work, if personality does not appear to be a fruitful area because of the uncertainty of evidence and difficulty of relating traits to specific types of behaviour, then attention might be better focused upon design and ergonomic issues (chapter 9). However, to ignore personality factors because of the problems of measurement and its ambiguous relation with behaviour would be a mistake in the long term. This is first of all because personality factors have been shown in many studies to be related to aspects of job performance which are relevant to safety and risk, and second because personality testing is extensively used in the selection process – which is a critical component of managing human resources strategically.

While there are a number of theories of personality, the trait approach is experiencing a revival at present, current research suggesting that personality can be described in terms of a relatively small number (e.g. five) of main factors or traits. Nevertheless, concepts which are familiar to the safety and risk professional generally do not figure in typical personality tests or theories – with the exception of the special case of accident proneness. The extent to which personality factors can predict safe performance has not yet been adequately assessed – relatively few studies have been done which are relevant to this issue – certainly not in a systematic manner.

Personalities of workers **and** managers is one component of that complex of factors which together are important in managing the risk and safety features of jobs and tasks. However, progress on the **specific** ways in which personality factors influence occupational health, safety and risk has not been spectacular. There is widespread agreement among trait theorists that extraversion–introversion and neuroticism (or anxiety) are two major dimensions of personality. There is also evidence that these two major dimensions interact to produce different types of behaviour which are likely to be relevant to safety, risk and accident behaviours. There is likely to be a growing consensus that three more personality dimensions are conscientiousness, autonomy and tough (tender) mindedness. Most, if not all of these traits could have implications for risk and safety in certain circumstances. A number of studies have shown that these personality traits do affect aspects of job performance which under some circumstances, could impact upon safety and risk taking.

Personality is conceived of, and usually defined as, a relatively enduring set of individual characteristics. Thus, there is no such topic area within psychology as 'personality change', unlike for example 'attitude change' (chapter 4, pp. 93–7). However, even those personality theorists who consider that a large percentage of the variance in personality is inherited (e.g. Eysenck), believe that behaviour which is attributable to personality can be modified and shaped by external influences – a view which would be shared, albeit for different reasons, by personality theorists of all persuasions. Therefore, when seeking to modify behaviour in the context of managing safety and risk, it would not be correct to think of an individual's personality as immutable. By shaping the environment in particular ways, both physical and social, we can influence behaviour in many ways (e.g. chapters 2 and 9). By using various personality measures (e.g. MBTI, OPQ) we can acquire information which can be used to counsel individuals, giving feedback on their strengths and weaknesses in order to encourage change from within. Some personality instruments (notably the rep grid test which is the methodology associated with personal construct theory – summary text 6.8) were specifically designed for this type of use and to monitor changes in the individual's way of looking at things over time. This instrument has also been used in the evaluation of individuals' perceptions of risk (see for example, Pérusse, 1980; Glendon, 1987b). Thus, where personality is likely to be important in the performance of a task or job, then it may be part of the role of the safety and risk professional to acquire expertise to assess the personalities of relevant personnel and to take action accordingly. One way in which this could be done is suggested in chapter 11, pp. 333–4.

In only a small number of cases is it likely to be worth trying to use personality tests to select out candidates for jobs involving specific safety or risk components. For example, in some jobs where decision making on risk could have critical consequences – particularly in some senior managerial jobs – it may be prudent to screen candidates so as to exclude those with certain combinations of personality traits – for example, a combination of high levels of extraversion, neuroticism, tough-mindedness and impulsiveness. However, a more proactive use of personality tests would be as a basis for assessing training needs for particular types of job, especially where the job incorporates safety critical functions.

One approach would involve developing highly specific personality measures (perhaps based upon the big five) linked to particular jobs and tasks – similar to Quenault's typology for drivers and analogous with Ajzen and Fishbein's approach to attitudes as predictors of behaviour when the conditions under which they operate are rigorously specified (chapter 4, pp. 82–8). For example, an organization with a large vehicle fleet is susceptible to losses which are to an extent outside its immediate control. While on the basis of some evidence it might be considered worth administering personality tests to existing and would-be drivers to select out those with a combination of high psychoticism, extraversion and neuroticism scores, alternative approaches include more specific personality measures related to driving and identifying driver training needs (chapter 2) as well as thorough analysis and individual feedback of personality test results.

In general the type of job (managerial, supervisory, operational, etc.) and its safety requirements and responsibilities should be looked at systematically, for example using job analysis. If personality tests are to be used as a selection device, then systematic job appraisal can be used to develop appropriate tests, particularly for safety critical jobs. For decision making jobs involving risk decisions (essentially managerial jobs), there is an alternative in respect of team working (chapter 7).

PART THREE
The Work Environment

7 GROUPS AND TEAMS

❏ This chapter is the first of the three which are concerned with human aspects of the work environment. After outlining the functions and benefits of groups, group formation and types of group are reviewed. Characteristics of groups are then discussed, followed by group influences, inter-group relations and group effectiveness, with particular attention to safety committee effectiveness. Measures of group interaction are described as are group decision-making and groupthink. Finally, team roles are considered.

INTRODUCTION

In chapter 6, we concentrated upon individual personality characteristics. In this chapter the focus is upon characteristics of groups, or teams – as they are increasingly referred to in organizational settings. A group may be described as a collection of people who consider themselves to be one – unlike mere aggregates of individuals (e.g. bus queues). Groups are in evidence in many occupational contexts, from the formal setting of a board meeting to the focused discussion of a task force, or from monitoring function of a safety committee or quality circle to the ad hoc spontaneity of a demonstration against a shared grievance.

Group activity, where a group may range in size from two (a dyad) to a much larger number, is central to organizational functioning. Increasingly, it is recognized that the effectiveness with which groups or teams perform is critical to the survival and success of an organization. Thus, it is important that anyone with an interest in extending motivation and reward features beyond the level of the individual has some appreciation of the role and function of groups within an organization – this includes safety and risk professionals.

In some cases, the terms 'group' and 'team' can be used interchangeably. However, 'group' is a more generic term which can be applied in a wider variety of circumstances. The term 'team' implies a more formalized or purposeful focus for a group activity, for example in respect of project work (e.g. development of a health and safety audit programme), strategic development (e.g. planning a five-year risk management policy) or problem-solving (e.g. how to reduce an organization's accident rate). Teams (or groups) may come together to undertake a specific range of tasks or a single task. This chapter considers how groups or teams operate, some of the things that can go wrong and some techniques for overcoming difficulties.

Although the chapter is concerned primarily with the ways in which people interact as part of a group, it will be seen that discussion of this phenomenon requires occasional reference to other chapters, particularly the chapter on personality as well as those on motivation and attitudes.

FUNCTIONS AND BENEFITS OF GROUPS

Functions and benefits derived from group membership can be identified as having individual and organizational aspects. These are described below.

Individual

As far as individual members are concerned, groups provide these benefits:

• satisfaction of social/affiliation needs (chapter 3, particularly pp. 42–4);
• help to establish self concept (chapter 6, for example pp.140–1);
• support for personal objectives and attitudes (chapter 4, pp. 88–9);
• sharing activities which are important to the individual.

These benefits are described in greater detail in summary text 7.1.

Organizational

The functions of groups as far as organizations are concerned may be summarized as being:

• distribution of work;
• management and control of work;
• problem-solving and decision-making;
• information processing;
• testing and ratifying decisions;
• information and idea collection;
• coordination and liaison;
• increasing commitment and involvement;

Summary text 7.1 Some benefits of group membership for individuals

• fulfilment of individual needs for friendship, love and support;
• in relating to others the individual has the opportunity to establish self-identity and to maintain self-esteem;
• use of discussion, questioning, listening and challenging on a variety of issues allows the individual to test their views and attitudes (chapter 4, pp. 88–9) and to note how other people define and explain events;
• when in a low state, a group can be a source of support in combating negative emotions (e.g. boredom, fatigue) as well as boosting morale and personal satisfaction;
• in organizations, it is not uncommon for individuals to feel insecure, anxious and powerless as a result of uncertainty and lack of support; a group can assist the individual in combating the worst effects of these conditions;
• a group can provide some protection from the hostile intentions of other groups or powerful individuals.

- negotiation and conflict resolution;
- inquest, investigation and inquiry.

It would not be appropriate to discuss all these functions in detail; however, a review of some functions of groups in task performance is shown in summary text 7.2.

FORMATION AND TYPES OF GROUPS

The traditional way of describing the life cycle of a group is as comprising four stages:

1. forming – group members come together;
2. storming – initial conflict and hostility, which may give way to trust;
3. norming – establishment of agreed norms and standards of behaviour (pp. 171–7);
4. performing – carrying out of tasks (pp. 168–9).

Traditionally, groups have been classified in various ways, depending on their nature and function. A **formal** group such as a safety committee is established to perform a particular type of task. Its goals or objectives are usually determined by the organization, as are aspects of the committee's structure, procedures and membership. Some formal groups may be relatively permanent – e.g. a board of directors; others are temporary, such as an inquiry panel or an accident investigation team.

Informal or **social** groups emerge spontaneously in workplaces, for

---

Summary text 7.2 Some task performance benefits of groups for organizations

- work can be distributed to a number of people to harness their unique set of skills and abilities; coordination and control is essential to ensure smooth group management;
- a forum can be created in which it is possible to draw on a set of skills and talents to enrich a solution to a problem on the basis that a number of informed individuals is better than one; in this process, information is exchanged, ideas are tested and the accumulated fund of knowledge and expertise of the group is increased (although an expert individual may outperform a group of less competent people);
- a group can generate new ideas and suggest creative solutions to complex problems (e.g. using brainstorming); in this process it is usual to delay critical evaluation until all ideas have been expressed;
- a group can be a useful vehicle for promoting commitment and involvement among members when people are encouraged and given scope to get involved in setting plans and running organizational activities;
- a group with experienced and skilled members could offer initiation and training to a new entrant;
- a group can be used to settle a dispute between parties and could thereby serve as a forum for reduction of conflict and for negotiation;
- a group has a role to play in the implementation of decisions as well as in decision making; in particular a group is more likely to carry out a decision which it helped to make rather than one which is imposed.

example, during meal breaks or on outside visits. Physical proximity is important in social group formation; employees working on the same shift or in a particular part of the premises associate to fulfil at least some of their social needs (chapter 3, pp. 42–4). Formation of social groups stems from common interest or friendship, and no formal rules govern the operation of these groups. Informal groups also occur within the boundaries of a formal group, as people develop relationships through their activities.

In a **primary** group there is much face-to-face contact and a high level of familiarity among members. The family and intimate work groups fall into this category. Although members of a **secondary** group share common values and outlook on a number of issues, they do not do so to the same extent nor interact as much as members of a primary group. Employees within an organization may constitute a secondary group, and within that group could exist a number of primary groups, e.g. works committee, quality improvement team, board of directors.

A reference group is a group to which a person aspires to membership (e.g. a higher group in the social stratum) and as such can influence an individual's outlook and behaviour without them being a member of it (although an individual **could** also be a member of his/her reference group(s)). For example, if a quality circle had developed a good reputation for efficient and effective operation then it could be predicted that the success of this group would influence non-members so that they wished to be associated with its activities. This desire to be associated with success could be used so that the influence of the reference group within a workplace could be reflected in improved safety performance as an adjunct to quality.

Reference groups may be positive or negative – i.e. there may be groups which an individual does **not** wish to be associated with! One way of distinguishing between the various types of reference group is:

- **normative** – the individual accepts the general values of the reference group and adopts its social norms as a basis for his/her own behaviour;
- **comparative** – the individual compares themselves with reference group members and imitates their behaviour;
- **status** – the individual seeks acceptance by group members and aspires to membership.

All types of reference group could be relevant to workplace health and safety.

Work groups

A work group is one in which inter-dependent individuals interact in the pursuit of a work-related task or goal. Work groups, rather than individuals, are often taken as the basic unit of analysis in organizations. As well as the traditional division between formal/informal and primary/secondary types of groups, a number of more targeted descriptions or work groups have been devised. One of these resulted from the work of Sayles (1958) who described four types of work group:

- **erratic** – characterized by: having short-term goals and shifting norms, and being unstable, short-lived and with low cohesion;
- **conservative** – these groups were: steady and traditional, usually composed of skilled craft workers and typically showed high member loyalty;
- **strategic** – these groups had high cohesion and were oriented towards advancing the interests of their members;
- **apathetic** – like the erratic groups, these were characterized by low cohesion and were unstable.

It is important for management, or for safety and risk professionals, to understand the type of group that they are dealing with, for example when introducing change through the medium of group acceptance and initiation. For example, strategic groups are likely to be favourably treated by management because of their cohesion and influence within a workplace. Other types of groups (e.g. those which are dependent, vulnerable or substitutable) are likely to be subject to higher degrees of management control. It should also be recognized that the goals of work groups will not be synonymous with management goals, or necessarily with the goals of other parties.

GROUP CHARACTERISTICS

To understand how groups function it is necessary to appreciate their internal dynamics. These will be examined with reference to norms, cohesiveness, discussion, social interaction and communication.

Norms are rules or standards established by group members to denote what is acceptable and unacceptable behaviour. Norms can cover a variety of situations; for example, quantity and quality of output, production methods, how individuals interrelate and appropriate dress. The relevance of group norms to safety related behaviour may be seen from the following example.

Group norms and expectations

As with other activities, our behaviour in respect of risk-taking is very much influenced by the company we keep – especially our peer group as well as by the norms of our wider society. Thus, while attitudes may be important in influencing our behaviour (chapter 4, pp. 76–84), the power of a group norm or a wider social norm to determine our behaviour should not be underestimated. Expectations of fellow workers as well as of management in adherence to safety rules can exert strong influences upon the way we act – this also relates to the safety culture of the organization (chapter 10, pp. 291–5).

Kelman (1958) expressed the extent to which an individual relates to the norms or expectations of a group or organization in terms of three levels. His theory of attitudes, already discussed in chapter 4 (pp. 89–90), can also be related to group behaviour. At the first level – **compliance** – the individual complies because of a rule of the organization to behave in a certain way (e.g. to wear a safety helmet) and because of the sanctions which will be applied if it is broken. The second level – **identification** – means that the worker wears the safety helmet because other members of the group do and no-one wishes to stand apart from the group. At the third level – **internalization** – the worker wears the helmet because s/he considers it to be the best way to behave in response to the risk.

Kelman's model illustrates that behaviour may be influenced by the organization imposing rules (and ensuring compliance among the workforce) or by groups of workers deciding to behave in a certain way (i.e. a norm) and encouraging identification with this behaviour among group members. However, only when individuals themselves believe (i.e. internalize the view) that to behave in a certain way is correct, is their own (safe) behaviour likely to be consolidated. Subsequently reinforcing individual behaviour or inducing behavioural change through organization rules and group norms which are consistent with this behaviour can then provide powerful support for an individual's behaviour.

Group norms are often not explicitly defined and it is only when they are breached that they become obvious. A worker who ignores a group safety norm by, for example, persistently ignoring safety rules is a deviant. Pressure can be put on deviants to conform using such methods as verbal or physical coercion, silence, black-listing or expulsion from the group.

Group norms were first described in an early classic US study of groups of production workers at the Hawthorne Western Electric works near Chicago (Roethlisberger and Dickson, 1939) in which informal norms were established to set an acceptable level of output. Sanctions were used to denote disapproval of deviation from these norms and pressure (e.g. name calling, ostracism or mild physical assault) was applied to deviants to encourage them to conform. The group also applied social pressure on the work quality inspectors and supervisors to get them to confirm to the group's standards.

Although these studies have been criticized (e.g. Franke and Kaul, 1978), they were very influential in giving rise to the human relations school of management – which is part of the lineage of the 'soft side' of HRM described in chapter 10, pp. 322–6. Specifically, the three main components were:

- recognition of the prime function of social interaction among group members;
- relevance of the informal group at work;
- the importance of taking an interest in workers (generalized as the 'Hawthorne Effect').

An early UK study of the effects of group norms on output levels found a restrictive norm in one factory aimed at regulating output and stabilizing income; this was referred to as the 'fiddle'. In another factory, no such 'restrictive norm' existed. The difference between the two situations was accounted for by economic and social influences, which dictated attitudes to productivity. In this study, group norms related to production levels were significantly influenced by the different orientations workers brought to their jobs (Lupton, 1963). An example of a social norm acting to the disadvantage of safe work practice is reflected in the experience of a worker in the telecommunications industry described in summary text 7.3.

Summary text 7.3 Example of a social norm being opposed by a single worker leading to norms changing (after Rosario del Grayham, 1984)

The worker insisted on wearing safety gloves during certain tasks, a practice not ingrained in established group norms. Pressure was put on this worker to change his behaviour and conform. At first disapproval took the form of remarks, such as 'sissy' and reference to how the gloves did not fit well. In fact it was possible to return badly fitting gloves and obtain gloves which fitted. The group foreman, who was a senior technician, prided himself on his speed and masculinity. He felt strongly about the worker wearing safety gloves and eventually instructed him to stop wearing them. A second line supervisor also passed derogatory comments about wearing the gloves, maintaining that the practice reduced productivity. However, it took a couple of incidents, in which splinters from a telegraph pole entered the glove rather than the finger, to convince other members of the work group of the value of safety gloves. Eventually, the foreman wore gloves during certain processes and it became a group norm to wear them.

Group norms are analogous with individual attitudes (chapter 4, pp. 72–6) and may be changed through similar types of process. Often, people's own experience is a powerful change agent – as in the example in summary text 7.3.

Cohesiveness

When group members share common values, beliefs and objectives this promotes sharing of similar ideas and their mutual acceptance, so advancing group cohesiveness. Members of a cohesive group agree among themselves how best to achieve group objectives, emphasize the need for close cooperation in order to complete various tasks effectively, and create conditions for satisfying members' personal needs. The more that members derive benefit from group membership, the greater will be cohesiveness.

Teamwork and cooperation are key features of cohesive groups and may be critical, for example in flight safety. Problems stemming from a good working relationship between an airline captain and first officer have been cited in a number of incidents and accidents. In the 1982 Boeing 737 air accident in Washington the Captain ignored the unassertive co-pilot's concern about the performance of the aircraft during take-off (Hawkins, 1987). A study of 249 airline pilots in the UK focused on flight deck communication. Nearly 40% of the first officers surveyed stated that on several occasions they had failed to communicate to the captain their legitimate doubts about the operation of the aircraft. The reasons for doing so included a desire to avoid conflict and deference to the captain's experience and authority. First officers in this study attributed arrogance, strongly held and intransigent attitudes to the captains. However, captains reported that domineering, aggressive or uncooperative behaviour were the most descriptive characteristics of their fellow crew members. Thus, attributed personality characteristics (chapter 6, pp. 142–7) were a significant source of interaction problems (Wheale, 1984).

Although group cohesion usually has positive associations, under some circumstances it can have an adverse effect on safety as illustrated in summary text 7.4.

Summary text 7.4 Illustration of negative impact of group loyalty upon safety (after Chapman, 1982)

'The function of a factory unit was to modify rod-shaped machine tools by cutting or bending them. Before modifying them one end of each pen-sized tool was dipped in a protective molten plastic substance. After modification some of the tools were sand-blasted to make them look better. Almost every one of these actions was undertaken in a grossly unsafe manner. One Monday, the manager told six of his subordinates to make the place presentable because the factory inspector was coming around. Three of them were asked to tidy up around the machines and the other three to pick up the boxes of tools from the gangway and place them on a long bench. The manager told the group that they could replace the boxes as soon as the visit was over, and gave them a wink, because the bench was required for other things.

'The factory inspector seemed to be viewed as an enemy. The men grumbled about the visit but the manager said: "Surely we don't want people, like factory inspectors, finding fault with our unit, lads!". This prompted jokes about setting booby traps for the factory inspector. When the factory inspector left, there was evidence of a lot of anti-safety behaviour. In this case the behaviour would suggest that there appeared to be mindless devotion to the group, particularly in the face of an outside authority figure with powers of sanction. The "them and us" sentiment was aroused by the factory inspector's visit, but the "them" in this case was the factory inspectorate.'

Group discussion

Decisions taken by a group are liable to have a greater effect on the individual's behaviour than if a decision is already made by, for example, a speaker who instructs an audience about the course of action to follow (Lewin, 1958). Lectures tend to result in passive listening, individual members of the audience using their experiences as a basis for accepting or rejecting the ideas suggested (chapter 4, pp. 93–7). Also, each individual is unaware of what other members of the audience are going to decide, and none is therefore exposed to a new social norm as a guide. However, in discussion, group members exchange views and consider advantages and disadvantages of various courses of action. Decisions emerging from such discussion become norms and if decisions are to be manifested in behaviour it is likely that most or all group members will act in accordance with group decisions.

The discussion group has been recognized as having value in an advisory and educational context (Zander, 1982) as follows:

• helping members to recognize what they do not know, but should;
• an opportunity for members to get answers to questions;
• enables members to seek and obtain advice on matters that they do not understand;
• provides opportunities for people to share ideas and take advantage of the shared wisdom of the group;
• gives members opportunities to learn about one another as individuals.

In summary text 4.12 in chapter 4 on attitudes, the use of group discussion as a means to change attitudes was described in which three companies in the explosives industry in Sweden experimented with group decision-making. The researchers were confident that positive efforts to reduce health and safety risks materialized, and that participants in the discussion groups benefited from greater awareness and understanding of problems connected with health and safety at work, and accepted the suggested remedies (Kjellén and Baneryd, 1983). Safety committees and quality circles are among the forums which provide opportunities for discussion/exchange of views on health, safety and workplace risk issues.

Before accepting too readily the advantages of group discussion it is worth noting circumstances under which group decision-making may be less effective, for example when:

- tasks or problems are simple or routine;
- problems have a correct solution;
- it is difficult to demonstrate solutions to group members;
- problems require subtle, logical reasoning.

Social interaction

A prominent characteristic of a group is the richness of social interaction. When we are with others, even in an ad hoc or very loosely formed group, this influences our behaviour. For example, when faced with an emergency we are more likely to respond quickly if we are on our own than if we are in the presence of others (Latané and Darley, 1968). If others do not react decisively, then it is likely that we will perceive the situation as not being serious, particularly if circumstances are ambiguous. This slowness to respond may occur in an emergency when life or property are at risk.

For example, if an individual alone in a room sees smoke coming from under the door, he or she is likely to respond quickly. However, a group confronted with the same situation reduces the likelihood of rapid response because of an inclination to discuss the nature of the threat and how best to deal with it (Latané and Darley, 1968). This may be a typical response during a fire on premises, particularly where fire drills are under-rehearsed and workers' attitudes reflect the sentiment that 'fire drills are a needless imposition'.

When frightened or threatened, people seek others' company – preferably those frightened by the same event so as to compare their feelings with others' to see if their fears are justified. Group support in reducing anxiety while waiting for a potentially painful experience (e.g. a diagnostic medical intervention or an injection) is critical, even in situations where group members do not communicate directly with each other (Wrightsman, 1960).

Communication

In a classic study of communication networks (Levitt, 1951) a group of five people was set simple problem-solving tasks in different types of interrelationships. Participants were only permitted to communicate using written notes. These situations are unlike a small group in which communication is face-to-face and where each member can see and hear every other member. The studies were more like situations in large organizations where a number of people in different parts of the organization are in touch with one another either indirectly, or if directly, then frequently only through a relatively impersonal medium such as telephone or memorandum. The different communication patterns are shown in figure 7.1.

Characteristics of the different communications patterns are described below.

Circle

- average member satisfaction;
- slow to reach a solution;
- erratic – poor coordination;

Conclusion – not a strong pattern, subject to informal group rumours and gossip.

Chain

- low member satisfaction;
- poor performance;
- minimal coordination.

Conclusion – not a strong pattern, typifies organizational hierarchy type of communication.

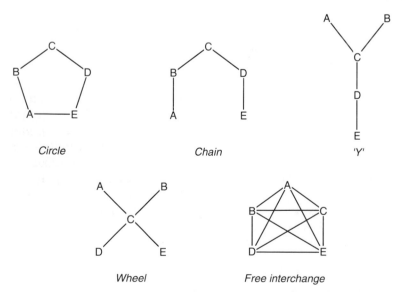

Figure 7.1 Communication patterns within groups (after Levitt, 1951).

Wheel

- quickest to solve problems;
- fewest messages required;
- very satisfying for central member – less so for others;
- could be inflexible if task changes – e.g. requiring different expertise.

Conclusion – most effective for simple tasks, classic group 'leader' emerges in centre of wheel.

The 'Y' pattern fell in between the chain and the wheel patterns.

Free interchange (e.g. working party, research team, consultative committee)

- best for solving complex problems;
- fairly high satisfaction for all members;
- doesn't stand up under pressure;
- can take a long time to solve simple problems.

Conclusion – important to select the right type of group structure for the task in hand.

Centralized networks, such as the wheel, lend themselves to efficient execution of simple tasks. However, complex tasks were found to be more effectively performed by less highly centralized networks, such as one in which all members can communicate with one another (Shaw, 1964). Complex tasks required more than the mere collection of information in exercises on sentence construction and solving arithmetic problems. In these cases the central person in a wheel could be overloaded with incoming messages and data manipulations in complex tasks, so a centralized pattern would be inappropriate.

GROUP INFLUENCES AND INTER-GROUP RELATIONS

Group membership increases the likelihood of having one's attitude or outlook changed as a result of exposure to group influences (chapter 4, pp. 93–7). This is particularly so when a reference group is taken as a guiding light by the individual. Many students at an exclusive residential college in the USA changed their attitudes as a result of their membership of the college, treating their contemporaries and senior staff as a positive reference point. However, some students behaved differently and did not succumb to the prevailing progressive attitudes because of their attachment to opposing attitudes derived from experiences outside the college or by remaining independent in outlook (Newcombe, 1943). Applying this finding to safety, it might be expected that a person with 'backward' views on safety who joins a group within an organization which has a high regard for good safety practices, experiences a shift in his or her attitude when the new group is used as a positive reference point. Whether a person changes his or her attitude as a result of membership of a group depends upon:

- the gulf between individual and group attitudes;
- the initial strength of the attitude (chapter 4, pp. 72–6);
- the individual's personality – e.g. how readily they may be 'reconditioned' (chapter 6, pp. 142–7).

Two important features of group influence are **social comparison** and **social control**. With regard to social comparison, we tend to compare ourselves with others to test our ideas in a variety of social situations. Sometimes this is to validate our beliefs when another person holds beliefs that are similar to our own; at other times we want to make the correct response in a particular situation – e.g. the best way to behave at an interview. We may investigate other people's views before considering the most suitable views to express on religious, social and political issues as well as the use of a particular vocabulary in conversation or the most appropriate clothes to wear at a social gathering. The safety and risk professional is continually comparing his or her views on professional matters with those of other experts in the field, as well as with those of line managers who are required to implement safety policy for example. People compare their own judgements on a particular issue with those of others in close proximity, so that they can check the validity of their judgements.

The influence exerted by a group is particularly apparent when people are conforming to norms. Two classic studies which examined the impact of group influence were conducted by Sherif (1936) and Asch (1958). In the Sherif experiment, participants were in a darkened room and were asked to estimate in what direction and by how much a single point of light moved. In reality the light did not move, but it appeared to do so – a visual illusion known as the autokinetic effect (chapter 5, pp. 112–14). The estimates made by individuals varied much more widely when they were on their own than when in a group in which others' judgements could be heard. In the groups, individual estimates tended to converge, thereby creating a norm.

This experiment exemplifies a highly ambiguous situation in which individuals feel unsure of their judgements. Ambiguity is reduced by information which the individual receives from other group members. An inference drawn from this finding in a safety context would be that a safety and risk professional faced with a major incident at work would find an exchange of views with interested parties at the very least valuable, before arriving at the most effective strategy for coping with the aftermath. This illustrates one advantage of a multi-disciplinary accident investigation team.

In the Asch experiment, groups of eight individuals were ostensibly given the task of comparing a series of standard lines with several alternatives to identify the correct match. This was essentially a simple task and you would not expect many mistakes if participants were to provide the answers acting alone. However, in this experiment a genuine participant was required to give a judgement after others who were confederates of the researcher and who had been briefed to give consistently wrong answers. When the colluders produced their consistently wrong answers, a surprisingly high percentage of genuine participants, who were unaware of the conspiracy, endorsed the group response in the face of evidence to the contrary from their own eyes. Even when genuine participants resisted the group influence, it was apparent that they felt uncomfortable about their isolation.

In this experiment, unlike the Sherif one, there is no ambiguity. What is happening is that the individual is giving way to social pressure and conforming to others' judgements – which happened to be wrong in this case. However, some strong-willed individuals who were confident in their judgements did not succumb to group pressure.

With regard to social control, influence is exercised from above rather than horizontally – as in social comparison. Experiments on obedience to authority have shown that a significant number of people are prepared to inflict harm on others because an authority figure instructs them to do so (Milgram, 1965). Other forms of social control are institutional control and brainwashing. In institutional control, the inmate of a prison is often stripped of personal props to his or her identity – e.g. removal of personal clothing and furnishing, control of mail and prevention of frequent association with relatives and friends. In brainwashing there is an attempt to undermine the individual's stability of mind and self-image by not permitting him or her to relate to friends or identify with his or her normal group. This is achieved by segregating group members, prohibiting group formation, formenting mutual distrust, manipulating news and exposing the individual to the desired message in a state of social isolation.

In the safety literature, various references are made to the influence exerted by different types of social groups. One writer mentions social class as a group factor (norms and values) to explain differences in accident rates. It is suggested that the upper and middle class child is imbued with respect for property and is taught to value intellectual rather than physical superiority in competition with others, to guard his or her health and to attend to his or her physical well-being, to conform to acceptable standards of behaviour and conduct and not to be too rash in his or her actions. On the other hand, less physical restraint is placed on the working class child; care of self is not so highly valued, nor is consideration for others a principal concern (Suchman, 1965).

This approach views differences in accident rates as attributable to cultural values acquired and nurtured within societal groups. The view seems to be that the middle classes are expected to take precautionary measures with respect to safety compared with the working class who are more likely to respond to peer group influence without analysing problems systematically. Such a simplistic view may be challenged by examples of cases in which working-class groups have struggled against the odds to provide for safety at work (e.g. Kinnersley, 1973; Stellman and Daum, 1973). In a broader social context, Roberts et al. (1992) report on parents' (mainly mothers') attempts to secure child safety against all the odds in an area of Glasgow. Their report is a powerful indictment of the adverse effects on safety within the built environment of the contributions of such (middle-class) agents as policy-makers, planners, designers and architects.

Inter-group relations

Membership of one group could predispose members to view other groups with suspicion. Experiments were conducted to reduce friction and prejudice between hostile groups (Sherif, 1967). Members of hostile groups were brought together socially, and accurate and favourable information about one group was communicated to the other. The leaders of the two groups were brought together to bring their influence to bear. However, taking these measures as a way of developing social contacts as a means to reduce conflict did not work; social contacts in these circumstances may serve only to intensify conflict because favourable information about a disliked group may be ignored or reinterpreted to fit negative stereotyped notions about the other group (see section on stereotyping in chapter 5, pp. 116–17).

A workable strategy for achieving harmony between groups in conflict in this case was found to bring the groups together to work towards a common goal (e.g. to work on a project which required active cooperation between the groups for successful completion). It is also necessary for successful completion of the task to have important outcomes for the groups involved.

In the 1986 Chernobyl disaster, a nuclear power plant was destroyed as a result of a combination of factors, including human error (Munipov, 1991). In his analysis of this event, Reason (1987) refers to two groups at the plant – the operators and the experimenters – and the relationship between them in trying to explain events leading up to the catastrophe. Key observations from his analysis are shown in summary text 7.5.

Summary text 7.5 A safety and risk example of groups in conflict (after Reason, 1987)

'The operators, probably all Ukrainians, were members of a high-prestige occupational group, and had recently won an award. They probably approached the task with a "can do" attitude with some confidence in their ability to "fly" the reactor. Like other nuclear power plant operators, they would operate the plant using "process feel", rather than a knowledge of reactor physics. Their immediate aim was to complete the test as quickly as possible, get rid of the experimenters and to shut down the plant in time for the start of the Tuesday maintenance programme. But they had forgotten to be afraid of the dangerous beast they were driving. As the Russian report put it:

'"They had lost any feeling for the hazards involved. The experimenters, akin to a development group, were electrical engineers from Moscow. Their aim was quite clear: to crack a stubborn technical problem once and for all. Although they would have set the goals for the operators before and during the experiment, they would not, themselves, have known much about the actual operation of a nuclear power station". The Russian report makes it evident that the engineer in charge of this group knew little or nothing about nuclear reactors.

'Together the two groups made a dangerous mixture. The experimenters were a group of single-minded but non-nuclear engineers directing a group of dedicated but over-confident operators. Each group probably assumed that the others knew what it was doing. And both parties had little or no understanding of the dangers they were courting, or of the system they were abusing.'

EFFECTIVENESS

The traditional view concerning group size is that generally between five and seven members is regarded as an optimum for group effectiveness. Beyond around 20 members, effectiveness is considerably reduced and there is a tendency to form sub-groups. In an analysis of various sizes of small groups, Belbin (1993a) observes that ideal size is a compromise between the conflicting criteria of maximizing participation (tendency to smaller) and breadth of experience, ability and knowledge (tendency to larger). While six members seems to meet this compromise, teams of up to 10 or 11 members would maximize the second criterion without jeopardizing the first **providing** that the group has a formalized structure to allow for adequate member participation. Group effectiveness is affected by a number of factors which are intrinsic to the group. An illustration of a traditional view is shown in summary text 7.6. Findings which relate specifically to safety committee effectiveness are considered on pp. 184–5.

Summary text 7.6 Characteristics of effective and ineffective groups (after McGregor, 1960)

Effective	*Ineffective*
Informality, relaxed atmosphere, involvement, interest	Formality, tense atmosphere, indifference, boredom
Much discussion, high contributions	Domination by few, contributions often irrelevant
Understanding/acceptance of common aims	Aims ill-defined/misunderstood, conflict from private aims
Listen, consider, forward ideas	Unfair hearing, irrelevant speeches, members fear ridicule/condemnation
Examine disagreements, dissenters not overpowered	Disagreements suppressed, large minority dissatisfied, disruptive minority imposes its views
Consensus, decision-making, members feel free to disagree	Lack of consensus, premature decision-making, formal voting
Constructive criticism	Personalized destructive criticism
Feelings and attitudes are aired	Feelings remain under the surface
Awareness of decisions/actions, clear assignments	Lack of awareness of decisions, unclear assignments
Leadership role undertaken by most suitable member	Leadership role jealously guarded
Frequent review of group operations	Not too concerned with group deficiencies

In response to criticisms that a lack of theoretical development has hampered understanding of work-team functioning, Kellett and Claytor (1993) developed a two-dimensional model of work-team effectiveness based upon organizational climate and goal setting which resulted in 16 team types. Thorne (1992) summarizes the fundamentals of teams that are to operate as effective problem solving units as the 'seven Rs' – raison d'être, rules, roles, relationships, rituals, reward, results. These are summarized in summary text 7.7.

In referring to evidence that an increase in team working can lead to productivity increases within organizations, Hackman (1994) warns that building effective teams is not easy and that it may be possible to obtain similar improvements in other ways. He also cautions that the use of teams is not an easy solution and that if carried to its logical conclusion, could well represent a revolutionary threat to the established management order. Hackman (1994) identifies five common mistakes made by organizations in installing teams – with the expectation that performance will thereby be enhanced. These are reviewed below.

1. **Call a performing unit a team but manage it as a set of individuals – for example in respect of work allocation, reward, selection and appraisal.** Hackman cites work undertaken by the National Aeronautical Space Administration (NASA) which indicates that teamwork among flight crews enhances safety (summary text 7.8 gives a brief description of this study). Traditionally, solutions to accidents or incidents have involved: technological 'fixes' such as warnings or interlocks, procedural changes or individual training – chapter 9, pp. 275–86. The first two of these at least are likely to decrease the amount of autonomy which individuals may exercise over their work. It is probable that there will be considerable scope for teamwork to enhance safety provision. It is interesting to note that participative safety is one of four sub-scales in a team climate inventory (Anderson and West, 1994), indicating that it is possible to measure this important aspect of team functioning within organizations.

Summary text 7.7 Seven fundamentals of effective teams (after Thorne, 1992)

1. **Raison d'être** – purpose, focus and function must be clear to all.
2. **Rules** (or norms) – formal or informal, extensive or single purpose, static or changing, new or traditional – should be followed.
3. **Roles** – e.g. task leader ('father'), emotional leader ('mother') are both essential for adequate team functioning (Bales' interaction process analysis, pp. 185–6 – share roles out among members (e.g. pp. 192–200).
4. **Relationships** – can help or hinder team functioning (e.g. sociometric assessment of team inter-relationships, pp. 186–8).
5. **Rituals** – rules (norms) in action, confirm the right of group/team membership.
6. **Rewards** – pay-off for membership (pp. 168–9 and summary text 7.1).
7. **Result** – added value of teamwork that could not be achieved by individuals acting alone.

Summary text 7.8 Teams and aircraft safety

A study was undertaken to assess the importance of fatigue among airline flight crews. Two sets of crews were tested. The first comprised crews who had just flown together for extended shifts, while the other was made up of crews whose members were well-rested but who had just been brought together. It was found that while the fatigued pilots made more **individual** errors, the fatigued **crews** made fewer errors than the rested crews did. The conclusion was that crews that fly together perform better than crews that don't fly together and that this higher level of performance can be sustained over time, even to overcome the fatigue factor. However, airlines continue to pursue policies which do not retain consistent flight crew membership. Despite the safety implications, both labour and management prefer individual rostering.

Source: research by NASA, cited by Hackman, 1994.

2. **Fail to maintain a balance between authority and democracy.** It is important to recognize that extremes of both authority and democracy are inimical to team effectiveness. Specifically, it is important to specify the ends or objectives of the group or team but also to allow the group to determine the means for achieving their objectives. This may be represented by a simple matrix, shown in figure 7.2. This shows that specifying neither the means nor the ends (complete 'democracy') can result in an anarchic state in which the team has no raison d'être. However, specifying both means and ends (extreme authority) is also a poor team management strategy because the team has no autonomy or opportunity to display creativity in achieving its objectives – thereby representing a waste of human resources. However, worst still is to prescribe the means (e.g. parameters and mode of operation) but not to give the group any indication of what its ultimate objective is. This is liable to leave the group frustrated and demotivated. The best option is to provide the group with its objective and leave it up to the members how to achieve it. This is most likely to result in an active search for solutions which will involve group members in enjoyable and effective problem-solving. Many 'outward bound' team building exercises are designed on this principle. The irony of such exercises is that while they are designed to develop teamwork, frequently they are used as a means of identifying **individuals** for development or promotion within an organization, for which there is no evidence of their validity.

3. **Organizational structures are left unchanged.** This is one component of the revolutionary aspect of teamwork because it means that traditional organizational structures need to be dismantled. However, it should be acknowledged that team members can reliably be left to work things out for themselves and that the role of the organization should be to provide an enabling structure.

4. **Skimp on organizational supports.** It is a common failing that once teams have been formed that they are left unsupported, when what is required are:

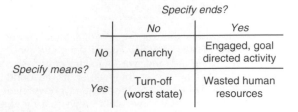

Figure 7.2 Specifying ends and means in group activity (after Hackman, 1994).

- rewards for the team not for individuals;
- adequate material resources;
- a system to provide relevant information to the team;
- a supportive educational system.

5. **Assume that team members are eager to work in teams and that they are already skilled in doing so.** In individualistic cultures (e.g. USA, and increasingly in the UK), people may be unused to doing this and therefore require expert coaching in teamwork.

Hackman (1994) concludes that conditions required for effective teamwork are:

- well-designed workgroup – in terms of task, composition and norms of conduct;
- bounded authority – i.e. specify ends but not means;
- clear, engaging direction – providing motivation;
- a supportive organizational context – rewards, resources, education, etc.;
- available expert coaching.

SAFETY COMMITTEE EFFECTIVENESS

Features of UK safety committees which were found to contribute towards effectiveness are reported by Coyle and Leopold (1981), Leopold and Coyle (1981) and Beaumont *et al.* (1982), and are shown in summary text 7.9.

Safety committees have also been studied in the USA. In one study (Kochan *et al.*, 1977) several factors were found to be associated with safety committee effectiveness. These were:

- number of recommendations for action made within the previous six months;
- frequency of meetings;
- cooperative behaviour by management and union members;
- input by rank and file workers to their health and safety representatives;
- active feedback to rank and file workers through local union meetings;
- pressure exerted by the Occupational Safety and Health Administration and its effectiveness.

> **Summary text 7.9** Features of effective safety committees (after Coyle and Leopold, 1981; Beaumont *et al.*, 1982)
>
> • senior managers are present to approve decisions and to indicate priority given to health and safety (the standing of a safety committee can be affected by senior managers failing to attend because of more important matters);
> • safety adviser's role should be ex-officio advisory to all members; equal member opportunity to contribute agenda items;
> • membership should reflect representation within the organization; trade union representation, where there is more than one union, should reflect risk areas; regular feedback to and from employees;
> • regular meetings at pre-arranged dates; maintain good minutes;
> • in larger organizations, separate committees should represent individual work areas; above these should be a coordinating committee to deal with issues of concern to more than one work area and with issues that cannot be resolved within local committees;
> • generally health and safety matters should be dealt with close to the scene of action where the response can be immediate; follow up recommendations and concentrate upon important issues;
> • committee members should be firmly committed to the objective of improving health and safety; set high standards for achievement;
> • regular attendance of all members is important in facilitating development of solid relationships;
> • effective health and safety training for all members;
> • compact but manageable size.

In another study a small non-significant decrease in lost time caused by injuries over a six-year period was associated with the establishment of a joint health and safety committee (Cooke and Gautschi, 1981). In a detailed study of health and safety committee members in 13 US companies, it was revealed that when members perceived safety committees as effective they also reported on management commitment to health and safety, the vitality of committee meetings, the impressive numbers of positive inspection reports and level of factory safety (Boden *et al.*, 1984). It appears that the existence of effective safety committees is associated with appropriate measures to confront hazards and increase safety (Sheehy and Chapman, 1987). However, it is unlikely that there is a straightforward casual relationship and it is more likely that safety committee effectiveness and safety improvements are both aspects of broader safety culture (chapter 10, pp. 291–5).

MEASURING GROUP INTERACTION

When people interact (e.g. at work) they engage in two types of activities; first, accomplishment of tasks and second, maintenance of the group's social fabric. A balance has to be struck between task-related behaviour and behaviour directed towards social maintenance of the group (known as the social-emotional area). A system for assessing these two types of activities was developed by Bales (1950a, b) and is called interaction process analysis. The 12 categories used to observe and code group behaviour under this system are

> **Summary text 7.10** Categories used to describe group members' behaviour (after Bales, 1950)
>
> **Social-emotional positive area**
> 1. Shows solidarity – raises other's status, gives help, rewards.
> 2. Shows tension release – jokes, laughs, shows satisfaction.
> 3. Agrees – shows passive acceptance, understands, concurs, complies.
>
> **Task area – attempted answers**
> 4. Gives suggestion – direction, implying autonomy for other.
> 5. Gives opinion – evaluation, analysis, expresses feeling, wish.
> 6. Gives orientation – information, repeats, clarifies, confirms.
>
> **Task area – questions**
> 7. Asks for orientation – information, repetition, confirmation.
> 8. Asks for opinion – evaluation, analysis, expression of feeling.
> 9. Asks for suggestion – direction, possible ways of action.
>
> **Social-emotional negative area**
> 10. Disagrees – shows passive rejection, formality, withholds help.
> 11. Shows tension – asks for help, withdraws.
> 12. Shows antagonism – deflates other's status, defends or asserts self.
>
> Headings for the various types of behaviour – which can be either positive or negative, with the category numbers given above, are:
>
> **Task area**
> (a) Communication   6 & 7
> (b) Evaluation   5 & 8
> (c) Control   4 & 9
>
> **Social-emotional area**
> (d) Decision   3 & 10
> (e) Tension reduction   2 & 11
> (f) Reintegration   1 & 12

shown in summary text 7.10.

Both verbal and non-verbal contributions made by group members can be classified by trained observers using Bales' system as an aid to interactive skills training. Group members can subsequently observe their interactions on video as a way of understanding their contributions to the group and as a prelude to discovering ways of improving these.

Sociometry

Other systems have been developed to assess group interaction and effectiveness. For example, sociometry, developed by Moreno (1953) and described by Bukowski and Newcombe (1984), uses preferences – likes and dislikes of group members for one another as the basis for describing the structure of a group in terms of relationships between its members. Asher and Gottman (1981) describe sociometry as the 'process of assessing and describing the interpersonal attraction among members of a group'.

Group members are asked to identify for themselves the two most liked and the two most disliked members of the group (usually phrased in terms of the two group members they most and least like to work with). Group relationships can then be represented in two ways – respectively showing positive and negative preferences among the members. The resulting diagrams can be used to determine where problems exist within the group and to monitor interventions made to improve matters (e.g. taking a particular member out of the group or seeking to repair relationships between certain members). Examples of sociograms – the output from this type of analysis are shown in figure 7.3. The main categories of group members which result from sociometric analysis are:

- popular (including 'stars' who receive many positive choices);
- rejected (receiving many negative choices);
- neglected (including 'isolates' who receive no choices of any type);
- controversial (who receive numbers of both positive and negative choices).

Figure 7.3(a) shows the positive preferences among a 6-member group. The two most popular members (known as 'stars') are A and C with four choices each, while the least popular members are E and F whom no other member has chosen. There are mutual choices between group members A/B, A/C and C/D and a clique which revolves around A, B and C – the most popular mem-

(a) *Positive preferences*

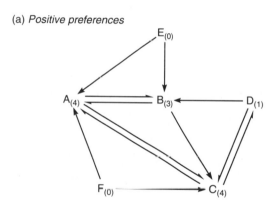

(b) *Negative preferences*

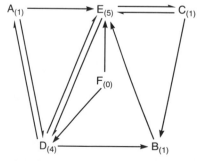

Figure 7.3 Examples of sociograms.

bers. However, to complete the picture, we also need to examine the negative choices in figure 7.3(b). This reveals that while E is disliked by every other group member (a possible case for removal from the group?), F is not selected by any other member once again. Such individuals are known as isolates and interventions might be directed at integrating them within the group. This diagram shows that D is an unpopular group member – a conclusion which could not be drawn from the figure showing only positive preferences. It can also be seen that while B likes C, C dislikes B – indicating a possible case for working on this particular dyad. Thus, useful information can be gleaned about a group's structure and inter-relationships from mapping the results of two simple questions in this way.

DECISION-MAKING AND GROUPTHINK

As stated earlier, a prime function of groups is to make decisions. The 'ideal' decision-making process, for example as espoused through a risk management tradition, might be identified as:

1. Identify problem – define and diagnose.
2. Generate alternative solutions.
3. Evaluate and choose solution between alternatives.
4. Implement chosen solution to control the problem.
5. Monitor, review and appraise the solution.

However, this ideal process ignores the fact that there will inevitably be different perspectives on a problem. For example, diagnosis and definition of a problem is subjective and interpretive in respect of any facts or other information to hand. Similarly, some alternatives will not be tolerated within the organization – for example, those which are not profit generating, and thus the reality is that a very restrictive range of alternatives is likely to be considered. Thus, rather than maximize the possibilities from group decision-making, groups tend to 'satisfice' – i.e. to find something that will work even if it is not the best possible option (March and Simon, 1958) with respect to problem solutions.

Thus, in contrast with the 'ideal' decision-making process, a **cycle of decision failure** may be more typical of many decisions made by groups, for example taking the form:

1. Problem arises.
2. Solution proposed (before options are considered).
3. Begin decision process towards this solution.
4. Further issues emerge (they are ignored).
5. Increase commitment to initial solution – try to eradicate problems.
6. Commit more resources (time, money, people).
7. Failure.
8. New problem(s) – cycle repeats.

If a group embarks upon the decision-making process with a ready-made solution which emerges simultaneously with defining the problem, then decision-making is very likely to be directed towards justifying that solution and the process is therefore liable to fail. The whole group may be involved in self-justifying behaviour. In a study of 150 strategic decisions within organizations, 60% were observed to follow the path of the decision failures cycle described above (Wilson and Rosenfeld, 1990). Organizations continue to survive despite poor group decision-making because of a degree of market tolerance for such decisions. However, once a satisficing decision is made, the tendency is for another problem to arise as a result of a poor solution to a previous one.

Risky shift

A number of studies have found that groups take riskier decisions than individuals do (e.g. Stoner, 1961) – the so-called 'risky shift' phenomenon. For example, when business executives made decisions on investment projects, they settle for more risky decisions as a group than they had chosen as individuals (Kogan and Wallach, 1967). This may be due to the fact that responsibility for any loss associated with the decision is spread among group members; thus, because each member feels less personal responsibility for the potential loss, consensus moves towards acceptance of more risk. However, it also seems that under some circumstances, groups could take less risky decisions than individuals acting alone, suggesting that a more general phenomenon of group decision-making is towards more extreme decisions (Semin and Glendon, 1973).

Groupthink

As noted already, an important characteristic of an effective group is cohesion. While some 'storming' (conflict of ideas) is necessary, too much confrontation could have adverse effects in being divisive and threatening group unity. However, there is a danger that too much cohesion could result in inadequate evaluation of issues confronting the group. A highly cohesive group may suffer the symptoms of 'groupthink' – a term introduced by Janis (1972) to describe decision-making within a small group in the US government during the 1960s Bay of Pigs crisis. Groupthink can occur whenever groups are involved in decision-making, particularly when the group is isolated from alternative views or external advice. Any of the processes described in summary text 7.11 may occur as a result of groupthink.

Consequences of groupthink include poor decision-making and inadequate solutions to problems. A limited number of alternatives are considered, potential gains from alternatives may be overlooked, and assessment of the cost of alternatives which are rejected by the group, are likely to be ignored. The group fails to obtain expert opinion on losses or gains; instead there is a tendency to use selective bias in evaluating expert opinion. Group members tend to display a positive interest in facts and opinions that support their preferred policy, but are hostile to information that challenges their

---

Summary text 7.11 Characteristics of groupthink (after Janis, 1972)

1. Excessive optimism leads to a tendency to take risks because of the shared illusion of invulnerability.
2. Warning signals which, if acknowledged, could lead to a reconsideration of policy are discounted or ignored.
3. Unquestioned belief in the morality or self-righteousness of the group, which provides scope for ignoring ethical consequences of decisions.
4. Tendency to underestimate the significance or strength of enemy or competitor groups – perhaps manifested in descriptions of leaders of these groups as weak or stupid.
5. Reluctance to deviate from what appears to be group consensus. A deviant may be listened to at first, then questioned before appeals to 'logic' and group loyalty are made. The deviant is then counselled and may capitulate at that stage. A persistent deviant is likely to be ignored and then ostracized. Cohesion is usually retained if there is only one deviant. If there is more than one, then the group might fragment as two or more can use their strength to influence others (in the Asch experiment on conformity, the presence of one other supporter for the true participant virtually guaranteed that the participant would stick with their view). A lone deviant will eventually fail to convince other group members of their case. Thus, any potential deviant remains silent about his/her misgivings or doubts and is capable of convincing themselves of a lack of substance in these doubts. In any case, there would be direct pressure on any member who expressed strong arguments against the group's position as being contrary to expectations of loyal membership. Thus, individuals self-censor contrary views.
6. Belief that judgements of members are unanimous, simply because members have subscribed to the majority view, creates an illusion of unanimity. Silence is taken as assent, along with the self-censorship. Being insulated from outside views assists in developing unanimity.
7. New information is likely to be rejected on the grounds that it might compromise or conflict with decisions already taken ('We've made up our mind; don't confuse us with the facts!')
8. Some members take it upon themselves to protect the leader and fellow members from adverse information about the morality and effectiveness of past decisions. Expert opinion which challenges the wisdom of the group's decisions may be subtly undermined.

---

views. There is a tendency not to have contingency plans to cope with set-backs.

In an analysis of events leading up to the Chernobyl disaster, Reason (1987) focuses on two perspectives. The first deals with the cognitive difficulties that people have in coping with complex systems. The second is concerned with the 'pathologies' of small cohesive groups as in groupthink. Reason (1987) identified five groupthink symptoms as being attributable to the Chernobyl operators and these are shown in summary text 7.12.

Summary text 7.12 Application of groupthink characteristics to the Chernobyl disaster (after Reason, 1987)

'The actions of the operators were certainly consistent with an illusion of invulnerability. It is likely that they rationalized away any worries (or warnings) that they might have had about the hazards of their endeavour. Their single-minded pursuit of repeated testing implied an unswerving belief in the rightness of their actions.

They clearly underestimated the opposition: in this case, the system's intolerance to being operated within the forbidden reduced-power zone. Any adverse outcomes were either seen as unlikely, or possibly not even considered at all.

Finally, if any one operator experienced doubts, they were probably "self-censored" before they were voiced. The above speculations suggest that the group aspects of the situation were prominent.'

Overcoming groupthink

The basic principle to apply in overcoming groupthink is to ensure heterogeneity of inputs in order to break the group norm of conformity. A number of approaches are possible, one of which is considered in more detail on pp. 192–200 which considers team roles. Other techniques for reducing homogeneity of thought among group members are shown in summary text 7.13.

A psychological approach to reducing the likelihood of groupthink is to ensure a plurality of cognitive decision-making styles among group members. In chapter 6, pp. 151–3, the notion of different personality types was introduced in the discussion on the Myers Briggs Type Indicator and the four Jungian dimensions which structure an individual's personality. From such analyses emerge two basic contrasting thinking styles used in decision-making:

- receptive (or intuitive);
- systematic (or preceptive).

Summary text 7.13 Means to reduce effects of groupthink and poor group decision-making

- build critical evaluation into the group discussion so that it is legitimate to disagree or be sceptical;
- encourage people to air doubts and uncertainties;
- leader tolerates criticisms of his/her judgements;
- leader avoids stating his/her preferences and expectations with regard to outcomes at the start of discussion;
- conclusions only arrived at after consideration of an adequate number of alternative courses of action (e.g. via brainstorming);
- test decisions against external, impartial parties;
- use external expertise in decision-making;
- ensure heterogeneity among members (i.e. individual differences).

Summary text 7.14 Plurality of cognitive styles for avoiding groupthink

1. **Receptive (intuitive) thinkers**
- keep overall problem in mind throughout ('helicopter' factor);
- redefine problem as they proceed;
- work from verbal cues and hunches;
- alternative solutions simultaneously considered (females generally better at this);
- jump from one step to another in the process and may go back many times;
- explore and abandon alternatives very quickly.

2. **Systematic (preceptive) thinkers**
- look for a method and make plans for solving problems;
- are conscious of their approach;
- define quality of solution in terms of decision method;
- define constraints early in process;
- conduct an ordered search for additional information;
- complete all analytical steps before they begin.

More detailed descriptions of these two styles are given in summary text 7.14.

If a group is dominated by receptive thinkers, then multiple solutions may be produced which bear little reference to the original problem. On the other hand a group composed entirely of systematic thinkers may fall prey to the groupthink phenomenon by failing to search for alternatives. A mix of thinking styles is required for effective group decision-making.

In making the primary decision in respect of whether to use groups for decision-making, the most important issues would be whether this would:

- improve the quality of the decision;
- increase the likelihood of acceptance of the decision by those in authority;
- be an efficient use of time;
- contribute significantly to subordinate development.

Other criteria to be aware of include, maintenance of group member interrelations and the ability to solve future problems, as well as the use of groups to improve member motivation (chapter 3, pp. 56–63). For the safety and risk professional, or any other decision-maker, the process of deciding on the use of groups to make any particular decision can be viewed as a simple series of steps – itself a decision-making process. This is shown in figure 7.4.

In general, groups outperform individuals in such activities as:

- problems that pose a challenge, requiring a variety of information, knowledge and skills in their analysis and solution;
- decisions that call for judgement rather than factual analysis;
- situations which call for the bringing together of different ideas and building on them prior to arriving at a decision;
- situations when it is necessary to gain employees' acceptance of a decision and commitment to its implementation (Cowling et al., 1988).

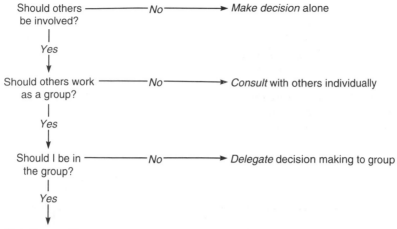

But also consider:

• can others provide leadership?
• can others answer unanticipated questions?
• would my involvement inhibit sensitive but useful information emerging?
• is this an effective use of everyone's time?

Figure 7.4 Decision process for use of groups in decision-making.

TEAM ROLES

During the discussions on group communication and conflict, the issue of leadership arose, and the problem of what constitutes a 'good' leader has taxed authors for some time. However, there is no simple formula to apply in assessing what constitutes a 'good' leader as circumstances may change so that different qualities are required on different occasions. Thus, what is required is either a leader who is sufficiently flexible to be able to change his/her style according to changing circumstances, or more than one person in the group who can perform a leadership role, depending upon circumstances. Thus, the idea that different group members are capable of performing different roles within a group is not new. A number of writers have extended this notion to incorporate roles for all members of a group if that group is to operate effectively. Such an approach is in marked contrast with the more traditional descriptive view of group effectiveness, for example as reviewed in summary text 7.6.

Although, as will be evident from references cited in this chapter, work into group functioning has been conducted over many decades, some recent work has focused upon characteristics of groups – or teams – which make them particularly liable to success or failure. Three of these efforts are represented respectively by the works of Belbin (1981, 1993a), Margerison and McCann (1991, 1992) and Davis *et al.* (1992). All these approaches are based on the premise that a heterogeneity of roles is required for successful team (or group) performance and each has emerged with similar models which identify a number of different roles required for effective team performance.

Belbin's model in particular has strong links with personality traits, as described in chapter 6, pp. 142–7.

Margerison and McCann (1991, 1992) identify eight major types of work to be carried out by a typical team, these being:

- advising – obtaining and disseminating information;
- innovating – creating and experimenting with new ideas;
- promoting – searching for and persuading others of new opportunities;
- developing – assessing and testing the applicability of new approaches;
- organizing – establishing and implementing ways and means of making things work;
- producing – operating established systems and practices on a regular basis;
- inspecting – checking and auditing that systems are working;
- maintaining – ensuring that standards and processes are upheld.

Margerison and McCann found that most people can operate in any of eight team roles which correspond with the various types of work but that they prefer some roles to others – the majority of people rate themselves as being quite strong in three or four areas and moderate to weak in the rest. They extend Jung's (1953) approach that there are four critical personality dimensions and use these to explain many differences in work preferences. These dimensions (Extraversion/Introversion, Sensing/Intuition, Thinking/Feeling, Judgement/Perception) were described, along with the Myers Briggs Type Indicator used to assess them, in chapter 6, pp. 151–3. Margerison and McCann noted that these four dimensions were often related to the types of work that people did and they began to associate these different types of work with the different personality types.

The result of this exercise was the Team Management Wheel, in which role preferences occupy particular areas. Each of the eight sectors was named to reflect the role and the behaviour pattern expected – for example, promoting is best carried out by the explorer personality type, innovating by the creative type, maintaining by the upholder type and so on. The complete Team Management Wheel is shown in figure 7.5. It will be seen that a ninth role has been added in the centre of the wheel – the linker. Linking is a set of skills which should be performed by all team members. The linker role is therefore a shared one rather than a role belonging to an individual.

The Team Management Wheel is used as a basis for such human resource management activities as: team building, cooperation and leadership, training and development, recruitment and selection, project management, counselling, performance review, organizational change management and career planning (Team Management Systems, 1992). Questionnaires have been developed to measure individuals' preferences for the team roles and their work preferences.

The typology devised by Davis et al. (1992) distinguishes five preferred primary roles, each of which has three secondary role preferences and a preferred communicating style. Use of the TEAMBuilder team development tool based on the work of Davis et al. (1992) also takes account of how role

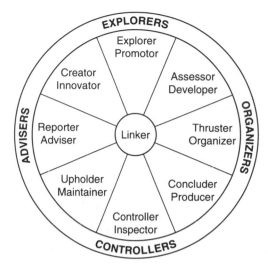

Figure 7.5 The team management wheel (after Margerison and McCann, 1991; reproduced by kind permission of TMS (UK) Ltd).

preferences can change under stress, leading to changes in team functioning and effectiveness (pp. 180–4). The topic of stress is considered in chapter 8. Davis *et al.*'s (1992) team role typology is shown in summary text 7.15.

Belbin's (1981) approach is that it is teams and not individual leaders which are critical to successful management. Central to his approach is the notion of a team role which defines the ways in which members with characteristic personalities and abilities contribute to a team. Thus, his approach also links the individual personality perspective considered in chapter 6 with the group theme of the current chapter. Some of the influences upon Belbin's work have already been reviewed in this chapter. For example, building on the ideas of such authors as Janis (1972) and the methodology of Bales (1950a, b), Belbin reached the early conclusion that teams composed entirely of very intelligent people don't necessarily win in a competitive situation. They may even come last because each member seeks to persuade the others that their own approach is correct and the result can be stalemate and no solution to the problem in hand. Such teams are characterized as:

- being difficult to manage;
- prone to destructive debate;
- having difficulty in making decisions;
- emphasizing analysis and counter-analysis ('paralysis by analysis').

Belbin points out that much of manager's job is typically more concerned with synthesis (of ideas, policies, strategies, competing claims, etc.) than with analysis. Furthermore, people with high mental ability are not necessarily creative (creativity being a separate dimension) and so teams composed of such people are unlikely to be effective.

Summary text 7.15 Team role typology (after Davis *et al.*, 1992)

Primary role preference	*Secondary role characteristics*
Driver	Developer, Director, Innovator
Planner	Strategist, Estimator, Scheduler
Enabler	Resourcer, Promoter, Negotiator
Executive	Producer, Coordinator, Maintainer
Controller	Monitor, Auditor, Evaluator

Belbin also experimented with teams comprised of individuals with similar personalities – the main findings are summarized in summary text 7.16. While each team type had its characteristic strengths and weaknesses, their effectiveness also depended upon the type of task set. In general, stable extravert teams were the most successful of the four basic types. Belbin also notes the links between personality types predominating and the culture of an organization, giving Mars as an example of a stable extravert type of culture.

Essentially, teams composed of 'pure' personality types, while they can perform well in circumstances which match their abilities, are prone to too many weaknesses to succeed across a range of tasks in the long run. Belbin used the 16PF (chapter 6, pp. 142–3) and other personality questionnaires (including the OPQ at a later date – chapter 6, pp. 151–3) to experiment with different combinations of personality types to form teams and to identify team roles. He noted for example, the ambiguities and complexities of leadership. Thus, where action is required, one type of leader emerged (called a 'shaper'

Summary text 7.16 Performance characteristics of teams comprised of 'pure' personality types (after Belbin, 1981)

Team composed of:	*Performance characteristics*
Stable extraverts	Pull well together, enjoy group work, versatile approach, use results well but inclined to be euphoric and lazy; good results on the whole, but individually rather dependent on one another
Anxious extraverts	Dynamic, entrepreneurial, good at seizing opportunities, prone to healthy altercation, easily distracted and liable to rush off at tangents; good results in rapidly changing situations but unreliable performance otherwise
Stable introverts	Plan well, strong on organization, but slow-moving and liable to neglect new factors in a situation; generally indifferent results
Anxious introverts	Capable of good ideas but a tendency to be preoccupied, lacking cohesion as a team; usually poor results

in Belbin's typology), but when coordination and control of team members was needed, a different type of leader was more effective (the 'coordinator').

In experimenting with different team role combinations to establish which were consistently successful and unsuccessful, Belbin found that while various combinations of roles could achieve success, the best teams were those which had a good spread of team roles represented – that is, they were composed of individuals whose preferences and abilities naturally led them to adopt different roles within a team.

Individuals who were considered to be 'good to have in a team' (in what ever role) had the ability to:

- time their interventions appropriately;
- vary their role;
- create roles for others;
- do some of the jobs that others deliberately avoided.

That is, someone who pulls their weight and does nothing to detract from the contributions of others.

The design of effective teams from the different roles depends to an extent on the task to be completed. Belbin designed inventories to measure individuals' team role preferences (later developed to measure other team members' perceptions as well). Eventually, nine team roles emerged and these are described in summary text 7.17. Furnham *et al.* (1993a, b) challenge aspects of the validity of Belbin's Team Role Self-Perception Inventory. It thus appears that debate on the precise nature of the variety of team roles will continue (Belbin, 1993b). However, the basic principle of the variety of roles required remains intact.

Belbin (1993a) summarizes the six factors underlying team role behaviour and these are shown in Figure 7.6. The first of these is personality, discussed in chapter 6, pp. 142–7. Like a large number of researchers, Belbin considers that the two key dimensions of extraversion-introversion and anxiety

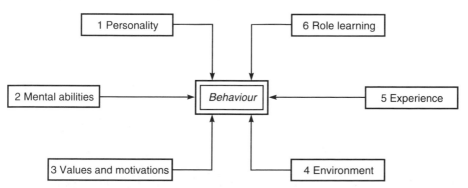

Figure 7.6 Factors underlying team role behaviour (after Belbin, 1993a; reproduced with kind permission of Butterworth-Heinemann Ltd and the author).

Summary text 7.17 The nine team roles described by Belbin (1993a)

Role	Description; (and allowed weaknesses)
Shaper	Challenging, dynamic, thrives on pressure, has the drive and courage to overcome obstacles, task leader who brings competitive drive to the team, makes things happen (can be abrasive and provoke others, hurts people's feelings).
Coordinator	Mature, confident, a good chairperson, clarifies goals, promotes decision-making, delegates well, sets team goals, coordinates team efforts, leads by eliciting respect (can be seen as manipulative, delegates personal work).
Resource investigator	Extravert, enthusiastic, communicative, explores opportunities, develops contacts, salesperson, diplomat, resource seeker, good improviser with many external contacts (can be over-optimistic, loses interest once initial enthusiasm has passed, may be easily diverted from task in hand).
Plant	Creative, imaginative, unorthodox, solves difficult problems, intelligent, source of the team's original ideas, concerned with fundamentals (may ignore details and be too preoccupied to communicate effectively).
Monitor evaluator	Sober, strategic, discerning, sees all options, judges accurately, offers measured, dispassionate and critical analysis, keeps team from pursuing misguided objectives (can lack drive and ability to inspire others or be overly critical).
Team worker	Cooperative, unassertive, mild, perceptive, diplomatic, likeable, good listener, builds on the ideas of others, averts friction, calms the waters, promotes team harmony (can be indecisive in crunch situations and be easily influenced).
Implementer	Disciplined, reliable, conservative, efficient, turns ideas, decisions and strategies into practical actions and manageable tasks, brings logical, methodological pursuit of objectives to the team (can be inflexible and slow to respond to new possibilities).
Completer finisher	Painstaking, conscientious, anxious, searches out errors and omissions, delivers on time, worries about problems, personally checks details, intolerant of the casual and the slapdash, sees projects through (may be inclined to worry unduly, reluctant to delegate, can be a nit-picker).
Specialist	Single-minded, self-starting, dedicated, provides knowledge and skills in rare supply (contributes only on a narrow front, dwells on technicalities, overlooks the 'big picture').

(neuroticism-stability) underlie behaviour. However, high intelligence (the second factor) can override any adverse personality traits to generate exceptional behaviour. The third factor is concerned with underlying values and motivations, described in chapter 3, pp. 36–8. Fourth are factors in the immediate environment which operate as constraints – e.g. resources. Fifth is personal experience and cultural factors which may serve to adapt behaviour to certain wider social norms for example. Finally, awareness and learning (chapter 2, pp. 15–23) of how to play a role improves personal versatility.

Many people performing work roles for which they are not suited may express their preferred role in activities outside work. Mismatches between individuals and work roles may result from confusion between the rather different notions of eligibility for a job (in the formal sense) and suitability – in a more direct, empirical sense. Eligibility, for example as assessed by qualifications, relevant experience, references and interview may be at odds with suitability – as determined by more incisive criteria of aptitude, versatility (in role), systematic assessments (e.g. psychometric tests) and role fit (with other team members) – summary text 7.18. Belbin's work has been extended to decision making in the selection process in terms of finding an appropriate type to fill a particular team role.

Belbin (1993a) examines various relationships between all nine team roles, particularly those which are most likely to succeed or fail. So called 'personality clashes' at work may more accurately be described as 'role clashes' – a less dramatic term, but one which describes more adequately the basis for interpersonal disharmony at work. Adapting behaviour is often possible as most people will have a second and third choice team role which they can adopt if necessary, for example in cases of conflict. An alternative is to use an effective third party to hold a work relationship together. However, it is particularly important for people to avoid team roles for which they are manifestly unsuited. It is also necessary to match individuals' own assessments of their team roles with assessments of others who have had adequate opportunities to observe them perform in a team. There may be concordance (agreement between self and other's assessments), discordance (disagreement) or confusion (incoherent – no real team role emerges). Least desirable in teams are individuals who have an incoherent profile of team preferences.

From his research, Belbin (1993a) describes the steps in building a strong team, and these are outlined in summary text 7.19. It will be seen that the principles espoused can readily be incorporated within accepted principles of risk management and of human resource management.

In respect of leadership – which may be described as 'a capacity to cause others to follow', Belbin distinguishes between 'solo leaders' and 'team leaders', the differences between these types are summarized in summary text

---

Summary text 7.18 Criteria of eligibility versus suitability (after Belbin, 1993a)

Eligibility – entry criteria	*Suitability – performance criteria*
• qualifications	• aptitude
• relevant experience	• versatility
• references	• assessments
• acceptability at interview	• role fit with those adjacent to job

---

Summary text 7.19 Stages in building a successful team (after Belbin, 1993a)

1. **Identify needs** – shapers and coordinators particularly strong at this stage.
2. **Find ideas** – plants and resource investigators have a crucial role to play here.
3. **Formulate plans** – weighing options to provide pointers to the right decision and making good use of all relevant experience indicates that monitor evaluators and specialists are likely to have a key part to play at this stage.
4. **Making contacts** – ideas and plans require champions and those who can persuade others of the benefits of a new approach; resource investigators and team workers are likely to be needed here.
5. **Establishing the organization** – plans need to be turned into procedures, methods and working practices and people need to be adapted to the system; this is likely to require implementers and coordinators.
6. **Following through** – it cannot be assumed that all will be well and completer finishers and implementers will be needed at this stage.

7.20. Belbin favours the team leader as being more appropriate ('first among equals') to the modern work enterprise. Such leaders are less likely to take personal credit for successes as they recognize that this could damage team relations. While solo leadership provides more scope for talent, it also offers more opportunities for making enormous mistakes (Belbin, 1993a).

Summarizing the advantages of a team based approach to group functioning:

• all individuals potentially have a role to play – the initial task is to match their strengths and preferences with a suitable team role;
• awareness of team roles by group members can help individuals to perform better within a group and the group to be more effective;
• work on team roles reinforces research that has demonstrated the importance of variety as an antidote to such dysfunctional aspects of group decision-making as groupthink and the cycle of decision failure;

Summary text 7.20 Contrasting leadership styles (after Belbin, 1993a)

Solo leader
• plays unlimited role – interferes in everything;
• strives for conformity – tries to mould people to particular standards;
• collects acolytes – admirers and sycophants;
• directs subordinates – they take their lead from the solo leader;
• projects objectives – makes it plain what everyone is expected to do.

Team leader
• chooses to limit role – delegates roles to others;
• builds on diversity – values differences between people;
• seeks talent – not threatened by people with special abilities;
• develops colleagues – encourages growth of personal strengths;
• creates mission – projects the vision which others can act on as they see fit.

- people readily adopt their preferred team role and experience conflict and discomfort in non-preferred roles – this is particularly the case when the team is competing with other teams;
- leadership is a multi-dimensional aspect of group activity, requiring a complex blend of skills and abilities, rather than a quality vested in an individual; however, individuals who are 'shapers' in the Belbin typology come close to the traditional view of a leader; nevertheless, they need to be in the correct type of relationship with other group members for their leadership qualities to be most effective.

CONCLUSIONS

The study of the dynamics of group functioning has developed from an essentially mechanistic approach which considered group members as players of a generally interchangeable or homogeneous nature, to a more sophisticated psychological approach which regards group members' personalities as well as tasks which the group (or team) performs as essential variables.

Because groups serve a variety of functions and provide benefits both for individuals and for organizations, it is not unlikely that conflicts could arise in the execution or appreciation of these functions and benefits. For example, an individual seeking to use a group to support his/her own objectives and attitudes could well be disappointed in a group designed to increase commitment to and involvement in the organization.

While cohesion is generally regarded as a positive feature of group functioning, in combination with inappropriate norms (e.g. opposed to safety) it can become a negative feature of group functioning. As far as group discussion is concerned, this is held to have a number of benefits for group functioning and for individual member satisfaction. However, for some types of problems, suitably able and qualified individuals acting alone may make better decisions. In any case, it is important to select the right type of group for the task to be undertaken.

While there is strong pressure to conform to group norms, there are always likely to be those (deviants) who can resist the pressure. This may be a positive asset if non-conformity brings new approaches to tasks or leads to the identification of risks (as in a HAZOP exercise for example) that others have overlooked. However, it is not likely to be acceptable in circumstances in which the group norm is positively related to safety.

Effectiveness of team functioning requires a variety of conditions to be met. Thus, the team needs to be well-designed in terms of its task, composition and norms. It should also have bounded authority so that ends or objectives are specified but not the detailed means to achieve them. The team should be motivated through having a clear, engaging direction. Finally, there should be a supportive organizational context in terms of rewards, resources and education, as well as expert coaching available. Thus, effectiveness when applied to group functioning, for example to a safety committee, can be problematic. Committees, like all groups, operate in a particular environment and the extent to which that environment is hostile or benign to their operation is important. This reflects the organization's safety culture (chapter 10, pp. 291–5). However, there are a number of established criteria which may be applied to maximize the effectiveness of safety committees.

While there are various ways of assessing group performance, it is generally accepted that there are two broad areas of group functioning. The **task** area deals with substantive topics, and the **social emotional** area is relevant to procedures and member inter-relations. Both are important and can be assessed in various ways – for example, sociometry (for examining member inter-relations), beating the competition (for determining task effectiveness) and interaction process analysis (to evaluate interactions across both areas).

Groups may well not follow an ideal route in making decisions, falling prey to such dysfunctional outcomes as the cycle of decision failure and groupthink – either of which could produce disastrous results, particularly in cases where decisions involving high risks are concerned. In order to overcome these types of failures and to increase the effectiveness of group decisions, it is important to build in procedural audits of the quality of decision-making and to ensure heterogeneity of personal styles and roles within the group.

Various studies suggest that in making decisions of various kinds, groups will tend to see the responsibility for the outcomes of those decisions to be shared among group members. This may result in groups taking riskier decisions than individuals acting alone. Some decisions are best made by individuals, perhaps in consultation with others, while in other cases groups offer a superior decision-making forum. It is possible to adopt a logical approach in deciding whether to use a group or an appropriate individual to make any given decision.

Leadership is a problematic concept – the qualities required of a group leader vary according to: the stage in the formation of the group, the type of task to be undertaken and the mix of personality types within the group or the organizational hierarchy. In general, it is very rare to find all the characteristics required of all styles of leadership in one individual. Generally, team leaders are preferred to solo leaders. It is easier to identify the characteristics of a good team member in that they know how to time their contributions and can vary their team role as well as creating roles for others and carrying out disliked but necessary tasks for the group.

Exploration in the building of effective teams has also contributed to the development of other human resource management techniques such as psychometric testing and person specification identification measures for use in selection procedures as well as tools for use in career development, organizational change and a variety of other circumstances.

8 STRESS, STRESS MANAGEMENT AND PSYCHOLOGICAL HEALTH

❑ This chapter considers a topic of widespread concern to many – that of stress and how to deal with it effectively. After reviewing a model of the stress process and ways of conceptualizing stress, a number of workplace stressors are considered. Both chronic (e.g. burnout) and acute (post traumatic stress disorder) forms of severe stress are discussed before revisiting the topic of chapter 6 in a review of personality factors and stress. The focus in the latter part of the chapter shifts to coping strategies, both individual and organizational.

INTRODUCTION

Why should safety and risk professionals be concerned with psychological stress (which can present a mental hazard) as well as with physical (e.g. visible hazards) and physiological (e.g. long-term damage) risks? First, psychological stress is a component of health, safety and welfare and there is thus at least a reasonable ethical requirement to safeguard this aspect of employees' well-being. As physical hazards decrease in importance, mental hazards are likely to become relatively more important.

A second reason is that beyond a certain point, individuals under stress perform less than optimally and that stress therefore has adverse effects upon productivity, quality and ultimately safety. Finally, it has been predicted that the UK will follow the US experience in respect of compensation claims against employers for illness resulting from work-related stress.

A distinction has been drawn between **eustress,** which is associated with positive arousal and motivation, and **distress** – which accompanies feelings of extreme anxiety, depression and low self-esteem. In this chapter, 'stress' assumes the more commonly used negative connotation. Under severe (di)stress, people are more likely to make poorer decisions as well as being more liable to error and to have accidents. For example, Matthews *et al.* (1994) report findings from a number of studies which suggest that stress may predispose drivers to heightened risk of motor vehicle accidents.

Conditions which predispose employees to experience stress, particularly those associated with organizational change resulting from mergers, relocations and staff reductions are likely to continue (Callan, 1993). Roles and role boundaries are likely to continue to become increasingly fluid while greater ambiguity and uncertainty means that individuals will need their own resources to deal adequately with effects of stress (Sykes, 1989; Shaw *et al.*, 1993). From an HRM and strategic business perspective, as numbers of employees within organizations reduce and employee productivity increases, it becomes increasingly important to protect employees' psychological as well as their physical health. Costs of stress-related illness associated with work have been variously estimated and some examples are illustrated in summary text 8.1.

Because a significant amount of stress is caused at work as a result of organizational culture and relationships, stress is a problem for organizations and not merely for individuals. Stress and its management or control is widely recognized as a workplace problem. For example, effective stress control is an EU goal and was a priority of the 1992/93 Year of Safety, Hygiene and Health Protection at Work. The UK government white paper, *Health of the Nation* (April 1992) identified mental health as one of five key targets and emphasized the need to implement workplace prevention strategies.

Stress is multi-dimensional and complex, having both objective (e.g. physiological measures) and subjective (e.g. cognitive appraisal or perceived) components. A definition which incorporates both these components is from McGrath (1970):

> A (perceived) substantial imbalance between demand and response capability, under conditions where failure to meet demand has important (perceived) consequences.

Summary text 8.1 Costs of stress at work – some estimates

- 100 000 cases of ill-health per annum are caused by or made worse by work;
- at least 40m working days lost per annum due to nervous and other ailments associated with or exacerbated by stress;
- 70m days work are lost annually through mental ill-health problems and stress (compared with 4m lost from industrial action in the same period);
- 270 000 people daily take time off work because of stress-related mental disorders;
- drink-related absenteeism which is related to stress costs industry an estimated £700m per annum;
- top management in Xerox (USA) estimate the cost of losing one executive with heart disease or other stress-related disease is $600 000;
- annual estimate of heart disease alone to a company with 10 000 employees is almost £2m;
- stress-related absenteeism and staff turnover alone costs UK industry around £1.3bn per annum;
- the cumulative cost of lost production, sick pay and NHS charges is in the order of £7bn per annum.

Sources: Jee and Reason (1988); Labour Force Survey (Department of Employment, 1990); The *Guardian*, 31.10.92; Thompson (1992).

Psychological stress is experienced as an individual phenomenon and has links with motivation and personality. However, many of the origins of stress (often referred to as stressors) are generally held to lie externally, although as will be seen, the issue is not clear-cut because stress is experienced as a result of interactions between individual variables (e.g. personality, coping style, attitudes, expectations) and environmental factors (e.g. organizational culture, rate of change).

A MODEL OF STRESS

Numerous models of stress have been proposed to describe the process involved. The basic engineering analogy – apply stress and strain results – needs to be modified to take account of individual differences in respect of reaction to stress. A general stress model which describes the main features of the stress process is shown in figure 8.1.

In the model shown in figure 8.1, stressors take the form of pressures which are mediated by various environments. Effects of stress (sometimes called strain) can take a variety of forms – psychological, physiological, behavioural, etc. In response to a threat from stressors, coping mechanisms serve to reduce their impact upon the individual. One way in which an individual may seek to cope is by tackling the causes of stress directly, known as problem-focused coping. An alternative approach is for the individual to change the way they feel about the situation – called emotion-focused coping.

Stress operates upon many physiological aspects of bodily functioning. When confronted with a perceived stressor, the hypothalamus and pituitary glands release a hormone (ACTH) into the blood. When this reaches the

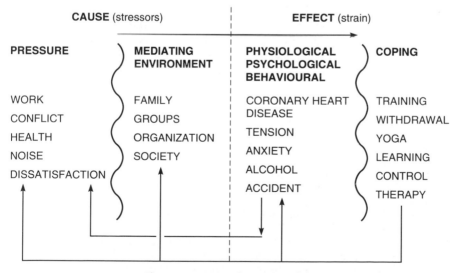

Figure 8.1 General stress model.

adrenal glands, adrenalin and related hormones are also released into the blood and flow to all organs, muscles and cells of the body, producing the activation ('flight or fight') response. This response results in a number of bodily changes, shown in summary text 8.2, which are designed to prepare the individual to meet the threat.

The human 'flight or fight' response evolved to meet environmental threats which required an immediate response (e.g. natural hazards, wild animals or hostile members of other groups) and thus the behavioural reaction usually occurred straight away. Because the rate of social change in human society has outstripped our evolutionary capability to adapt to all these changes, most of the threats which we encounter do not require an immediate response. Thus, the evolved response is often blocked and we are obliged to find other ways of coping with threats. Experiences which result from blocking of the 'flight or fight' response are commonly referred to as 'stress'.

To counterbalance the stress response, evolution has also provided us with a relaxation response. This becomes operational when a threat passes and the body reverts to more normal functioning through a relaxation process in which the phenomena described in summary text 8.2 are reversed. Generally, both the stress response and the relaxation response are not under voluntary control, being governed by the involuntary (or autonomic) nervous system which has two branches. The sympathetic branch governs the stress response and the parasympathetic branch controls the relaxation response. The voluntary nervous system activates all the behaviour which we choose to undertake – including putting ourselves in stressful situations. However, various coping responses, described later in this chapter, can be brought under voluntary control so that they can influence the stress and relaxation responses.

One problem with a multi-dimensional concept such as stress is the large number of variables that can be associated with it. For example, almost anything we encounter in life may be considered to be a potential stressor – depending upon our perception or attitude to it at the time. This 'rag bag' approach to stress has been criticized by some writers (e.g. Briner, 1993) on the grounds that there are too many variables for sensible study and that causal links between them are either very small or impossible to detect.

Summary text 8.2 Characteristics of the 'flight or fight' response

- pupil dilation and increased sensory perception (increases the capacity to take in relevant stimuli from the environment);
- involuntary vocalization (crying out – as for a warning);
- reduced salivary secretion (dry mouth) and inhibited gastric activity (to conserve blood for the muscles);
- hyperventilation and irregular breathing (increases the amount of oxygen required to run away or fight);
- increased blood pressure, pulse rate and peripheral circulation plus reduced bleeding (increases the flow of oxygenated blood to the muscles);
- increased muscular tension, capacity and activity (state of readiness for action).

However, some examples of variables which have been associated at some time with stress are given in summary text 8.3. Clearly, not all the features described will affect everyone, but a combination of some of these, together with others not mentioned, are likely to be experienced by most people for at least some of the time.

An attempt to allocate 'points' for life events (e.g. bereavement, marriage, divorce, moving house) which could produce stress in people was developed by Holmes and Rahe (1967) to produce a cumulative score which would indicate a person's critical stress level. However, it was subsequently found that daily hassles such as household concerns, time pressures, inner concerns, financial and work issues, etc. – produced more stress than the much less common major life events (Lazarus *et al.*, 1981).

Moving to the other side of stress model in figure 8.1, there is a wide variety of possible ways in which stress can be exhibited, both short-term and long-term. In the short term, the effects may be annoying but in the long term, chronic stress effects are most likely to be damaging. Effects of stress are generally identified as being: physical/physiological, psychological (cognitive), emotional, behavioural and medical and some of the main ones are identified in summary text 8.4.

Stress indicators are many and varied, affecting individuals and organizations as well as families and other groups. As far as long-term medical effects are concerned, the process which seems to operate is that the stress response, if unrelieved over time, can eventually reduce the effectiveness of the immune system, so decreasing our defences against cancer (Finch and Marshall, 1983;

Summary text 8.3 Pressures that can act as stressors

Life pressures from:
community (keeping up with neighbours), noise (e.g. traffic, aircraft, neighbours), marital disharmony, sex (or lack of it), conflicts with children, ethnic relations, gender relations, medical condition, finance, diet, inadequate housing, bereavement, traumatic experience, driving, physical danger, etc.

Organizational pressure from:
role ambiguity, role or interpersonal conflict, role overload (too much work), responsibility for others, size of organization, abilities inadequate for task, task makes too few demands, lack of opportunities for self-development, fluctuating workload, lack of control over job, lack of participation, poor communication, poor relations with colleagues, discriminatory practices, unsettling IR problems, lack of feedback on work performance, not appreciated, not promoted, too little scope for initiative, position in hierarchy, organizational culture, change processes, threat of/actual redundancy, etc.

Job pressure from:
ambient environment (too hot/cold), other physical hazards, others smoking, harassment, overcrowding, workplace layout, workplace design, job design, poor welfare facilities, excessive workload, unreasonable production targets, machine pacing, repetitive work, long working hours, restricted social contact, shiftwork, conflict with superior, work group demands for conformity, having a sedentary job, heavy work, vibration and motion, pollution, perceived dangers, etc.

Summary text 8.4 Indicators of stress (strain)

Physiological
increased secretion of – catecholamine, adrenalin and cholesterol, raised blood pressure (hypertension), increased heart rate, dryness of throat and mouth, loss of/excessive appetite, hyperexcitation ...

Physical
increased muscular tension, changes in breathing rate, elevated pulse, cold hands and feet, perspiration, sleeplessness, constant tiredness, headaches, backaches, indigestion, nausea, trembling, frequent urination, diarrhoea, elevated voice pitch, circles under the eyes, restlessness, blurred vision, skin rashes, colds and minor illnesses, change in sexual response (e.g. impotence) ...

Emotional
greater displays of emotion, depression, irritability, anger, low self-esteem, apathy, anxiety (state), development of phobias (irrational fears), nervous laughter, defensive reactions to other people's remarks, more judgemental of self and others, emotional withdrawal, emotional outbursts, crying, hostile feelings, frustration, tension, boredom, irritability, monotony, unreality ...

Psychological (cognitive)
inability to concentrate on tasks, sudden change in ways of thinking about or dealing with tasks, tendency to make more mistakes, difficulty in making simple decisions, increased forgetfulness, general decrease in performance, tendency to lose perspective, excessive 'daydreaming' and fantasizing, less rational thinking, reliance on old programmes, inability to concentrate, increased caution, poor judgement ...

Behavioural
sudden changes in (e.g. work, personal) habits (e.g. hygiene), lethargy, nervous laughter, increased use of nicotine/alcohol/other drugs, increased absenteeism, poor timekeeping, increased labour turnover, increased requests for early retirement, increased accident rate, increased disputes/strikes, refusal to take orders, alienation, speeded up (manic type) behaviours, avoiding work and other obligations, speech difficulties, increased clumsiness, increase in compulsive behaviours (e.g. shopping, cleaning), change in food intake, impulsive behaviour, easily startled, taking too little exercise, taking short cuts, loss of interest in work, decrease in work performance, petty theft and vandalism (e.g. at work), sabotage, short tempered, inefficiency and incompetence (e.g. at work), inability to maintain personal relationships (at home and at work), low morale, reduced product quality, low productivity, marital and family breakdown, social isolation ...

Medical
coronary heart disease (CHD), hypertension, stroke, ulcers (gastric, intestinal), colitis, irritable bowel syndrome, constipation, migraine headaches, allergies, asthma, hay fever, skin conditions (e.g. dermatitis), cancer, rheumatoid arthritis, multiple sclerosis, myalgic encephalomyelitis (ME), diabetes mellitus, accidents, obesity, (various) mental disorders (e.g. neurosis, mental breakdown), chronic insomnia, nightmares, panic attacks, suicide ...

Cooper, 1984), diabetes mellitus (Kisch, 1985) and a variety of other conditions. Cohen *et al.* (1991) found that people were more prone to catching colds when under stress, suggesting impairment of the immune function. Other studies have also found reduced immune system effectiveness to be associated with stress (e.g. Kiecolt-Glaser *et al.*, 1987, 1988).

The transactional model of stress

A widely accepted model of stress which is a specific instance of the general model discussed above, is the transactional model (Lazarus and Folkman, 1984; Folkman and Lazarus, 1988). The transactional model posits a dynamic relationship between the individual and the environment. Stress is experienced when a situation that is valued and significant to the individual is appraised as exceeding the individual's coping capacity – for example starting a new job. In this model, there are two stages to appraisal of the threat (potential stressor). In the primary appraisal stage the individual asks, 'Is this situation important to me?' and 'Is it challenging or threatening?'. If the situation is appraised as being important, than at the secondary appraisal stage the individual asks, 'How can I cope with it [options are considered – e.g. using past experience of similar situations]?' 'Can I affect the situation [control]?' and 'What resources [e.g. social support from colleagues] have I got available?'

In reality, secondary appraisal (perceived coping ability) affects primary appraisal (perception of threat) because a potential stressor that can be readily dealt with will not remain a threat. For example, if the individual is confident, on the basis of their past experience, that they can cope with the situation, it will not be considered to be threatening. The issues of coping and control are taken up again on pp. 224–32 after a consideration of work stressors and personal aspects of stress experiences.

WORK STRESSORS

As will be seen from summary text 8.3, the organization and work environment together provide many opportunities for stressful encounters and ill-health ranging from working conditions to the role of the individual within the organization (e.g. Cooper, 1986). This section considers some of these.

Machine-paced and repetitive work

The nature of repetitive work varies between jobs as do individuals' susceptibilities to stress from such work. Cox (1985) describes repetitive work as a discrete set of activities, repeated over and over again in the same order without planned interruptions by other activities or tasks. The activities are simple and unskilled, often with a short time cycle. Features of repetitive work are 'switching off' and 'letting your mind go blank' – strategies used for example by car assembly workers for coping with repetitive and monotonous tasks. A source of dissatisfaction and stress could be lack of control over the task (pp. 224–32), with the worker enjoying little autonomy or responsibility. Under-utilization of skills and knowledge are frequently associated with repetitive work, as are high levels of machine pacing, often at a relatively isolated work station with reduced social contacts, low job complexity and a lack of participation.

It is maintained that workers engaged in repetitive work suffer poorer health than other occupational groups, which could be exacerbated by shift-work which involves night working (Cox, 1985). One research study into repetitive work, pacing and short time cycle at a large car factory (Broadbent and Gath, 1981), used the following health indices:

- anxiety (feelings of tension and worry);
- depression (lethargy, inability to make an effort);
- somatic symptoms (e.g. stomach upsets, giddiness);
- obsessional problems (e.g. perfectionism, failures in control due to un-wanted thoughts).

The main findings from this study are outlined in summary text 8.5. From the findings, it seems that pacing rather than short cycle times, is a health hazard, and that people can become stressed without being dissatisfied with the job.

Working conditions

Poor physical working conditions, including poor ergonomic design of equip-ment, postural problems, noise, extremes of temperature, pollution and a wide range of hazards can contribute to stress at work. Ergonomic issues are dealt with in chapter 9.

Shiftwork

A number of studies have found shiftwork to be a stressor, particularly where this involves night work, the most obvious manifestation being disturbance of sleep patterns. For research findings on effects of sleep and circadian rhythms on performance, see Campbell (1992), effects of time of day and performance (Smith, 1992), sleep deprivation (Tilley and Brown, 1992), vigilance (Nachreiner and Hänecke, 1992) and acute and chronic fatigue (Craig and

---

Summary text 8.5 Findings from a study of repetitive work among car workers (after Broadbent and Gath, 1981)

1. Workers doing repetitive work disliked the job but were not necessarily unhealthy.
2. Workers who were well paced in their work showed a higher level of anxiety.
3. Workers with a pronounced obsessional personality (i.e. meticulous, conscien-tious and precise) were not less satisfied than others but they suffered more anxiety when they worked in paced jobs. Thus, it seems that those with an obses-sional personality type (or trait) are unsuited to paced jobs. A worker who likes to check his/her work meticulously is likely to become anxious if s/he has no control over the speed of work.
4. Short work cycle times (under a minute) were not connected with either job dissatisfaction or ill-health when compared with work cycles of up to half an hour in repetitive jobs.
5. A slightly higher proportion of workers in paced jobs, compared with those in other jobs, may require psychiatric help.

Cooper, 1992). Other effects include: disturbance of neurophysiological rhythms (e.g. blood temperature, metabolic rate), blood sugar levels, mental efficiency and work motivation, which may ultimately lead to stress-related disease (Monk and Tepas, 1985). Shiftwork may be exacerbated by repetitive tasks, one outcome of which may be accidents. In a review of shiftwork and accidents, Carter and Corlett (1981) suggest that minor accidents were more likely to be due to over-arousal or hyper-alertness – associated with careless and disturbed behaviour. More serious accidents and errors of omission tend to be due to low levels of alertness and automatic cerebral functioning, for example as in monotonous tasks. There are a number of reviews of the effects of shiftwork on health (e.g. National Institute for Occupational Safety and Health, 1976; Harrington, 1978).

Job overload

This might be represented as having too much to do or having to perform tasks which are too difficult. While some people put great pressures on themselves and others, overload can result from insufficient delegation and poor time management. An extreme instance of job overload is trauma associated with work. Some illustrations are given in summary text 8.6. The more specific topic of post-traumatic stress disorder is dealt with on pp. 217–19.

Job underload

This may be associated with some factors reviewed above, such as repetitive, boring, routine and under-stimulating work. There may be inevitable periods in many jobs when boredom has to be accepted, even those in which task performance is critical for safety – for example, pilots, air traffic controllers. Boredom and disinterest in the job may adversely affect employee responses to emergencies.

Role

Various aspects of role have been identified as sources of occupational stress. For example, role ambiguity (being unsure of what you are supposed to be doing), which may result from communication failure, can be distressing because it can lead to feelings of being out of control, or being controlled by others. Role conflict (e.g. expected to do two or more incompatible things) and role strain (e.g. doing something you feel you ought not to be doing) can also be stressful. Problems connected with role conflict were demonstrated in a study of dentists (Cooper et al., 1978). The dentists considered themselves to be 'inflictors of pain' rather then 'healers' and felt that their clinical role clashed with other non-clinical roles such as performing administrative duties and building up their practice. In addition, their work roles interfered with their private lives. One adverse health outcome associated with the dentist's role was abnormally high blood pressure.

Summary text 8.6 Illustrations of job overload and trauma

A former junior hospital doctor, backed by the British Medical Association, sued his employer – a London health authority – for stress-related symptoms arising from being required to work an 88-hour week. His claim was that the stress was caused by unreasonable working hours; conditions which left him exhausted and depressed as well as endangering the health of his patients.

Awards of £34 000 to a fireman and £65 000 to two booking clerks for trauma following the Kings Cross underground railway fire which claimed 31 lives in November 1987 (Department of Transport, 1988) signifies that the UK judiciary are prepared to award substantial damages in certain cases. Suing for stress and trauma may be relatively recent in the UK, but it has been a feature of the US scene for 30 years.

The trauma referred to above relates to workplace accidents such as fires, crashes or other disasters. By contrast, cumulative trauma arises out of such factors as adverse working hours or conditions, consistently unpleasant superiors and blocked careers, and frequently occurs over a considerable time period. Approximately 11% of all occupational disease claims in the US relate to cumulative trauma.

In an attributed interview, Professor Cary Cooper of the University of Manchester Institute of Science and Technology maintained that the UK was swiftly moving towards US levels of occupational stress and he personally is increasingly receiving letters from solicitors who have clients pursuing stress-related claims. He attributed increased occupational stress in the UK to: (i) the drive by industry for increased competitiveness, (ii) technological change, and (iii) the growth of dual-career families. Poor handling of such issues can cause problems.

Sources: Frost, B. (1990) Fireman awarded £34 000 for trauma after Kings Cross. *The Times*, 19.12.1990, p. 3; Summers, D. (1990) An act of faith that can reap rewards. *The Financial Times*, 23.11.1990; Summers, D. (1990) Testing for stress in the workplace. *The Financial Times*, 7.12.1990.

Where a role entails responsibility for people and their safety, there is potential for occupational stress. For example, responsibility for people's safety and lives was identified as a major source of long-term occupational stress for air traffic controllers (Crump *et al.*, 1981).

Carrying out work roles often involves developing relationships with others. Poor relationships with one's superior, colleagues and subordinates have been related to occupational stress which may result in psychological strain and job dissatisfaction. Good work relationships tend to have the opposite effect.

Other considerations affecting movement between roles in the organization hierarchy, or the lack of such movement, hinge upon career development. People may experience occupational stress as a consequence of being over-promoted or failing to obtain a job promotion, or they may experience confusion about their status in the organization or feel a lack of job security. Individuals are liable to experience these feelings differentially, depending upon their career anchors – their fundamental career motivation (e.g. security, autonomy, entrepreneurship) (Schein, 1978, 1990).

Blockages to career development may be particularly pronounced among women managers (Davidson and Cooper, 1983). The most adverse health and job satisfaction factors were associated with career development and related issues, for example sex discrimination in promotion, inadequate training, insufficient delegation of assignments to women and male colleagues being treated more favourably.

Interactions between work and home roles have also been studied. Employees under stress could find the home a refuge from a competitive and demanding work environment. However, there is a danger of spillover of tensions from the work role to the family environment with detrimental consequences. This may be aggravated in the case of dual career partners in a situation where both are experiencing occupational stress. Inability to balance competing demands of home and work successfully can be a major source of stress for some managers – particularly evident when work is taken home frequently and the full holiday entitlement is not used.

Work with visual display screen equipment

Computer technology advanced rapidly through the 1980s to find applications in a wide range of industrial and commercial operations. Although some early health fears about display screen equipment (DSE) operation appear unfounded (e.g. radiation exposure), health problems relating to ergonomic factors (e.g. visual, postural, fatigue) can persist (Mackay and Cox, 1984). Display screen equipment can impact upon work in a number of ways, as described in summary text 8.7.

Summary text 8.8 outlines some measures which can be adopted to tackle the type of problems identified as arising from DSE operation. A more com-

---

Summary text 8.7 Some features of display screen equipment (DSE) work

Underload
Being under-stretched is a prime characteristic of many repetitive work practices, particularly machine-paced assembly lines and is now associated with DSE operation where simple clerical tasks are computerized. Following computerization, these tasks may retain their monotonous and repetitive features.

De-skilling
When a job is changed to accommodate new technology, some de-skilling can occur. If this happens then it represents a loss of some of the organization's past investment in skills development. If existing patterns of skills are not fully utilized then job interest and motivation may well decline.

Control
An important factor determining stress-related symptoms among DSE operators is lack of control. In some computerized systems, the machine is able to monitor the operator's performance, for example in respect of keying-in data. This information can often be used to determine remuneration levels, for example through payment-by-results systems. Understandably, this type of machine control is often resented and regarded with suspicion by many computer operators as well as being associated with feelings of fatigue and stress.

Summary text 8.8 Steps to reduce negative outcomes from display screen equipment (DSE) work

1. Repetitive aspects of the task should be minimized by introducing a variable workload throughout the day. It is also helpful for operators to know what is in store for them.
2. In allocating tasks over a period of time, allow the operator some discretion as to how work is allocated, thereby offering some potential for use of individual skills.
3. Seek to avoid treating the DSE operator essentially as a machine minder. Where possible, design jobs to be mentally challenging, but within the operator's abilities.
4. If the equipment is intensely and continuously used, then optimum screen features and good workplace conditions are required.
5. Improvements in ergonomic aspects of the DSE will have little overall effect if staff are demotivated and experience low morale. Attempts to enrich operator's jobs should involve both designers and system users.
6. Natural breaks or pauses are features of many jobs and help to prevent the onset of fatigue. Such informal breaks need to be frequent with certain types of DSE work, for example data entry tasks requiring continuous and sustained attention, concentration and high rates of data entry. In such cases, introducing formal rest breaks helps to maintain attention and concentration. Mackay and Cooper (1987) provide guidance as shown below.
   (i) Arrange rest pauses prior to the onset of fatigue and not as a means of recuperating from it. Rest pauses should be introduced when performance is close to the maximum – i.e. before a productivity decrease sets in.
   (ii) Short, frequently occurring rest pauses appear to be more satisfactory than longer breaks taken occasionally.
   (iii) Ideally, breaks should be taken away from the location of the DSE.
   (iv) In considering the nature of the work, rest pauses are more effective for work which requires concentration than for work that is more or less 'automatic'. The latter allows the operator some discretion in respect of 'daydreaming', conversing with others or other monotony-reducing strategies.

---

prehensive risk assessment approach is given in the guidance associated with the Health and Safety (Display Screen Equipment) Regulations 1992 (HSE, 1992a).

Burnout

The term 'burnout' dates back to the mid-1970s and rapidly gained acceptance in the literature of the 1980s. A scale to measure burnout (the Maslach burnout inventory) was developed by Maslach and Jackson (1981). According to Maslach and Jackson (1981, 1984), burnout is a multi-dimensional construct comprising three related, yet independent components:

1. emotional exhaustion – feelings of fatigue that develop as one's emotional energies become drained;
2. depersonalization – development of negative and uncaring attitudes towards others;
3. reduced personal accomplishment – deterioration of self-competence and dissatisfaction with one's achievements.

The existence of these three factors has been validated for large samples of teachers (Byrne, 1993) – a group particularly prone to burnout and stress (e.g. Travers and Cooper, 1993). Thus, burnout can be described as a state of physical, emotional and mental exhaustion marked by physical depletion, chronic fatigue, feelings of helplessness and hopelessness, a negative self-concept and negative attitudes towards work, life and other people. Burnout is also associated with people feeling that nothing they do is rewarded or encouraged and they have no control over whether others are pleased or not with their work.

Burnout, which results from prolonged exposure to stress, seems particularly likely to occur in individuals and professionals who are characterized by a high degree of investment in their work and who have high performance expectations. There has been particular interest in burnout in the caring and health-related professions (e.g. Cherniss, 1980; Naisberg-Fennig and Giora, 1991). Burnout has also been observed to affect counsellors, teachers, childcare workers, nurses, police officers (Cook, 1988) and psychotherapists (Grosch and Olsen, 1994). The work of such professionals is often characterized by stressful shift rotas, excessive workload and responsibilities, extremely long hours and resource deficiencies (Rudner, 1985).

Matteson and Ivancevich (1987) describe burnout as occurring in five stages:

1. Involvement – a period of excitement and high job satisfaction which may hide unrealistic expectations by the job incumbent.
2. Stagnation – gradually satisfaction decreases, efficiency falls off and mental and physical fatigue may set in. The individual shifts attention away from work to non-work areas such as family or hobbies.
3. Detachment – may be the first stage when people realize that something untoward is happening. The person begins to withdraw physically, exerting only minimal effort necessary to maintain their position. At this time, they may experience chronic exhaustion, illness, depression and anger.
4. Juncture – is an extremely serious stage of burnout where behavioural and physical symptoms become critical, thinking becomes permeated by self-doubts and an escape mentality becomes the central focus. The results of this stage may be devastating as individuals may be unable to function on or off the job; they may leave their jobs and families, or even contemplate suicide.
5. Intervention – is the attempt to break out of the burnout cycle, but in a more positive way than might have been contemplated previously, for example by changing jobs within the organization or leaving the organization altogether. Intervention may also be on-the-job in respect of modifying job responsibilities or relations with others, including clients. Ideally, intervention would occur before stage 4 is reached.

Unemployment

For those without work, even the stress of employment could seem like a price well worth paying. Redundancy and unemployment generate their own stress (see for example, O'Brien, 1986; Fryer and Ullah, 1987; Warr, 1987; Fryer, 1992a, b). One view is that for many people unemployment for more than a very short period can result in psychologically destructive behaviour, quite apart from difficulties arising from financial and social problems. A key factor is the absence of latent benefits associated with employment (Jahoda, 1981, 1982), described in summary text 8.9.

Psychological effects of unemployment have been described by Eisenberg and Lazarsfeld (1938) as:

1. shock on losing the job;
2. optimistic, exemplified by job hunting;
3. pessimistic, when efforts to find another job fail – a crucial stage because active distress and anxiety can occur;
4. fatalistic, where the unemployed person adapts to the situation by accepting unemployment.

In a small-scale UK study of unemployed managerial staff it was concluded that although the men passed through the first two stages, they delayed entry to the pessimistic and fatalistic stages by using various strategies to confront the negative effects of unemployment (Swinburne, 1981). Warr and Jackson (1984) suggest that the negative mental health consequences of unemployment occur within the first three months of a job loss and remain fairly stable thereafter.

In an overview of a number of studies, Fryer and Payne (1986) conclude that compared with employed people, those who were unemployed experience:

- higher levels of strain and negative feelings;
- lower levels of happiness and present life satisfaction;
- lower levels of pleasure and positive feeling;
- higher levels of depression;
- higher suicide rates;
- cognitive difficulties.

Summary text 8.9 Benefits of employment (after Jahoda, 1981, 1982)

1. **Time structure** – imposed on the working day appeals to our need for order and continuity.
2. **Enforced social contact** – amounts to the sharing of experiences and the development of regular contacts outside the nuclear family on a regular basis as well as appealing to our need for affiliation.
3. **Enforced activity** – means we are forced to be active and satisfies our need to expend energy.
4. **Status and identity** – work provides the opportunity to define aspects of personal status and identity which is related to our need for personal accomplishments.
5. **Purposefulness** – a sense of practical purpose behind our contributions is linked to the achievement of overall goals and purposes of the organization. This satisfies our need to make some personal contribution.

In respect of the last point, Fryer and Warr (1984) found small percentages of a group of unemployed working-class men who reported taking longer over doing things, having difficulty concentrating and making mistakes in shopping or understanding written material. While Fryer and Payne (1986) found few differences between professional/white collar and semi-skilled/blue collar workers in terms of reactions to unemployment, working-class unemployed people reported greater anxiety over financial difficulties and more problems in occupying their time.

It has been suggested that unemployment is associated with increased family stress, particularly among the long-term unemployed and those in lower occupational groups (Fagan and Little, 1984). However, other evidence indicates the opposite effect and emphasizes the resilience of the family. For example, it has been asserted that 'unemployment actually reactivates dormant family ties, and for a majority of families... crisis does not accompany the husband's unemployment' (Fryer and Payne, 1986). Strains could nevertheless result from a reduction in activities in which expenditure is involved and effects upon children have included pressure on their social relationships, poorer school performance, deterioration in physical and emotional health and physical abuse (Madge, 1983).

POST-TRAUMATIC STRESS DISORDER (PTSD)

A syndrome which is increasingly recognized as requiring expert attention is post-traumatic stress disorder (PTSD). PTSD may be described as a set of symptoms following a psychologically distressing event that is outside the range of usual human experience. Thus, events such as normal bereavement, chronic illness, business loss and marital conflict, although potentially stressful, would not be regarded as experiences which could result in PTSD.

PTSD can follow extreme experiences such as war, being a hostage, torture, rape and other assault, or involvement in serious accidents. Usual PTSD symptoms include:

- being numb to the world – lack of interest and depersonalization of experience;
- reliving the trauma – in memories (e.g. 'flashbacks') and dreams;
- adrenalin releases and associated features – e.g. anxiety, palpitations, accelerated pulse, heightened perception and bowel upsets;
- sleep disturbances, difficulty in concentrating, over-alertness, hyper-arousal;
- feelings of guilt or self-blame – e.g. that they survived when others did not, depression, suicidal tendencies;
- social dysfunction – e.g. hatred of others which would normally be considered irrational, withdrawal, isolation.

PTSD is not a newly discovered disorder. Veith (1965) claims that its description can be traced to the first Egyptian writing of around 1900 BC. Homer describes it in the Greek warriors Achilles and Odysseus after the

Trojan wars. Shakespeare described the symptoms in *Macbeth*, while Samuel Pepys noted it in reactions of Londoners after the Great Fire in 1666. Figley (1988) charts its more recent development over the past 100 years since the time of Freud.

There are many reports of PTSD from observers of war victims at different times; often the symptoms were regarded as 'cowardice' and those reporting them were executed. The diagnosis of PTSD among American Vietnam war veterans was probably a milestone in the general acceptance of PTSD as a medical condition. However, PTSD was not introduced into the *Diagnostic and statistical manual of mental disorders (DSM-III-R)* (American Psychiatric Association) until 1980 (Rowe and Mink, 1993). An important development in the field of PTSD was in January 1988, when the new *Journal of Traumatic Stress* was launched. At that time, the Society of Traumatic Stress Studies had just under 1000 members and has grown considerably since that time.

Summary text 8.10 relates an example from Schottenfeld and Cullen (1986) of an accident victim who experienced the dramatic PTSD symptoms described. In a study of underground train drivers who had been involved in others' suicide attempts from station platforms, Farmer *et al.* (1991, 1992) found that variables indicating poor prognosis – e.g. PTSD or taking prolonged sickness absence after the incident were:

- body of victim mutilated;
- driver of non-UK ethnic origin;
- pre-incident average annual sickness absence > 20 days;
- high scores on mental and behaviour disengagement scales.

Summary text 8.10 PTSD symptoms resulting from a workplace accident (after Schottenfeld and Cullen, 1986)

Mr Jones, a 55-year-old married man, had a perfect work record as a labourer in a factory until he suffered a severe crush injury to his legs while he was at work. After more than one year off work, a series of orthopaedic operations and a painful rehabilitation, he returned to work.

About six months later, he began to experience recurrent episodes of apprehension, light-headedness, dizziness and nausea. Eventually, during one of these episodes, he was rushed to a nearby hospital emergency room. Subsequently, he was classified as disabled because of the repeated episodes, although no abnormalities were identified following medical evaluation.

He was then referred to the occupational medicine clinic. Prior to the clinic's evaluation of his condition, the possibility of PTSD was not considered because there was no recognized connection between his occupational trauma and the subsequent delayed appearance of his symptoms.

In the clinic he reported that his recurrent episodes were triggered by reminders of the accident. He first experienced the episodes at work when the man responsible for his accident returned to the worksite. The symptoms would then appear whenever he walked by the plant. He was severely depressed and plagued by nightmares about the accident and often became obsessed by it while awake. He would suddenly see the load of steel that had crushed his legs rolling towards him. He desperately attempted to avoid any reminders of his workplace and made sure that he never walked by the plant.

The effects of PTSD are not restricted to those who are victims or otherwise present at accidents or incidents, for there is evidence that there may also be 'peripheral victims' (e.g. police, helpers) who may not even have been present when a disaster occurred. Documented accounts of workers who have been traumatized while performing their work, include: emergency workers (Hartsough, 1985; Mitchell, 1985), police officers (Kroes, 1976) mental health workers (Rippere and Williams, 1985) and physicians (Lipp, 1980; Rose and Rosnow, 1973). Dixon *et al.* (1993) report PTSD in fourteen cross-channel ferry workers following the deaths of 193 people on 6 March 1987 at Zeebrugge on the *Herald of Free Enterprise.* The 14 workers were found to be suffering severe depression, social difficulties, anxiety, insomnia and somatic symptoms as a result of their involvement in the aftermath of the disaster. PTSD symptoms reveal that the long-term psychological impact of an accident can be far more debilitating than any immediate physical injuries. It is esti-mated that up to 70% of those exposed to a dramatic and frightening event will experience PTSD.

A few organizations have recognized that resources devoted to the support of PTSD victims is justified not only on ethical, but also financial grounds. Early diagnosis and commencement, within one to two days of the event, of support activities such as counselling is important. As part of a programme of rehabilitation, PTSD sufferers are likely to be debriefed on their symptoms and taught coping mechanisms for dealing with them. Without therapeutic interventions, symptoms are likely to persist indefinitely. Coping mechanisms might include a form of self-hypnosis in which the victim can learn to cope with the experience through a form of grieving process (Spiegel, 1988). Specialist texts provide details of therapies (e.g. Kroll, 1993).

PERSONALITY AND HEALTH ISSUES

Chapter 5 considered personality factors in relation to risk and safety and it is useful in this section to extend this theme by exploring some of the links between personality, stress and health.

Type A behaviour

Probably the most studied personality factor in the context of stress is type A behaviour (Friedman and Rosenman, 1974). Type A behaviour is typified by high achievement orientation – seeking to achieve more and more in less and less time. People who are characterized as being Type A are easily provoked and always concerned with meeting deadlines. Summary text 8.11 outlines a range of Type A behavioural characteristics. Type B behaviour is the opposite of Type A.

Individuals who are susceptible to Type A behaviour tend to be profes-sional/managerial (typically white and male), aged 36–55 years and living in urban environments. Type A personalities show a tendency to suppress stress symptoms and fatigue because they believe that illness might interfere with

---

Summary text 8.11 Type A behaviour characteristics

- extreme competitiveness;
- striving for achievement;
- aggressiveness;
- haste;
- impatience;
- restlessness;
- hyper-alertness;
- explosiveness of speech;
- tenseness of facial muscles;
- feelings of being under time pressure;
- feeling challenged by responsibility;
- committed to work so that other areas figure little.

---

the completion of important tasks. Where the Type A person feels a lack of control at work, conflict can ensue. This conflict can give rise to stress which in turn contributes to some uncertainty in the setting of work goals, handling information and task performance (Davidson and Cooper, 1981).

Adverse factors associated with the Type A disposition include conditions related to coronary heart disease (CHD) such as hypertension, increased cholesterol and norepinephrine levels, strokes, accidents, lack of exercise, smoking and poor family relations. Although prospective (considering data from one point in time to another point in the future, usually with some intervention) as well as retrospective (considering only historical data) studies have found a relationship between Type A behaviour and CHD risk factors, there are confounding factors in respect of the direction of causality. For example, Type As are less likely to stop smoking and may seek out work. Furthermore, although a large number of studies show that Type A behaviour is a risk factor for CHD, some studies challenge the link. For example, there is an absence of data on the association between Type A behaviour and CHD in women, blacks, Hispanics and young adults. Neither have sufficient data been accumulated to show conclusively which particular aspects of Type A behaviour are CHD risk-related (Matthews and Haynes, 1986). Thus, Dembroski and Costa (1987) sought to break down the Type A personality into its constituent parts, identifying:

- achievement;
- aggression;
- time consciousness;
- inhibition of expression of feelings.

Kasl and Cooper (1987) sought to establish the contribution of each of these to CHD and other stress-related illnesses.

Reviewing evidence from a number of studies, Cooper (1989), notes that Type B coronary patients could in one sense be more at risk from heart disease than Type As if they had inherited predispositions to CHD which were unrelated to lifestyle or behaviour patterns. However, while Type A behaviour is strongly implicated in a first heart attack, if they survive this, Type As are more likely to avoid a second one.

Cooper (1989) notes that it should not be assumed that Type A behaviour cannot be changed, as some efforts to change the characteristic behaviour pattern have been successful. Efforts to change Type A behaviour have included behaviour modification programmes involving:

* relaxation exercises;
* changing the spread of behaviour;
* attending fewer meetings;
* finding more free time;
* regulating telephone calls;
* counselling.

The beneficial effects of counselling on Type A behaviour have been endorsed (Gill *et al.*, 1985). It has also been maintained that more should be done to change the socialization process which may underpin Type A behaviour which appears prevalent in white, urban, middle-class home environments (Davidson and Cooper, 1981).

The Type A/B approach to personality factors emerged from a different tradition to those discussed in chapter 6, Type A being more of a type (i.e. recognizing discrete personality types on the basis of one or two main factors) rather than a trait approach (i.e. one which identifies individuals' personalities on the basis of their position on a number of dimensions). The trait approach arose from a psychoanalytical, academic, empirical lineage, while the Type A/B approach reflects more of an organizational, applied, medical tradition. Among the problems posed by Type A/B explanations for CHD is that these personality types may be culture-bound – i.e. found mainly in the USA where they have mostly been studied. Furthermore, the behaviours observed may be reactions to certain environmental 'triggers' (e.g. work expectations) rather than immutable personality factors. Thus, a number of studies have sought to relate CHD to personality characteristics as measured on various standard scales and some of the findings from these studies are outlined in summary text 8.12. One problem with many of these studies is that because they are retrospective, anxiety or neurotic symptoms could be reactions to CHD and other stress-related illnesses, rather than antecedents (things which precede something). However, some prospective studies have found similar associations.

It may be concluded that any link between Type A behaviour and CHD is not straightforward. A number of factors are involved, and because most people display a mixture of Type A and Type B behaviours and it is known that such personality attributes can change, it may be more worth while seeking links between stress and personality traits. Deary and Matthews (1993) argue that much of the variance in disease proneness (e.g. to CHD, asthma, arthritis, ulcers, headache – Friedman and Booth-Kewley, 1987) is more likely to result from neuroticism (Suls and Wan, 1989) than from Type A behaviour. It seems that Type A behaviour is likely to be associated with distress rather than with disease (Watson and Pennebaker, 1989; Stone and Costa, 1990). Consistent

---

Summary text 8.12 Individual personality characteristics associated with CHD

On the Minnesota Multi-phasic Personality Inventory (MMPI) – a scale used in clinical diagnosis:
- hypochondriasis (thinking that you're ill);
- depression;
- hysteria;
- neuroticism.

On the 16PF:
- emotional instability;
- high conformity;
- high submissiveness;
- high self-sufficiency;
- shyness;
- introversion;
- apprehensiveness.

---

relationships between Type A behaviour and neuroticism, and sometimes extraversion have been found (Eysenck and Fulkner, 1983; Wong and Reading, 1989; Friedman, 1990; Deary *et al.*, 1991; Deary and Matthews, 1993).

Neuroticism and similar traits

Neuroticism, discussed in chapter 6, in particular has been associated with psychological distress (Ormel and Wohlfarth, 1991) as well as with driver stress (Matthews *et al.*, 1991). McCrae and Costa (1986) and Endler and Parker (1990) found that neuroticism was associated with the use of emotion-focused coping strategies such as escapist fantasy, self-blame and withdrawal. Ways of coping with stress favoured by neurotics were judged as being generally ineffective. Parkes (1984) found that student nurses who were high on neuroticism and low on extraversion coped less well than others with stress in their new jobs. Neuroticism was also found to be related to doctors' ratings of patients' stress-related symptoms such as stomach disorders, headaches, insomnia and tiredness (Wistow *et al.*, 1990). In a study of over 9000 UK adults, Griffiths (1993) found that neurotics were more likely to have heart disease and to have a low fibre diet. Thus, there is the possibility of an association between personality, diet and physical health.

A concept which appears similar to neuroticism and depression is negative affectivity (feelings) (Watson and Clark, 1984). Individuals with high negative feelings are more likely than others to respond negatively to almost anything and to report stress even in the absence of any objective stressor or health problem, suggesting that this is an enduring personal trait. The existence of such a personal disposition among some people poses problems for identifying and eliminating stressors in the environment as it cannot be assumed that this process will eliminate, or even reduce stress for such people (Watson *et al.*, 1987).

A number of other personality traits have been linked with coping, for example self-esteem has been found to be important and is positively associated with dealing effectively with stress (e.g. Ashford, 1988).

Locus of control

Another approach to personality which was not discussed in chapter 6 is locus of control – which if anything is more of a type theory, although is perhaps better described as a continuum of attitudes to life events. Locus of control has been considered in both a general sense (Rotter, 1966) and as related specifically to issues such as health (Calnan, 1988; Niven, 1989; Schank and Lawrence, 1993). In going through life, some people make their way by reacting to situations as if they were ruled by fate. Other people, in similar situations, strive to control events to their personal advantage. In the former case, it is as if these individuals felt that the outcome of their efforts are controlled by forces and events external to themselves, while in the latter case the prime belief is that one can exert internal control to exploit situations so that outcomes result from the application of personal characteristics and effort. This view of personality is known as the internal–external locus of control, developed by Rotter (1966). Internals consider themselves to be authors of their own destiny so that their health and safety would be regarded as dependent upon their experience, skill and judgement. In contrast, externals consider that whatever experience, skill and judgement they possess could easily be counteracted by the many factors that are outside their control. Either powerful others (e.g. God, employers, politicians, decision makers) or fate (luck, chance, pre-determination, etc.) are considered by externals to be the main architects of their future.

A prevailing view of the relationship between locus of control and life stress maintains that people who define events in their lives as being outside their control (external locus of control) will be less able to cope effectively with stress, and are therefore more likely to experience physical and psychological distress than people with internal locus of control beliefs. Externals tend to see themselves as relatively powerless to influence events.

On the other hand, if people define stressful situations as amenable to their own control (i.e. have an internal locus of control) then it is possible that they have sufficient confidence in themselves to deal with stressful situations in a way that minimizes the negative impact (Krause and Stryker, 1984). A study of student nurses confirmed that internals were more adaptive at modifying their coping strategies after having appraised a stressful situation. This flexibility was not displayed by externals, who appeared to alter little their mode of coping (Parkes, 1984). Other writers have also regarded internal locus of control as assisting coping, as a person with this style is more likely to appraise ambiguous situations as controllable by them (Folkman, 1984). Internals have been found to use more problem-focused strategies and fewer emotion-focused strategies than externals do (Callan, 1993).

Internal locus of control dispositions can be traced to childhood health habits, including regular visits to medical practitioners for check-ups and vaccinations. These habits, more likely to be found in higher socio-economic groups, appear to contribute to the development of beliefs that underpin sound preventive health-related behaviour (Lau, 1982). Specific behaviours where locus of control is related to health include: seeking information on health hazards and remedies, taking medication, keeping appointments with physicians, maintaining a diet and giving up smoking. With regard to these types of behaviour, while externals showed positive interest and action, internals fared better (Wallston and Wallston, 1978).

Phares (1976) suggests that both extreme internals and extreme externals may be particularly vulnerable to life stress. The extreme internal confronting very stressful conditions may be so overcome with a sense of personal responsibility for its occurrence that they may experience anxiety and depression as a result. In a study of men aged 45–54 and their attempts to deal with stressful life events which included financial loss, unemployment, increased job pressure and retirement, it was found that extreme internals were gripped by feelings of guilt because they felt personally responsible for the initial event and did not cope well. However, moderate externals were also vulnerable to stress because they felt that their best efforts could not influence such events. The group which coped most effectively with a range of stressful events were moderate internals as they felt that they could exercise at least a certain amount of control over events (Krause and Stryker, 1984). The issue of control is considered in a broader perspective in the following section.

COPING AND CONTROL – INDIVIDUALLY ORIENTED STRATEGIES

Coping

Most people use a number of types of coping strategies to deal with stress (e.g. Folkman and Lazarus, 1980). A popular distinction is between problem-focused (which involves dealing directly with the problem) and emotion-focused (this involves dealing with your feelings about the problem) strategies. Active problem solving is held to have a positive effect upon personal well-being (Folkman *et al.*, 1986), while emotion-focused coping has been linked with poorer psychological adjustment in the long term (Billings and Moos, 1984; Terry, 1991). Another distinction that has been made in respect of coping resources is between those that are internal and relate to the personality and those that are external and relate to social situations or organizational strategies. In this section individual approaches to coping are dealt with, while pp. 232–40 address social and organizational approaches.

People in stressful situations may resort to maladaptive behaviour, such as smoking or drinking alcohol to excess, or to inappropriate responses such as working harder but making more mistakes or unrealistic promises. In contrast, adaptive responses would include: planning, organizing, prioritizing assignments and enlisting others' support (Murphy, 1985). Avoidance of maladaptive behaviour is one way of reducing the level of stress and job dissatisfaction (Parasuraman and Cleek, 1984). In one study of managers' attempts to cope with tension and anxiety, coping behaviour was categorized as:

- talking to others;
- working harder and longer;
- changing to a non-work or leisure activity;
- adopting a problem solving approach;
- withdrawing from the stressful situation.

The effectiveness of the different coping strategies varied depending upon the stressful situation (Burke and Belcourt, 1974). Personality type could also determine the effectiveness of the coping strategy used. Workers classified as Type A tended to use coping behaviour which was the least effective for reducing stress symptoms, for example changing to a different work activity (Howard *et al.,* 1975).

Cox and Ferguson (1991) note that in using coping strategies we seek to:

- problem solve;
- reappraise a (potentially stressful) event;
- avoid stressful encounters.

In adopting an avoidance strategy, individuals heed the warning signs of stressful episodes and side step the potential encounter. Avoidance can be acceptable in the short term, but in the long term it can mean that the individual loses touch with reality and suffers poor psychological adjustment (Fleishman, 1984). This strategy could be expected to leave people in a neutral position with respect to stress and coping (i.e. neither more nor less able to cope with future stress) because they have not addressed the stressor as such. In a longitudinal study of 79 social workers, Koeske *et al.* (1993) found that control-oriented coping strategies clearly acted as work stress buffers, while those who used avoidance coping strategies reported higher levels of negative consequences three months later.

Problem solving or the problem-focused approach to coping represents a learning style in which the individual seeks to acquire abilities to control outcomes, thereby leaving them better able to cope with future stressful encounters. Thus, while the learning task itself may be stressful, due for example to trial and error, the objective is to avoid or to mitigate future stress rather than to avoid current stress.

Event reappraisal corresponds with an emotion-focused coping style (Folkman and Lazarus, 1980) in which the individual changes their attitude or perception of the way they feel about a stressful encounter. In practice, coping strategies are likely to be used in combination; for example Glendon and Glendon (1992) found that ambulance drivers' use of problem-focused and emotion-focused coping strategies for dealing with stress were significantly correlated. Defence mechanisms, such as those outlined in chapter 6 (pp. 140–1, summary text 6.1), may also be used, particularly in response to substantial acute stress (e.g. denial on receiving news of the death of a loved one). Thus, defence mechanisms are likely to be used to some extent by everyone under certain circumstances and serve to protect the individual in the short term to allow more long-term strategies to come into play. However, if used as a prime or long-term strategy, defence mechanisms could lead to inappropriate behaviours and leave the person less able to cope with future stress, for example because people adjust their perception of reality to preserve inner balance.

In a review of over 60 studies on individual strategies, Dewe *et al.* (1993) note that the transactional process for stress involves:

• stress as a dynamic cognitive state;
• this represents a disruption in homeostasis or imbalance;
• which gives rise to a requirement to restore homeostasis.

The process is analogous with the notion of risk homeostasis (e.g. Wilde, 1982; Hoyes and Glendon, 1993) in which a posited target level of risk is maintained by individuals continually adjusting their behaviour in respect of the risks they take in relation to the environment.

In the transactional model of stress (Folkman and Lazarus, 1988), environmental demands are perceived as threatening the individual's coping ability and thus require resolution. Coping is thus:

• relational – i.e. reflects the relation between the individual and the environment;
• a process – i.e. continuous over time and not a discrete event;
• integrating – linking other stress process components.

Cox and Ferguson (1991) consider that all types of coping aim to deal with emotions associated with stress and seek to create a sense of control for the individual.

Control

As will have become evident from parts of the discussion so far, control is widely regarded as a central concept in the stress and coping process. Thus, it is appropriate to devote space to a consideration of some features of control. Based on a study of nearly 5000 workers, Karasek and Theorell (1992) conclude that workers whose work combines high demands with low control have up to three times the risk of heart attack than do professionals and executives who are also in stressful jobs but who have some degree of control over them. Whereas objective (i.e. behavioural) control over a situation may be very limited, perceived (or even actual) control over your own behaviour, even in a very restricted situation, is theoretically limitless. Thus, self-control over one's reactions is widely regarded as being beneficial.

Over the past 20 years there has been a shift in focus from environmental factors which affect individuals' behaviour to the study of processes by which we control our own behaviour. Self-control refers to the conscious decision to take charge of our own behaviour, particularly when new challenges arise (Bandura, 1977; Rosenbaum, 1990; Kanfer and Gaelick-Buys, 1991). For example, Bandura (1977) found that self-belief was important in a wide range of human motivations (chapter 3) and actions – i.e. belief in yourself does make a difference to what you can achieve. Similarly, people's beliefs in their coping capacity affects the level of anxiety, stress reaction and depression that they experience. This reinforces the point in the transactional model that it is our perception (or appraisal) of a threat which is critical.

Rosenbaum (1993) considers that self-control has three major functions:

1. Redressive – aimed at controlling responses such as anxiety and pain that interfere with a person's normal functioning and which are important in coping with stress.
2. Reformative – facilitating the adoption of new behaviours with low likelihood, for example those which have a delayed effect outcome such as dieting or stopping smoking.
3. Experimental – to allow for the experience of pleasurable activities – held to be important for individual growth and development – e.g. enjoying a party. This function is more positive and proactive than the other two and might involve using relaxation techniques, hypnosis or absorption (e.g. in music or a hobby) and is associated with the openness of experience dimension of the big five (see chapter 6, pp. 147–9). Whereas the first two are cognitive in orientation, this last is essentially emotionally directed.

In using the redressive component of self-control, skills – for example, acquired through relaxation and various thought control methods – are required to regulate pain and emotion. The reformative approach requires problem solving skills (D'Zurilla, 1986) in order to:

1. define the problem (e.g. 'I am overweight');
2. generate alternative solutions (e.g. reduce various forms of intake);
3. evaluate alternatives ('which would be the best to carry out?');
4. implement chosen solution ('I'll do this').

Generally, these two types of self-control are mutually supportive and a measure of individuals' ability to be able to use these approaches has been developed by Rosenbaum (1980, 1988, 1990) termed 'learned resourcefulness'.

How well does the notion of 'learned resourcefulness' predict individuals' abilities to employ various self-control strategies? In answering this question, it is instructive to record that a prime technique directed at improving self-control, cognitive behaviour therapy (e.g. Ellis, 1973; Meichenbaum, 1977; Beck and Emery, 1985) (e.g. rational emotive therapy), has been criticized for not dealing adequately with emotional aspects of coping. A paradox is that on the one hand high resourceful people have been found to respond better than low resourceful people to cognitive treatments and they tend to use redressive and reformative self-control skills (Achmon, 1987). However, on the other hand low resourceful individuals learnt better than high resourceful individuals how to control their heart rate using biofeedback techniques (biofeedback is a principle by which body temperature, heart rate and other organic functions can be brought more under conscious control – e.g. Rogers, 1980). Furthermore, low resourceful people could achieve deeper relaxation (Lowenstein, 1991).

Thus, it seems that use of analytical thinking can be very helpful in coping with difficult life events, but could be a drawback when seeking a more general experimental approach to coping, for example through relaxation or biofeedback (Rosenbaum, 1993). Therefore, it seems that in order to achieve the benefits of experimental self-control, it may be necessary to relinquish those cognitive control processes that are most frequently used in response to stressful situations. A dilemma which this poses for treatment (for example of phobias) is that individuals with anxiety disorders are particularly fearful of losing control of well-rehearsed (cognitive) coping strategies and feel threatened by a possible loss of control, for example during relaxation or hypnosis (Chambers and Gracely, 1989).

Decision latitude and job control

Decision latitude refers to the opportunity for the significant use of judgement and discretion in a job. When this factor is high and combined with a demanding job, people experienced job satisfaction and reduced depression. The opposite appeared to be the case, particularly with respect to satisfaction, when jobs were rated low in terms of decision latitude and demands posed by the task (Karasek, 1979). To relieve job strain, it is suggested that employees should be given greater scope for decision-making and use of discretion at work but at the same time not to overreach individual capabilities in the quest to obtain more substantial job responsibilities. Karesek and Theorell (1992) developed a model based upon the dimensions of decision latitude (high or low) and (job) demands (high or low), resulting in the 2×2 matrix of behaviours shown in figure 8.2.

In another study, positive health implications (i.e. a reduction in illness among full-time workers, including heart disease among males) of greater control in one's job, together with greater opportunities for democratic participation at work, are endorsed (Karasek, 1990). Karesek points out that one of the most disturbing conclusions of his study is that current changes to

		Large	Small
High Demands		Active	Tension
Low		Relaxed	Passive
Decision latitude		Large	Small

Figure 8.2 Demands and decision latitude matrix (after Karasek and Theorell, 1992).

white-collar jobs often involved less opportunity to exercise control at work, especially for older workers and women. Added to this is the stressful experience of lack of employee involvement in processes leading up to job reorganization and change. It should be noted that change is potentially stressful because people feel less secure in unpredictable environments. Individuals may be able to take one or two changes fairly readily, but too many changes at the same time could result in them becoming stressed and defensive. Fisher (1985) maintains that compared with white-collar workers, blue-collar workers experience less control in their work – the alleged disadvantages are shown in summary text 8.13.

Coronary heart disease (CHD) risk, stress and exercise

Of all diseases associated with stressful experiences, that between CHD and various stressors is among the most studied. For example, Siegrist *et al.* (1990) found that status inconsistency, job insecurity, work pressure and need for control, all predicted CHD.

Exercise (aerobic) is generally regarded to be a valuable technique in combating stress, and it is interesting to note that many body movements imitate the body's natural response to stress, i.e. action based on 'flight or fight'. Certainly, the pursuit of various lifestyle and health habits (e.g. physical

---

Summary text 8.13 Disadvantages of low job control in blue-collar work (after Fisher, 1985)

1. Working directly on the line, handling a product or process, blue-collar workers are more likely to feel helpless in that they are less able to avoid unpleasant conditions, and have less control over how their time is spent at work. In contrast, many of those in staff or managerial positions are more likely to have the opportunity to avoid circumstances they do not like, although may need to be aware of not being penalized for such behaviour.
2. Because their work is generally well-defined and integrated in an overall production process in a systematic way, blue-collar workers have less scope to modify their task. Should there be unpleasant conditions in the job, usually typified by a greater range of industrial hazards and uncomfortable working conditions than experienced by white-collar workers, they may have few options available to them for coping. The discussion on cognitive dissonance (pp. 80–2, especially summary text 4.5) reveals that behavioural options may reduce to complaining – and risking sanctions – or leaving the job, always assuming that there is another one to go to. Changing your attitude to the hazards, i.e. putting up with them, may be the line of least resistance.
3. Continuing the above point, from a market perspective, compared with white-collar workers, it is usually less easy for blue-collar workers to change jobs because of the lower transferability of their skills, lower income (and consequent lower savings to act as a buffer between jobs), and reduced opportunities.
4. Opportunities for social activity at work are greater if the worker enjoys greater discretion. In this sense, the blue-collar worker is also at a disadvantage as s/he can less readily counteract unfavourable conditions at work by exercising control outside mainstream work activity.

fitness, sleeping) has been found to be associated with reducing the impact of work stress (Steffy *et al.*, 1990). Exercise has also been found to be helpful in improving self-esteem and mastery and thus can also contribute to problem-focused coping in the future (Long and Flood, 1993). However, individual differences mean that regular exercise can help some, but not necessarily all, individuals.

In a review of 95 studies of links between physical activity and CHD risk, van Doornen and de Geus (1993) report that heart disease is almost twice as prevalent in inactive compared with active individuals. Long and Flood (1993) point out that exercise is an emotion-focused coping strategy. While a causal link between physical activity and CHD risk has been found (Powell *et al.*, 1987), the results are not overwhelming and van Doornen and de Geus (1993) consider that the effect of fitness upon stress is only modest. They conclude that individuals do have control over a number of CHD risk factors, although exercise has to be combined with other beneficial actions (e.g. diet, attitude to life) to reduce CHD risk significantly.

Stress and lifestyle

Different approaches to stress reduction strategies based upon self-control may be related to lifestyle and values in society. Skills and attitudes which are typically valued in Western society tend to be associated with productivity improvements, measuring outcomes, ambition and achievement (chapter 3, pp. 44–6, particularly summary text 3.5). These are the constellation of values which are typically associated with Type A behaviour. An alternative is to pursue a lifestyle which can accommodate these values within a broader perspective – for example by acknowledging their existence – but not giving them first call on the attention.

An important ingredient of a personal stress management programme is an appropriate diet. This means eating a variety of the correct foods in moderation. Most of those who smoke are aware of the associated health risks but can find it difficult to give up the habit without help. An increasing number of employers are introducing no-smoking policies in the workplace.

A potent cognitive approach to coping with stress is to isolate 'faulty thinking' which leads to harmful or unpleasant consequences. Techniques which are used to combat this include rational emotive therapy, which seeks to influence the way we think and feel about stressors in daily life. It involves taking responsibility for our feelings – such as anger or frustration – rather than allowing them to be controlled by others' behaviour. We cannot change the world, but it is possible to focus on changing ourselves so as to promote greater harmony with our environment.

A frequently undervalued approach to stress management is the use of humour. This can be a powerful weapon in combating stress because it eases the build up of tension. Without humour, people tend to be more stressed and when people are stressed, they lose their sense of humour (Foot, 1990).

In dealing with stress, two types of strategies have been identified which correspond with the hemispheres of the brain. Thus, they are referred to as 'left brain' and 'right brain' strategies. It should be pointed out that this categorization should not be taken to imply that the two hemispheres of the brain operate independently or are exclusively responsible for particular types of activity. It has been pointed out that the 'right brain for emotion' and 'left brain for cognition' is too simplistic (e.g. Davidson, 1992; Jones and Fox, 1992). Rather, it is a shorthand description of two distinct types of measures which it is possible to adopt to cope with stress.

One approach is to seek to reorder or redefine those aspects or symptoms of our live that are causing us distress. Thus, we may pursue a range of rational 'therapeutic' strategies which include:

- organizing – improving organizing ability;
- time management – improving use of time so that you can cram in even more activities!;
- calculating costs and benefits – so as always to make 'rational' decisions;
- goal setting – clarifying objectives;
- prioritizing – making clear what is really important;
- delegating – passing work on to others so that you can take on different activities e.g. more work!

These techniques reinforce our reliance upon 'left brain' strategies and represent attempts to improve our functioning by toning up existing patterns of behaviour. They are reflected in 'hard' HRM approaches to various forms of performance measurement, for example appraisal. A less familiar (to many) but alternative route is to adopt the softer approach – which may be referred to as 'right brain' – analogous with the 'soft' approach within HRM, and which is much less amenable to measurement in quantitative terms. The type of techniques, attitudes and experiences which may be subsumed under this heading are shown in summary text 8.14.

Summary text 8.14 'Right brain' coping strategies (after Nash, 1992)

- listen to your body;
- heed your emotions and be aware of intuition;
- listen to others;
- learn to 'open up' a little more;
- reduce defensive behaviours and shutting off feelings;
- establish a core of central stillness;
- play, laugh and wonder more – free up the child within;
- enjoy **being** as much as doing;
- deliberately choose to mobilize:
  - parasympathetic relaxation,
  - abdominal breathing,
  - deep relaxation,
  - meditation,
  - yoga.
- i.e. exercise the 'softer' and (for many) the less familiar side.

There is a substantive basis for a 'right brain' approach to stress reduction and coping – scientific evidence is available for the beneficial effects of a change in lifestyle. For example, Kiecolt-Glaser *et al.* (1987) found that immunological functioning among a group of older adults improved as a result of relaxation. Ornish *et al.* (1990) assigned 28 coronary patients to an experimental group involving a low-fat, low/no alcohol, vegetarian diet, no smoking or caffeine, stress management and moderate exercise condition. Another 20 patients were assigned to a usual medical care group. Ornish *et al.* (1990) found, from zero disease differences at base line, significant differences between the groups after one year in:

- cholesterol levels;
- weight and other heart disease risk factors;
- reported frequency, duration and severity of angina.

Those patients who made the greatest lifestyle changes showed the biggest improvements. Whereas patients in the experimental group showed significant regression of CHD, the usual care group patients showed significant progression in their disease. It was concluded that comprehensive lifestyle changes can begin to reverse coronary heart disease in only a year.

PREVENTION STRATEGIES – SOCIAL AND ORGANIZATIONAL

Strategies for coping with stress, for example arising from organizational change are usually categorized as either individual or organizational in origin. An effective stress management programme is likely to involve both types of strategy. Callan (1993) identifies strategies under these headings, his classification is shown in summary text 8.15. Individual strategies were considered in the previous section and this section reviews a sample of organizational strategies.

A range of booklets and other publications offer practical guidance on reducing stress at work. For example, Jee and Reason (1988) suggest the following principles for tackling stress at work;

- treat the cause, not the symptom;
- accept that work stress is a problem for the organization, not the individual;
- tackle taboo topics using alternative approaches as necessary;
- involve everyone;
- be realistic – don't try to do too much at once.

Jee and Reason's (1988) ten areas for action are shown in summary text 8.16.

Stress management programmes

As noted already, a fair range of stress management or stress reduction strategies is available for organizations and books are available on this topic (e.g. Quick and Quick, 1984). Stress management programmes were underway in a number of organizations in the 1970s (Hackman and Suttle, 1977) and the 1980s witnessed a proliferation of such programmes (Manuso, 1982). US

Summary text 8.15 Strategies for coping with organizationally induced stress (after Callan, 1993)

Individual coping strategies
- use of problem-focused and emotion-focused coping;
- reliance upon internal resources (personality traits, internal locus of control, hardiness, sense of mastery – see also chapter 3, pp. 44–56 on the basic motivation to achieve mastery or control over events);
- use of external resources and social supports (spouse, family, friends, managers, colleagues).

Organizational strategies
- empower individuals to take control of change;
- provide timely and accurate communications (figure 5.1 in chapter 5 for further details);
- training in communications (chapter 2, pp. 15–23 for information on learning and training principles);
- use transformational leaders;
- promote unlearning programmes to remove old organisational culture – e.g. workshops;
- job related activities – clarify roles and responsibilities, establish support teams, improve person-job fit, job enrichment, etc.;
- stress management – e.g. fitness and wellness programmes.

---

companies have led the way in the provision of employee health care, stress management and fitness programmes. However, with increases in worker compensation claims for stress-related accidents and illnesses, more of these programmes are likely to be seen in UK industry. There is evidence that they are associated with reduced absenteeism and medical costs (Cooper, 1986). The principles of such programmes include:

- create an environment for maximum participation;
- build bridges between home and work for greater understanding of domestic and family needs;
- use training to increase skills, awareness and interpersonal relations;

Summary text 8.16 Areas for action on organizational stress (after Jee and Reason, 1988)

- improve the physical work environment;
- analyse job organization and redesign jobs where appropriate;
- clarify job roles;
- overhaul organizational culture;
- review management styles and practices;
- encourage participation and control in all areas of work;
- assess coordination and communication systems;
- encourage development of good personal, professional and industrial relations;
- value and give recognition to employees;
- make adequate preparation for planned change.

- create an organizational culture of openness, communication and trust so that inability to cope can be expressed and help requested.

Apart from the coping behaviour adopted by individuals, organizations can offer a range of techniques, frequently involving relaxation, under the 'stress management' label. These techniques include:

- biofeedback,
- muscle relaxation,
- meditation,
- counselling,
- cognitive-based methods developed from clinical psychology.

When applied to a work situation, stress management techniques may emphasize prevention and imparting skills to health employees rather than treating stress-related problems. Thus, health promotion and disease prevention are key themes.

Most stress management programmes acknowledge relaxation skills to some extent. Some people have to learn how to relax, but the value of relaxation is unchallenged. High blood pressure, activated by stress, can be significantly reduced by using a relaxation programme. Breathing control is also a useful relaxation technique, breathing being a function over which we can exercise some control. Using such relaxation techniques enables us to confront maladaptive stress responses.

However, effectiveness of stress management techniques as a solitary weapon has been challenged. It is suggested that stress management training should only be used to supplement organizational change or job redesign programmes in order to deal with stressors which cannot readily be designed out of the job (e.g. seasonal workloads) (Ganster *et al.*, 1982). This view seeks to address the contention that stress management techniques inappropriately focus on trying to change the employee rather than the work environment. This stems from a view that stress is a phenomenon which is peculiar to the individual and emphasizes that a lifestyle change is necessary to cope with it. In contrast, trade unions attribute stress as springing from adverse working conditions, lack of worker control, unrealistic job demands and lack of understanding by management. They consider that use of stress management techniques were the easy option adopted by management who did not do enough to remove work stressors (Murphy, 1985).

Health promotion programmes

Changing attitudes and behaviour in respect of health has already been discussed in chapter 4 (pp. 84–8, particularly figure 4.7), the health belief model being a prime example of such an approach. Health promotion programmes are broader in scope than the preventive strategies outlined above. They range from purely educational schemes to promote health to learning to take one's own blood pressure, using stress management techniques or altering one's lifestyle. Recent years have seen a steady growth in employee health programmes. US employers generally take greater responsibility for paying workers' health insurance costs, principally because of the absence of a national health service. However, many larger companies offer more comprehensive programmes. There are signs that this trend is increasing in the UK, partly because of the increasing provision of a private medical insurance by employers. Paternalism and philanthropy may have a part to play in this development in some large and long established companies. However, increasingly employers adopt the HRM position that investing in employees' health produces dividends. These could include increased productivity, lower medical and disability costs, reduced absenteeism and staff turnover and improved satisfaction and morale among employees (Murphy, 1984).

The substantial increase in medical care expenditure in the US has helped to generate interest in ill-health prevention programmes. US employers are also more vulnerable to legal action in respect of occupational stress when they have failed to take preventive measures. Hence, they are motivated to do so. In the UK, workplace health promotion programmes are viewed by many employers as a very promising strategy for coping with rapidly increasing healthcare costs. For many employers, this could be the primary justification for embracing preventive measures (Ashton, 1990; Jenkins and Warman, 1993).

In recent years major UK healthcare specialist insurance companies have promoted preventive measures such as health screening, stress management programmes and occupational health advice, doubtless believing that healthier workforces will result in fewer claims. For the companies, this could mean reduced future premiums. However, such a fall in premiums may be forestalled if screening leads to the diagnosis of illness requiring medical attention and consequent claims. Some examples of activities in this sphere are given in summary text 8.17.

Social support

Although 'support' as a concept has had a place in social science for some time, the study of social support with a 'group' emphasis emerged more strongly during the 1970s. In studies of participative management, the principle of supportive relations was recognized as a core element in effective supervision, when supervisors related to subordinates in such a way that the individual's sense of personal worth and importance was enhanced. Supportive behaviour assumes a central position in certain branches of psychotherapy and counselling (House and Kahn, 1985).

External support networks can buffer individuals during times of crisis (Rodin and Salovy, 1989). Individuals with external support rely more on active coping strategies than do those without such support (Billings and Moos, 1984; Holohan and Moos, 1987). Those without external support tend to use avoidance strategies to cope with stressful events (Callan, 1993).

Social support refers generally to the existence or quality of social relationships, and could specifically refer to a marriage, friendship or membership of

---

Summary text 8.17 Preventive health measures in some companies

The headquarters of the Marks & Spencer organization in London has facilities such as a gym, dentist, doctors, nurses, osteopath, physiotherapist and health administrators. According to the company's deputy head of health services, the service reduces absenteeism, increases the efficiency of the workforce and is an example of the organization's commitment to its staff (*Source:* Summers, D. (1990) An act of faith that can reap rewards. *Financial Times*, 7.12.90).

The Post Office takes its mobile clinics and health education roadshows to its widely dispersed workforce of 120 000. Scottish and Newcastle Breweries undertook a stress audit (see for example, Sutherland and Davidson, 1993) among its 24 000 blue-collar workers. According to the company's chief medical officer, the results might indicate the need for a range of improvements in organizational practices from encouraging managers to improve the way they work with people to the overhaul of production methods.

Du Pont, a major US corporation with UK operations, has a scheme called 'Health Horizons'. There is a belief that employees can learn to extend their life expectancy by adopting improved lifestyles. Employees complete a lifestyle questionnaire, analysis of which will show employees where to concentrate their efforts to improve their health. Self-help kits are available, and incentives (e.g. free track suits) are provided to encourage appropriate behaviour.

(*Source:* Summers, D. (1990) Testing for stress in the workplace. *Financial Times*, 8.12.90.)

To date, few scientifically valid assessments of UK health promotion programmes have been undertaken. The most comprehensive and well researched health promotion programme in the USA – STAYWELL – was developed by Control Data Corporation, and covered 22 000 employees and their spouses in 14 US cities (Cooper, 1986). Free (to employees) company benefits included programmes on: stopping smoking, weight control, cardiovascular fitness, stress management and improved dietary control – particularly reducing cholesterol, salt and sugar.

The steps involved and significant outcomes of the Control Data Corporation health promotion programme were:

- a confidential health risk profile is provided for all employees (management and blue-collar) following a comprehensive physical examination, employees also giving information confidentially on lifestyle and health related behaviour;
- employees receive their personal results and action plans to reduce their own health risks;
- employees select appropriate programmes to follow on the basis of their risk profile;
- employees who were encouraged to stop smoking spent half the number of days in hospital and had 20 percent less health care costs, compared with smokers;
- compared with the sedentary group, employees who had exercise training had 30 percent fewer claims and spent half the number of days in hospital;
- employees who entered the cardiovascular fitness programme and reduced their hypertension levels, had less than half the health care costs of those who did not;
- high risk employees in terms of health (weight, stress, fitness, nutrition, smoking) were twice as likely to be absent from work due to sickness and be half as productive as the low risk, physically fit group.

Source: Cooper, 1986.

---

an organization. It is highlighted in the give and take of personal relationships – i.e. giving and receiving at an emotional level, particularly when help is needed. The popularity of social support has been partly promoted by recognition of the part it can play in reducing the impact of stress, both inside and outside work (see for example, Veiel and Baumann, 1992). The manner in which supportive social relationships alleviate stress at work, according to Williams and House (1985) is:

- support can directly enhance health by creating a setting in which needs for affection, approval, social interaction and security are met;
- support can directly reduce levels of stress and indirectly improve health by reducing interpersonal tensions as well as having a positive effect generally in the work environment;
- support acts as a buffer between the person and health hazards – as the level of social support increases, health risks decline for individuals exposed to stressful conditions; conversely, with the decline in social support the adverse impact of stress on health becomes increasingly apparent.

Caution needs to be exercised in respect of alleged beneficial effects of social support, because there are occasions when social interaction (and even inappropriate counselling) can have a detrimental effect upon an individual's health, for example where conflict and strife is inherent in social relationships.

Social support processes vary between groups. In one study, it was concluded that compared with their male counterparts, female managers were more likely to use social support to deal with job-related problems (Burke and Belcourt, 1974). Women have been found to be more likely to be the providers of support (Belle, 1982) and can become more emotionally affected by the problems of others, and as a consequence incur higher psychological costs.

Social support has also been considered in a racial context. The relationship between occupational stress, health and social support among 90 black and 93 white clerical employees in nine government agencies in South Africa was examined. The study found that social support reduced the negative effects of job stress among blacks, but not among whites (Opren, 1982).

Measures which have been forwarded to enhance social support and improve the flow of supportive behaviour among blue-collar workers have been identified by Williams and House (1985). These measures, which are relevant to other occupational groups, are described in summary text 8.18.

Health promotion programmes, considered above, are another avenue for delivering social support. They could be concerned with stress management and are often group-based rather than individual-based. Thus, they can serve as social support interventions and as stress-reduction techniques.

A social support scheme was developed by a large UK chemical company. An employee counselling service with a full-time counsellor having a psychiatric social work background, was established. The objectives of the service were to provide a confidential counselling service to all employees and their families, to work with outside agencies for the welfare of employees and to provide other activities that are likely to improve the quality of working life.

About half the employees who availed themselves of the service came for

Summary text 8.18 Measures to improve social support (after Williams and House, 1985)

1. **Structural arrangements**: work is organized in such a way as to facilitate stable interaction between employees in the performance of various tasks, as well as maintaining social ties. Here the importance of social interaction is emphasized as a means to reduce stress at work (Alcalay and Pasick, 1983). It is suggested that people who had a constant set of colleagues had lower cholesterol levels than did those whose colleagues changed frequently (Cassel, 1963).

The above finding is interesting in the light of evidence from the functioning of large Japanese organizations, in which a high level of job security results in membership of a group throughout a person's career. A cohort of workers who enter an organization together develop strong feelings of group solidarity over time. As a consequence, individual interests are at least partly absorbed into the work group interests, the work group offering satisfying emotional support and social ties in a friendly atmosphere (Matsumoto, 1970; see also chapter 7, especially pp. 168–9 and pp. 171–7). The importance of emotional support is recognized elsewhere. For example, in a sample of social workers the provision of empathy, caring, trust and concern by colleagues and supervisors was beneficial in helping each individual to cope better with stress at work, although was not viewed as a total stress-reduction process (Jayaratne and Chess, 1984).

2. **Other organizational change processes**: participative management schemes – including quality circles – broadly conceived, have potential not only to improve the quantity and quality of production, but also to increase social support, reduce stress and as a consequence to enhance health and well-being (Cobb, 1976). Participation in the management process is said to enhance employees' psychological and social functioning in ways that make them more effective as spouses, parents and members of the community. This experience teaches employees new skills and attitudes which are capable of improving the giving and receiving of social support (Crouter, 1984).

Central features of the quality circle are the emphasis given to the group process and effective teamwork (chapter 7, pp. 177–80 and 192–200), with scope for provision of social support. It is suggested that social needs are met in quality circles where an outlet is provided for grievances and irritations, and immediate recognition is given for members' abilities and achievements. Quality circles can thus provide a sense of dignity and assist in maintaining high morale. In addition, there is a good chance that group cohesiveness developed at work spreads to non-work activities as circle members engage in social activities outside the workplace.

Participative management is not without its potential downside and can have unanticipated negative effects. For example, employees may feel more responsible for problems on the job and worry about these problems may result in new stress in their non-work lives. There is also evidence to suggest that marital relationships can suffer when employees' wives transfer their new independence and competence learned at work to the home environment (Crouter, 1984).

3. **Facilitative supportive supervisory behaviour**: this type of behaviour is endorsed by a number of studies. Proponents argue that it should be encouraged and expanded, and be adopted at all levels in an organization, and that managers and supervisors who use it should receive appropriate recognition and reward for doing so.

advice on education, family matters, work-related housing problems, separation, divorce, children, ageing parents and consumer issues. The other half received longer-term counselling on fundamental personal and relationship problems. Over a four-year period, roughly 10% of all employees per annum took advantage of the service. This is the type of programme that some argue should be encouraged to deal with pressures of modern society (Cooper, 1981). In the absence of a formal social support system, an informal approach for the individual experiencing stress is outlined in summary text 8.19.

A human resource management approach to stress management

Callan (1993) notes that one organizational response to change is via HRM practices such as recruiting individuals who are able to cope with life in a changing organization and who will meet the challenges encountered (chapter 6, pp. 149–55 on personality tests at work). Similarly, training (chapter 2) can be oriented towards developing a 'cross-cultural' type of manager who responds well to ambiguity and change and is prepared to be involved in change processes. Burke (1993) describes a range of organizational interventions to reduce occupational stress. Other HRM strategies include:

- improving the job-person fit (e.g. Caplan *et al.*, 1975);
- job enrichment (Hackman and Oldham, 1980);
- stress management aimed at modifying employees' appraisal of threat (e.g. Ivancevich *et al.*, 1990);
- employee assistance programmes (EAPs).

Berridge and Cooper (1993) describe the history, coverage and operation of EAPs. A 1991 CBI survey revealed that 94% of member companies thought that stress and mental health should be of concern to them, yet only 10% had a programme for dealing with it. In the USA, over 75% of the *Fortune 500* companies and around 12000 others have EAPs (Feldman, 1991). With

---

Summary text 8.19 An informal approach to stress reduction (after Cooper, 1981)

1. Select a person at work you feel you can talk to, someone you don't feel threatened by and to whom you can reveal your feelings. Don't select someone who you may be using on an unconscious level at a manipulative level in organizational politics.
2. Approach this person and explain to him/her that you have a particular problem at work or outside that you would like to discuss. Admit that you need help and that he or she would be the best person to consult because you trust his/her opinion, like him/her as a person, and feel that s/he could identify with your circumstances.
3. Try to maintain and build on this relationship, even at times of no crisis or problems.
4. Review, from time to time, the nature of the relationship to see whether it is still providing you with the emotional support that you need to cope with difficulties that arise. If the relationship is no longer constructive or the nature of your problems changes, so necessitating a different peer counsellor, then seek another person for support.

employees increasingly prepared to take legal action against employers as a remedy for suffering job-related stress (summary text 8.6), EAPs and stress management programmes will make increasingly good business sense. Summary text 8.20 summarizes experiences from a few organizations in this area. However, in evaluating a number of studies of EAPs, Shapiro *et al.* (1993) conclude that 'the cost-effectiveness of EAPs while promising, cannot be taken for granted'.

CONCLUSIONS

Research on stress has revealed a considerable number of potential stressors, to the extent that it has become difficult, if not impossible, to make specific predictions about whether any particular type of event will result in a given individual experiencing a range of physical, psychological, behavioural or medical conditions. This 'rag bag' approach to stress has been criticized for a lack of explanatory and predictive utility. One problem in considering stress is the circularity of definitions in respect of cause and effect – for example 'a stressor is something which causes stress; stress is caused by stressors'.

It is likely to be more profitable to concentrate on the processes involved in the stress reaction, for example addressing the issue of continuous challenge to the human immune system. While humans are generally remarkably resilient, being 'designed' to withstand varying amounts of stress, beyond a certain point stress can, through various possible pathways, increase mortality and morbidity (e.g. through heart disease, cancer, suicide, alcohol-related problems or greater accident propensity through increased cognitive lapses).

Summary text 8.20 Employee assistance programmes (EAPs) – some companies' experiences.

- US companies offering EAPs get $3 return for every $1 invested;
- United Air Lines claims $17 return for every $1 invested in their EAP;
- 1988 Whitbread EAP involves:
  - free confidential telephone helpline,
  - individual counselling – first three sessions free,
  - covers financial, marital, other domestic, alcohol, drugs, etc.,
  - about 10% of workforce participate – 5% of these take advantage of programme,
  - costs about £15 per annum per employee,
  - substantial reduction in pub managers' turnover;
- UK Post Office has an extensive stress counselling service for its 120 000 employees – pilot study showed reduced absenteeism;
  - Midland Bank EAP involves stress counselling;
  - seen to enhance caring organization image,
  - lifts pressure on managers – who are not qualified to deal with staff problems,
  - improves productivity,
  - at least one suicide prevented.

Source: Guardian, 31.10.92.

Greater understanding of the pathways – for example, immune system effectiveness – through which the stress process operates would aid both theoretical and intervention studies. It might also be posited that stress has a natural selection function – individuals who are better equipped to cope with stress are more likely to survive and to transmit their genes to the next generation.

The human stress experience in a general sense may also be considered from an evolutionary perspective, as being a component of the natural selection process. Bandura (1989) maintains that there would not be an evolutionary advantage to humans if acute stressors always impaired the immune function because of their prevalence in everyday life. This would mean that we would be continually vulnerable to illness. However, Bandura (1989) contends that stress which is aroused in the coping process over a period of time as a result of dealing with stressors, actually enhances the immune function. That is to say, the more effective our coping in respect of stress becomes, the more robust is our immune system. From a functional perspective, experience of stress may serve to discourage us from continuing to engage in damaging activity.

The inverted 'U' has been a long serving model for stress, as it has for environmental demands, motivation and arousal (with which stress is frequently confused) in respect of performance level. It is frequently asserted that a 'certain amount' of (eu)stress is required for motivation and arousal and to meet extreme demands. Given that stress (like motivation) is a multi-dimensional concept, it is probably apposite to question the validity of this model also. One alternative would be a catastrophe theory model (e.g. Jones and Hardy, 1990), to reflect at least one further dimension and to accommodate the possibility of catastrophic events (for example, burnout, PTSD or mental breakdown) occurring beyond a certain point. Even such a model may prove to be unsatisfactory, as many variables require to be represented in a truly multi-dimensional model of stress. Because of the complex nature of the concept, we may learn more by continually seeking a satisfactory model than in ever designing one.

Not everyone suffers from work related stress and individual differences, such as personality factors, play a part both in the perception of stress (being in the eye of the beholder) and in stress-related behaviours and conditions, including illness. However, while personality is generally considered to be a relatively immutable association of traits or characteristics (chapter 6), there is evidence that behaviours associated with personality characteristics which affect the stress experience (e.g. Type A behaviour) can be influenced to benefit the individual. There is a suggestion that while Type A behaviour is likely to be associated with feelings of (di)stress and that there are links between Type A behaviour and neuroticism in particular, it is neuroticism which is associated with disease proneness.

The coping component of the stress process needs to reflect individual aspects as well, and there is scope for linking personal coping styles with personality theory. A promising route in this field is through the notion of cognitive architecture – which emphasizes the way in which people think

(Fletcher, 1993). Fletcher maintains that psychological factors play a major role in disease and life expectancy, while work stressors can also be transmitted to marital partners. The work that people do in turn influences the way they think and their consequent proneness to disease. Certainly, it can be argued that a more complete understanding of stress cannot be achieved unless we can obtain a picture which goes beyond the workplace, important though this environment is. To appreciate the stress response of an individual, we need to consider the person's total environment.

The notion of control is widely regarded as being central to individual stress management. This is in respect of perceived control over a set of circumstances (as in internal locus of control) or control over one's feelings about a situation (as in emotion-focused coping strategies) to actual control – as in the case of individuals who have powerful roles in organizations or who have high autonomy over their work and other aspects of their lives. It would be useful to develop the notion of control to be more specific in respect of skills and abilities in relation to various types of stressors and behaviour outcomes.

A range of potential integrating features which reflect analogous components at different levels – e.g. between individuals and organization, intra-individual and intra-organizational – may be discerned. These offer an opportunity to relate coping styles and control to personality dimensions or traits (chapter 6, pp. 142–9) as well as to human resource management practices (chapters 1 and 11). The concepts are shown in summary text 8.21.

Summary text 8.21 Analogous dimensions of personality, coping style and organization

Dimensions	*Origins*
Cognitive (redressive, reformative) vs experiential	Self-control (e.g. Rosenbaum, 1993)
Problem-focused vs emotion-focused	Coping style (e.g. Folkman and Lazarus, 1980)
'Left brain' vs 'right brain'	Stress management (e.g. Nash, 1992)
Sensing vs intuition	Personality type (Jung/MBTI)
Thinking vs feeling	Personality type (Jung/MBTI)
Judgement vs perception	Personality type (Jung/MBTI)
Extraversion vs introversion	Personality type/trait (Jung/Eysenck/Cattell/Big 5)
Practical vs open to experience	Big 5 (e.g. McCrae and Costa, 1989)
'Hard' vs 'Soft'	Human Resource Management (e.g. Storey, 1992)

9 HUMAN ERROR AND HUMAN FACTORS

❏ This chapter completes the trio of chapters concerned with different aspects of the work environment. Here the focus is upon physical aspects of workplaces and in human responses to them. The topic of human error is dealt with first before a broader discussion of human factors – or ergonomics. This is followed by a consideration of interface design issues and a review of some techniques used to reduce human error, including detailed examples.

INTRODUCTION

The man who makes no mistakes does not usually make anything
(William Conor Magee)

This chapter first considers a fundamental aspect of human behaviour, that of making mistakes or errors. This discussion is then taken into the area of some of the techniques which have been developed to address human error – under the general heading of 'human factors', or ergonomics. To address such topics in the context of human resource aspects of safety and risk management should hardly require justification. It is widely acknowledged that some understanding of human error and human reliability, as well as a sound grasp of ergonomic principles and practice should be part of the repertoire of the safety and risk professional. The objectives of the chapter are to explain different types of human error and to show how selected human factors (ergonomic) interventions can be used to diagnose and provide guidance for reducing either the likelihood or the consequences of human error.

Human errors may be complex phenomena, whose description, like motivation (chapter 3) and personality (chapter 6) can be traced at least back to Freud (1975), from whom the expression 'Freudian slip' has entered the language, particularly relating to slips of the tongue which have sexual connotations. Freud's view was that erroneous actions resulted from some underlying need or purpose.

However, human error – and its complement, human reliability – has only been investigated as an identifiable field of study since the 1970s and the contemporary orientation is essentially cognitive. Thus, Reason and Mycielska (1982) and Reason (1990) for example argue for a cognitive interpretation for most (if not quite all) human errors. Reason (1990) defines human error thus:

a generic term to encompass all those occasions in which a planned sequence of mental or physical activities fails to achieve its intended outcome, and when these failures cannot be attributed to the intervention of some chance agency (ibid, p.9).

Cognitive factors which relate closely to human error include attention and control mechanisms, concepts which have been introduced in earlier chapters. Empirical data on human errors have been collected through questionnaires and self-report diaries (see Reason and Mycielska, 1982; Reason and Lucas, 1984) as well as from case studies.

The study of human error has both theoretical and practical implications – both of which will be considered in this chapter. The other main component of this chapter is human factors – or ergonomics as it is also known. This is a well-established discipline which has widespread applications in the safety field and those which are particularly relevant are dealt with in this chapter, especially those concerned with human reliability.

HUMAN ERROR

This section seeks to:

- provide an outline appreciation of what human error is and why it occurs;
- explain the main types of human error;
- illustrate how different types of human error may be addressed.

Errors as a learning tool

Let us begin with the well-known saying 'to err is human'.* Why then do humans make errors? This question may be answered from an evolutionary perspective in that making errors has been functional – i.e. necessary for our survival as a species.

From a contemporary point of view, it is similarly necessary for all of us to make errors in order to learn – especially as children, but also once we are adults. Therefore, it is important to recognize that making errors – and acting on the feedback we get from so doing – is essential for human learning to occur. Thus, from an early age, error performance is how we learn not only about hazards in our environment – i.e. from direct experience – but also about aspects of our social world – about what is correct or expected behaviour in a wide range of situations. In this way we learn what is appropriate in different contexts – for example, how to treat other road users and how to behave at work.

Much of our early learning in these – and all other – environments is developed in part by us making errors and **being able to learn from them**. Thus, the reason that human errors are important in a functional sense is that they

---

*Alexander Pope (1711) *An Essay on Criticism,* 1.525. The extended quote is 'To err is human, to forgive, divine'.

provide the feedback which is essential for learning to occur – see also chapter 2 (pp. 15–23) on learning principles, particularly feedback. This principle can usefully be extended to learning situations. For example, Rubinsky and Smith (1973), during training in the correct use of grinding wheels, used a jet of water aimed at the trainee's forehead to warn the person that they had made an error. Frese and Altman (1988), in a word processing training study, found that trainees who were allowed to make errors performed better than those who were denied this opportunity.

Why then is human error such a problem in many modern industrial systems? From a human evolutionary perspective, learning took place over a lengthy time scale. Many generations of hunter-gatherers had to learn – initially through trial and error – which roots, berries and other naturally occurring plants and animals were edible and which were to be avoided. Once learnt, this important survival information was passed on to subsequent generations by word of mouth and became part of societal knowledge – i.e. known by all. Thus, trial and error learning has been functional for human evolution. Also functional was the inherent variability in human behaviour, and therefore in error making. This feature of our behaviour enabled generations to learn from a large variety of errors over a long period.

However, because of the massively harmful consequences that can sometimes result from certain types of human error, it is no longer the case that trial and error learning, or the inherent variability of human propensity for error making, is necessarily the most appropriate way of learning. As Reason (1990) notes:

> Whereas in the more forgiving circumstances of everyday life, learning from one's mistakes is usually a beneficial process, in the control room of chemical or nuclear power plants, such educative experiences can have unacceptable consequences (p.183).

Thus, in respect of complex work activities (as well as some other tasks, like driving), humans have to collapse their learning into an increasingly short period of time. During this time, the possibilities of making errors may be small, and correspondingly the opportunity to **learn** from making errors is much reduced. Thus, an important **feedback** element of the learning process may be considerably reduced.

Attempts to improve opportunities for experimental learning, including making errors and learning from them, may involve using simulators – for example as used in the civil or military aircraft industry, or in process control room operation. Managers who feel secure in their positions may be willing to let their subordinates 'learn from their own mistakes' – acknowledging the potency of this form of learning. Unfortunately, it is not possible to simulate all aspects of work behaviour or all situations in which human error might lead to disasters or other undesired consequences. Thus, it is impossible in systems which are complex and tightly coupled (linked with many other aspects of the system) to simulate all possible combinations of events (even if these are known) and which might lead to disaster, for example in the nuclear power generation industry (see Perrow, 1984 for a more detailed exposition of this point). The speed of our industrial advance has not allowed human ability to learn from making errors to keep pace so that an aspect of human behaviour, which was once functional for survival, under different circumstances can become part of a potentially dangerous system.

It should also be noted that because humans learn from their errors, they are also quite good at detecting certain types of errors and correcting them. Thus, it is likely that it will always be necessary to have humans within complex systems in order to solve problems when they arise. However, notwithstanding the necessity for humans to be located within complex systems, much of the energies of safety and risk professionals, designers and manufacturers must be devoted to attempts to eliminate, or at least to mitigate:

• the chances of human error occurring, and
• adverse effects of human errors that do occur.

For example, in the operation of complex systems, it is important that human operators have an adequate and accurate representation of what is happening in the system as a whole, or at least that part of it for which they are responsible. In a number of nuclear power plant accidents, for example Three Mile Island (Kemeny, 1979), an important aspect of the incident was that the operators did not have an accurate view of what was happening in the plant.

Categorizing human error

A first essential step towards ameliorating effects of human error within any organization is to understand it. Thus, we need to know what **type** of errors are occurring and **where** they are happening before we can begin to address them. In risk management terms, it is necessary to:

• **identify** errors;
• **assess** the risks which they pose before being able to ...
• **control** the behaviour which gives rise to errors and to ...
• **monitor** the control measures taken.

'Human error' is a term which can include a wide variety of human behaviour and therefore as a sole descriptor of an act or series of events, is not particularly useful. What is needed is a way of analysing the scope and nature of human error. There have been a number of attempts to classify human error. For example, Miller and Swain (1987) adopt an outcome-oriented approach in which errors are of:

• commission (adding or including something that should not be there);
• omission (missing something out, for example from a sequence of steps);
• selection (incorrect choice from a range of options);
• sequence (incorrect serial positioning of actions or events);
• time (too late or too early with an action);
• qualitative (not performing an action properly).

Another taxonomy of human error is that of Bryan (1989) and is shown in summary text 9.1.

Most human error classifications are likely to have some degree of validity, particularly if they are based upon a study of errors in a particular environment. Transport environments have been frequently studied in this respect. For example, Mashour (1974) found that the most frequent causes of train accidents were failures to confirm a signal, types being:

- detection errors;
- perceptual errors – especially those due to characteristics of signals;
- recognition error – problem of meaning or interpretation.

Similar categories were obtained from work by Taylor and Lucas (1991) on signals passed at danger (SPADs) in which misreading, disregard (driver didn't see signal) and misjudgement (usually involving braking failure) were primary types (Taylor and Lucas, 1991). Kellett *et al.* (1994) report results indicating that work sample tests of speed and accuracy of reactions to visual and auditory stimuli discriminated significantly between train drivers who made SPAD errors and those who did not (for a review of ability testing and other selection techniques, see chapter 6, especially pp. 149–55).

In a study of road accidents, Rumar (1985) found the most frequent human errors to be concerned with recognition (information acquisition) and decisions (information processing). Of 100 marine accidents studied by Wagenaar and Groeneweg (1987), only four did not involve human error; most were characterized by more than one error made by one or two individuals. The most frequent error types were 'false hypotheses' (incorrect assumptions about the state of things) and 'dangerous habits'.

However, while these various studies find different types and causes of human error, as Lourens (1989) notes, the allocation of 'causality' to 'human error' is problematic because there is no universally agreed classification system, also pointing out that definitions of 'human error' differ depending upon who is doing the judging. Thus, it is likely to be more useful in general to seek a classification which has a strong theoretical basis so that generic categories can be derived which will advance understanding of relevant phenomena and as a foundation for appropriate interventions across a range of circumstances.

Summary text 9.1 Taxonomy of human error (after Bryan, 1989)

- **substitution** – wrong selection due to habit intrusions;
- **selection** – among choices, not governed by habit;
- **reading** – e.g. altimeters, often a design problem;
- **forgetting** – cognitive failure, use a checklist;
- **reversal** – wrong direction, especially under stress – design issue, e.g. warning labels;
- **unintentional activation** – need controls to be locked off so that this is impossible;
- **mental overload** – fatigue, training and design could all be important here;
- **physical limitation** – e.g. due to physique, perception, design, placement, layout.

Reason (1990), in his generic error modelling systems (GEMS) follows Rasmussen's skills-, rules- and knowledge-based performance levels, which were introduced in chapter 2 (pp. 18–27, summary text 2.7 and summary text 2.11). The error types are:

- **skill-based:** unconscious, automatic actions resulting in slips (observable – at action stage) and lapses (inferred – at storage stage, e.g. memory failures); many of these being monitoring failures – either inattention or overattention;
- **rule-based:** following a series of steps and making a mistake – either applying good rules incorrectly or applying bad rules to a situation;
- **knowledge-based:** learning from the first principles – mistakes made during problem solving, for example those subject to attributional biases (chapter 3, pp. 48–56).

Reason (1990) distinguishes between these three types of errors within the GEMS decision-making sequence in which skills are accessed first, then if a problem cannot be solved using these routine level actions, rules and knowledge levels are respectively accessed until the level required to reach the solution is reached. Figure 9.1 summarizes the different error types.

Reason (1990) also distinguishes between:

1. failure of actions to go as intended, resulting in slips and lapses – i.e. **execution stage** failures (skill-based errors) which are usually readily detected;
2. failure of intended actions to achieve their desired consequences, resulting in mistakes – i.e. **planning** failures (at either the rules- or knowledge-based level) which are usually much harder to detect.

In addition, there are violations (typically at the rules-based level, but which could occur at the knowledge-based level), which Reason (1990) describes as:

deliberate – but not necessarily reprehensible – deviations from those practices deemed necessary (by designers, managers and regulatory agencies) to maintain the safe operation of a potentially hazardous system (p. 195).

As well as being subject to adherence to rules, policies and procedures, for example through selection and training processes, violations are also subject to individual differences. For example, in driving, males report more violations than females do and violation rate declines with age (Reason *et al.*, 1988).

At the skill-based level of performance (e.g. an experienced driver driving a car, a skilled operator carrying out tasks on a machine or tool at work, using computer software that you are very familiar with), according to Reason, errors result from either **inattention** to the task in hand or to **overattention** to the task (i.e. monitoring skill-based behaviours too closely – like the centipede who was asked to state which leg came after which and ended up not being able to walk!). An example of an inattention error is an omission associated with an interruption or distraction. For example, you may be interrupted by someone speaking to you in the middle of carrying out a familiar task and when you return to the task you forget where you were and miss out a step.

Usually, these types of errors are quickly spotted and corrected by the person doing the task and, even when they are not immediately seen and corrected, rarely have serious consequences.

However, occasionally, a missed step is not noticed and thus not recovered and serious consequences result. For example, a busy plant operator is about to make an important 'phone call to correct a malfunction, is interrupted by a colleague with an urgent problem just before making the call and on returning to the work station forgets to make the call until it is too late.

An example of an overattention error is a repetition of an already completed part of a task – for example a toggle switch or a valve lever which has been operated once for a sequence of events to occur, is operated a second time to end up in the wrong position. In most cases, following the sequence of tasks through will reveal such an error, but occasionally it will not and now and then serious consequences could ensue.

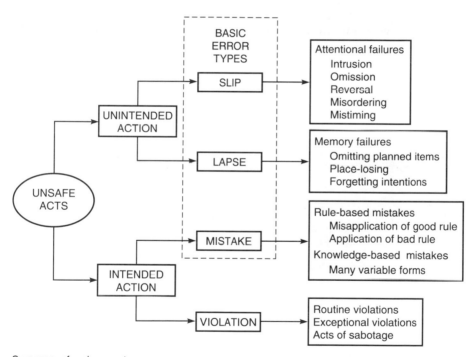

Summary of main error types:
- *slips* – skill-based, actions not as intended, perpetrator is unaware, task-execution failures;
- *lapses* – skill-based, unconscious mental errors, perpetrator may become aware of later, storage-stage (memory) failures;
- *mistakes* – rule-based or knowledge-based, perpetrator unlikely to be aware of unless deliberate (violations), planning stage failures;
- *violations* – deliberate deviations from standard practices, carried out to maintain safe operation.

Figure 9.1 Human error types (after Reason, 1990; reproduced by kind permission of Cambridge University Press and the author).

Error occurrence and detection

As already indicated, errors at the different levels are not equally likely to occur, nor are they equally likely to be detected or recovered from. A common way of designating human error probability (e.g. Miller and Swain, 1987) is:

$$\frac{\text{number of errors}}{\text{number of opportunities for error (i.e. exposure)}}$$

In numerical terms, the range of probabilities for making errors at the three levels has been calculated (Rasmussen, 1980). At the skill-based level the probability of making an error (depending on the type of task, stress level at the time, etc.) varies between something less than 1 in 10000 to something greater than 1 in 100. The comparable range for rule-based errors is between less than 1 in 1000 and greater than 1 in 10 (depending on the rules and the circumstances in which they have to be executed). At the knowledge-based level, the lower limit of the range is below 1 in 100 while at the other end the probability is 1. This means that for a novice performing certain tasks it is certain that they will fail (imagine someone who has never flown an aircraft before trying to land one unaided). These error probability ranges are summarized in figure 9.2 along with average error occurrence, detection and recovery rates given by Reason (1990) from reviews of a number of studies.

Error type	Probability of occurrence	Proportion of all occurrences	Detection rate (by perpetrator)	Recovery rate
Skills	<1 in 10 000 to >1 in 100	61%	86%	69%
Rules	<1 in 1000 to >1 in 10	27%	73%	35%
Knowledge	<1 in 100 to 1 (certain)	12%	71%	23%

(a)

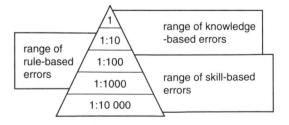

(b)

Figure 9.2(a) Error occurrence, detection and recovery rates
(after Rasmussen, 1980; Reason, 1990).
Figure 9.2(b) Probability ratios for different error types.

As far as error detection is concerned, because of the evolutionary learning function of human error, we are reasonably adept at correcting errors. A number of possibilities exist. First, there is self-monitoring – or feedback control, itself an error-prone process. Slips and lapses are more likely to be detected than mistakes are, although any type of error, unless it is detected immediately by the perpetrator, is likely to remain undetected by them. However, certain types of error are known to be particularly resistant to detection – for example, omitting steps in a calculation sequence. A second possibility is error detection by others. This is likely to be particularly helpful in respect of diagnostic errors and when the operator is under stress – for example, when driving in a strange town to a location when you are under time pressure, it is very helpful to have a companion with a map. A third possibility is that the system responds to an error in some way, for example by flagging up a warning or locking up the system until a correct response is obtained. Lewis and Norman (1986) present a number of other possible ways for systems to respond to human operator errors. A final possibility is to use a **forcing function**.

A forcing function is 'something that prevents the behaviour from continuing until the problem has been corrected' (Lewis and Norman, 1986) and is a standard way of preventing some skill-based errors from occurring, for example in the operation of machinery and plant. Forcing functions thus operate to prevent a sequence from continuing unless all previous actions have been performed correctly. Examples include interlocked guarding mechanisms (described in summary text 9.12, along with other types of guards), bolts which only fit one way and machinery which it is only possible to (re)assemble in the correct way. However, forcing functions may be seen as a challenge – a barrier to be overcome (e.g. an interlocked guard which is designed to prevent access to moving machinery or a 'deadlock' system designed to deter a would-be car thief) rather than as a safety provision. Notwithstanding this problem, it is impossible to prevent all skill-based errors by forcing functions and it is necessary to rely on the fact that:

- most are detected and corrected by the perpetrators;
- in most cases the consequences are not severe.

Where the consequences could be severe, either in safety or cost, then there are grounds for installing some form of forcing function within a system. Further illustrations of human errors at the skill-based level, with examples are given in summary text 9.2.

From the descriptions outlined in summary text 9.2, it will be clear that outcomes of most cases of human error will be benign – that is, they will result in no more than trivial or temporary annoying conditions. Thus, as inherently error-prone systems, humans will not be strongly motivated to avoid errors in most situations because the costs of seeking error-free performance (for example, loss of speed in using a computer) will not be off-set by the benefits derived. In any case, checking routines (e.g. spell checks in word processors, formulae checks in spreadsheets and logic checks in databases) can now be built in to most automated systems. Also, as noted earlier, a vital component

Summary text 9.2 Types of skill-based errors (after Reason)

Repetitions – an action carried out more than the required number of times, for example a toggle switch which is pressed one more time than is required may be annoying if you find that you have typed the last two lines of text on your word-processor in capitals, but could be critical if it is a design fault in at two-handed control on a power press.

Wrong objects – actions carried out in relation to the wrong object. It may be very inconvenient if you have brought your reading spectacles by mistake to the conference session where you are sitting at the back and cannot see the presenter's poorly prepared slides, but bringing the wrong spectacles to a job which requires precision engineering for safety to be ensured could result in more than mere inconvenience for those ultimately affected. Another case involved an elderly woman's daughter mistaking a super glue dispenser for her mother's eye drops, with excruciatingly painful results for the poor old lady.

Intrusions – unintended actions are incorporated into a sequence of behaviour (sometimes called errors of commission). These usually take the form of **strong habit intrusions** in which one sequence is 'captured' by another, perhaps more familiar sequence. Thus, adding sugar to your tea when you only take sugar in coffee may result in a displeasing taste, although adding water to concentrated acid in the belief that you are dealing with a different chemical could leave more than a nasty taste in the mouth!

Omissions – intended actions are left out of a sequence of behaviour. Forgetting to pack your personal organizer for a business trip could result in embarrassment; forgetting to check the setting before replacing the grinding wheel could result in a bad accident.

Reason (1984) summarizes error data on action slips as follows:

1. Slips of action most likely to occur in relation to familiar things in familiar surroundings.
2. Preoccupation/distraction associated with error.
3. Up to 40% of absent-minded slips involve strong habit intrusions.
4. More specific situations in which strong habit intrusions are likely include:
   - change of goal demands departure from well-established routine;
   - changed circumstances require modifications to an established action pattern;
   - when a familiar environment is entered in a reduced state of 'intentionality' (attention not remaining fixed on what you intended to do);
   - when features of our present circumstances contain elements common to those in highly familiar environments.
5. Other classes of action slips are:
   - place losing errors – mostly omissions and repetitions;
   - blends and reversals – 'crosstalk' between two currently active tasks.

of learning is to make errors and use the feedback on our performance to adjust subsequent behaviour, i.e. error-making is essential for us to learn. Problems arise when the consequences of our errors are severe and it is on such occasions that the design of automated checking systems is necessary. In exploring the links between everyday lapses and those which have resulted in some catastrophic accidents, the difference usually lies in a unique **combination** of factors (which often include errors) and an unforgiving environment (Reason and Mycielska, 1982).

The middle level of performance is rule-based, which involves behaviour in which we follow a series of steps in a conscious fashion. This contrasts with skill-based behaviour where we are operating on 'automatic pilot' and remain essentially unconscious of the skilled behaviour. Examples of rule-based behaviour include: following instructions in the assembly of some machine (or piece of self-assembly furniture) which we have not previously encountered, carrying out a series of diagnostic checks on some plant using a checklist, driving to a novel location using a road map or set of instructions. Each of these behaviours involves a set of rules which need to be followed for the desired outcome to be achieved.

According to Reason, there are two types of error which might occur during rule-based behaviour – either good rules may be applied wrongly or bad rules may be applied. Examples of the latter include instructions which are incomplete, difficult to understand or ambiguous. In this case, the 'human error' may be attributable to the party who prepared the rules, or to the fact that there are no effective rules, as well as to the person(s) executing the action. For example, the Kegworth air crash pilots followed the 'trial and error' rule for determining which engine had failed (Department of Transport, 1990). The feedback which they received gave the appearance that the problem had been solved, whereas the problem had been exacerbated as the wrong engine was shut down. The rule was a bad one and the consequences were disastrous. A summary of events preceding the crash is given in summary text 9.3.

Although there are other documented cases of aircraft crashes which have resulted from pilots shutting down the wrong engine (Reason and Mycielska, 1982) these are sufficiently rare for the rule not to have been challenged. Thus, opportunities to learn from such occurrences – and thereby to improve the safety of systems such as civil airlines – are lost if attributions are made exclusively to 'human error' on the part of the pilots. Reason (1990) explains that in a world which has both regularity and uncertainty, people tend to gamble in favour of high frequency alternatives (e.g. events that we know have happened before) and that this is generally an adaptive – i.e. successful, strategy. However, like any gamble, there is always a downside.

An obvious way of countering the possibility of bad rules within a system is to review all rules systematically at intervals. However, in complex systems with large numbers of rules and procedures, this may be a gigantic task, particularly when the systems to which the rules apply and therefore the rules themselves, are continually changing. The cost-effectiveness of undertaking such an exercise needs to be carefully considered. A first step is to ascertain the extent of the problem, i.e. find out what proportion of human error results from the application of bad rules. If it transpires that this is significant then a review of rules and procedures may be desirable.

The other type of rule-based error is incorrect application of good rules. Again, this may occur in various circumstances, one instance of which is information overload. This might result in operator stress and, as for skill-based behaviour, an important step in a sequence may be omitted or two steps reversed. During emergencies, there is usually additional pressure on

Summary text 9.3 Summary of the Kegworth air crash

On 8 January 1989 at 20.25 a British Midland Boeing 737-400 series crashed into a bank alongside the M1 motorway at Kegworth, just short of the East Midlands Airport runway. A total of 47 passengers died from their injuries and most of the remainder who were on board suffered serious injury.

The active failure was that the flight crew shut down the No. 2 engine after a fan blade had fractured in the No. 1 engine. This engine subsequently suffered a major thrust loss due to secondary fan damage after power had been increased during the final approach to land. Factors which affected the incorrect response of the flight crew included:

- symptoms of engine failure – heavy vibration, noise and smell of smoke were outside their training and expertise;
- previous experience of vibration gauges on other planes – which, unlike the 737-400 gauges, tended to be unreliable;
- secondary position of the vibration gauges and absence of any warning light or labelled 'danger zone';
- lack of familiarity with the automatic fuel system which meant that when the healthy No. 2 engine was throttled back, the automatic fuel system was shut off thereby resulting in a normal flow to the damaged No. 1 engine, persuading them that they had (by trial and error) correctly identified the defective engine;
- no cabin crew or passengers who could see the flames emanating from the No. 1 engine, informed the flight crew which engine was involved. The flight crew had no means of seeing which engine was faulty and their instruments gave no strong clue that the No. 1 engine was faulty, even when No. 2 engine had been shut down.

When the flight crew were about to review the action they had taken, they were interrupted by messages from flight control and did not return to the review process. Although the flight crew were primarily blamed for the crash, other contributory factors were:

- the design, manufacture and inadequate testing of the engine – a new design;
- inadequate training on the new aircraft;
- inadequate procedures for determining which engine to shut down;
- position and display features of critical instruments.

Source: Department of Transport, 1990.

operators – for example in the form of large number of alarms going off, as at Three Mile Island (Kemeny, 1979), with the operators being unable to deal with them all satisfactorily.

While skill-based behaviour errors are usually revealed immediately, because of rapid feedback, it is much more difficult to diagnose rule-based errors because the consequences may not be obvious. Thus, it is much more difficult to control situations which result from the misapplication of rules which in themselves are satisfactory, but which may be misapplied for various reasons – in the extreme case in the form of violations. Violations are deliberate breaches of rules, which may be justified by those in charge of a system on the grounds that it is necessary to test the safety of the system. Such a violation was among the factors characterizing the Chernobyl disaster (Munipov,

1991 and the two outline descriptions of this incident in chapter 7 – summary text 7.5 and summary text 7.12).

Summarizing the two types of errors discussed so far, those at the skill-based level are referred to as either slips (actions not as intended of which the perpetrator is aware) or lapses (unconscious mental errors such as forgetting to do something – which the perpetrator may become aware of at some later time). Errors at the rule-based level are referred to as **mistakes** and occur at the **planning** stage of a task or sequence of events. In contrast, **lapses** occur at the **storage** stage – putting something into memory so that it is accessible when we need it, and **slips** are a result of failure at the **execution** stage – doing something which we did not intend. Both these are examples of errors which result in **active** failures – it is usually clear what has gone wrong and who is involved. A more insidious type of error results in **latent** failures – those which exist within an organization or system until triggered by some event.

Latent failures occur at the third level of human error, which is the most important of all from a total potential loss point of view, and this is the knowledge-based level. The knowledge-based level of performance is the one at which we first learn a task – for example the new worker on his or her first day in a workplace has to learn about the new environment, the learner driver who sits in the driving seat for the first time, or our efforts to solve a novel problem – all illustrate knowledge-based learning. Here, opportunities for error are considerable because we are often trying out things for the first time – for everything we know we have had to go through this learning stage.

An example of the type of error which can occur at this level is over-confidence that we have selected and performed the correct action when in fact we have not done so. For example, if several people have made an input to a problem to be solved, then the group is more likely to be confident of the situation than is an individual acting alone who arrives at the same solution. This particular type of error – 'groupthink', is described in chapter 7 (pp. 189–92), especially summary text 7.11). It may occur when a group of like-minded people with similar backgrounds and interests tackle a problem – they are likely to see the problem in similar terms and arrive at similar conclusions, especially if unchallenged from outside (a characteristic of groupthink). Antidotes to this particular type of error-prone behaviour were also reviewed in chapter 7 (summary text 7.13 and summary text 7.14).

Thus the distinction drawn by Reason (1990) between **active** and **latent** errors is useful. The former are generally made by front-line operators, e.g. pilots, drivers, control room staff and machine operators. The latter are perpetrated by those whose activities are removed in time and space from operational activity – e.g. designers, decision-makers and managers. Latent errors pose the greater threat to the safety of complex systems. In particular, the more removed individuals are from the front line, the greater is their potential danger to the system. Mason (1992) identified the following examples of latent failures:

- poor design of plant and equipment;
- ineffective training;
- inadequate supervision;
- ineffective communications;
- uncertainties in roles and responsibilities;
- management failure to provide adequate safeguards.

Summarizing the two types of failures:

- **active failures** – proximal and not recoverable;
- **latent failures** – distant but recoverable – usually hidden within an organization until triggered by some event, hard to detect, likely to have serious consequences.

In addition to these two types of failure, there are also triggering events or circumstances which could, in combination with active and latent failures, produce a serious accident. Reason (1990) likens such triggering events to 'resident pathogens' within the human body, which when combined with other agents – e.g. stress, emergencies, organizational change – result in accidents or even large-scale disasters. Resident pathogens are most likely in complex, interactive, tightly coupled, opaque systems (Perrow, 1984). For example, a resident pathogen in the human body might be a predisposition to cancer. A latent failure could be smoking and the active failure, developing cancerous cells.

As individuals behaving at the knowledge-based level we make assumptions about a new task or problem to the extent that we infer that it is like some other task or problem with which we are familiar. We might focus our attention on certain features of it and ignore others – which might be very important. For example, we might assume that a new car, a different control panel or a novel flightdeck, is sufficiently similar to the one we last used that our behaviour in respect of it can safely remain unchanged. Because of the great diversity of knowledge-based learning, the potential for human error at this level is considerable and is the most difficult to correct.

Because most forms of work activity involve behaviour at all three levels (skills, rules and knowledge), errors can be compounded. Nearly all disasters involve errors of various types – typically three or four in combination, whose coming together could not reasonably have been foreseen (Perrow, 1984). Examples include the sinking of the ferry ship the *Herald of Free Enterprise* (Department of Transport, 1987) and the Kings Cross Underground station fire (Department of Transport, 1988). Brief summaries of the human factors components of these accidents are given respectively in summary texts 9.4 and 9.5.

Error reduction strategies

As general strategies for reducing human error, Sanders and McCormick (1987) identify training, selection and design approaches. Training was considered in chapter 2 (see in particular, pp. 23–7) and selection to a limited

---

Summary text 9.4 Sinking of the ferry ship *Herald of Free Enterprise*

On 6 March 1987, the roll on/roll off passenger/freight ferry, *Herald of Free Enterprise* sailed from Zeebrugge inner harbour at 18.05. The ship capsized rapidly about 23 minutes later, just after it had left the confines of the harbour: 188 passengers and crew were killed and many others were injured.

It was revealed that both inner and outer bow doors had been left fully open and that water entering the ship through the doors had resulted in the capsize. The most immediate cause was that the assistant bosun, whose job it was to close the doors was asleep in his cabin, having just been relieved from maintenance and cleaning duties. His immediate superior, the bosun, had seen that the bow doors were still open, but did not close them as he did not consider this to be his duty.

The chief officer, responsible for ensuring that the bow doors were closed was also required to be on the bridge, 15 minutes before sailing time. He thought he had seen the assistant bosun going to close the doors. There was pressure from management on the first officer to sail early (15 minutes), to avoid delays. Company procedures appeared to require 'negative reporting' only – i.e. unless informed to the contrary, the master assumes that all is well. The chief officer had not made such a report on this occasion.

Despite repeated requests from the masters to the management, no bow door indicators were available on the bridge and the master was unaware that he had sailed with the bow doors open. It was also the case that the design of the ship was inherently unstable, once water entered. Thus, it may be seen that a combination of factors or 'human errors' – individual, management and design, combined to produce the disaster.

Source: Department of Transport, 1987; Reason, 1990.

---

extent in chapter 6 (pp. 149–55). As illustrations of selection criteria to reduce errors, Sanders and McCormick (1987) suggest perceptual and intellectual abilities and motor skills. However, they caution three provisos:

1. that it is possible to identify the skills and abilities required (for example, using task analysis – see pp. 275–7);
2. that reliable and valid tests exist to measure these abilities;
3. that there is an adequate supply of qualified people.

Of the design approach, Sanders and McCormick (1987) note the following alternatives:

- **exclusion** design – makes it impossible to make errors;
- **prevention** design – makes it difficult (but not impossible) to make errors;
- **fail-safe** design – reduces consequences of errors (without necessarily affecting their likelihood).

Other alternatives, such as the use of procedural checklists, depend upon the operator actually using the checklist correctly on every required occasion. Overall, Sanders and McCormick (1987) consider that the design approach is usually the most cost-effective as it only has to be done once, whereas selection, training and other solutions require continuous maintenance and support. Lourens (1989) is among other authors who commend the primary means of reducing slips through improved equipment and job design. As

---

Summary text 9.5 Kings Cross Underground station fire

On 18 November 1987 at 19.25, a discarded match or cigarette end (most probable cause) set fire to grease and rubbish on the Piccadilly line ascending escalator running track. Running tracks were not regularly cleaned because of ambiguous responsibilities. Smoke detectors were not installed on cost grounds and water fog equipment was infrequently used due to rust problems.

A booking clerk is alerted to the fire by a passenger (at 19.30), although only four of the 21 station staff on duty at the time had received any training in evacuation or fire drills. At 19.34, railway police evacuate passengers via an alternative escalator, although no evacuation plan existed for the station and no joint exercises had been conducted between London Underground staff and the emergency services.

A relief inspector, not regularly based at Kings Cross and without any fire training, enters the upper machine room at 19.38 but cannot get close enough to the fire to use a fire extinguisher and does not activate the water fog equipment.

At 19.39, police in ticket hall begin evacuation of area and request that trains on Piccadilly and Victoria lines do not stop at Kings Cross, although trains continue to stop there. At 19.41, metal gates to ticket hall are closed by police and soon after, first fire engines arrive. At 19.45, flashover occurs and the whole ticket hall in engulfed in intense heat and flame: 31 people are killed and many others are seriously injured.

The tragedy is aggravated by the lack of evacuation plan, escape routes blocked by locked doors and metal barriers, outdated communication equipment, no access to station public address system by headquarters controller, non-functioning of cameras and TV monitors, lack of public address system on trains and absence of public telephones at the station.

A combination of factors resulted in a disaster made worse by a variety of behaviours and circumstances.

Source: Department of Transport, 1988; Reason, 1990.

Sanders and McCormick (1987) note, it is 'easier to bend metal than to twist arms'.

Comparable error reduction strategies are recommended by Mason (1992), who uses Reason's error typology, and these are outlined in summary text 9.6. In general terms, the way to reduce or minimize knowledge-based performance errors – which, like rule-based errors are also mistakes because they occur at the planning stage of behaviour – is in principle for the organization or individual to become an effective learner. What this means for organizations is that they should develop systems which enable them to identify and control errors – at all levels. This has also been found to be an important feature of safety culture (Ryan, 1991) and means that the organization must be able to respond appropriately to human error occurrences. An outline example of how such a programme could operate in principle is outlined in summary text 9.7.

It is important that such an exercise – the examples in summary text 9.7 are but illustrative – is carried out in an open way, that all employees have an opportunity to become involved, and that it is – and is perceived to be – quite separate from any element of blame, i.e. that it is most definitely not linked with any form of disciplinary procedure. This may be quite difficult for an

Summary text 9.6 Error reduction strategies (after Mason, 1992)

To reduce **slips and lapses**:
• design improvement route is most effective, plus training.

To reduce potential for **mistakes**;
• training – team and individual, overlearning, refreshers; duplication of information, clear labelling, colour coding.

To reduce **knowledge-based** errors:
• hazard awareness programmes, supervision, work plan checks, post-training testing.

To reduce **violations** address:
• motivation, underestimation of risk, balance between perceptions of risks and benefits, supervision, group norms, management commitment.

Summary text 9.7 Identifying and controlling errors within organizations

1. Institute a system for reporting and recording all near miss incidents on a sample basis – e.g. for a fixed period of time (e.g. using 'human error diaries' in which all human error incidents are recorded).
2. Analyse the incidents recorded in an objective way to establish antecedents (direct causes or other relevant circumstances) – e.g. by interviewing personnel to follow up reported incidents.
3. Involve personnel at all levels within the organization in a continuing improvement programme to address the issues revealed by the exercise. This in itself should be a joint problem-solving exercise which should address a further important aspect of safety culture – that of shared perceptions of goals at all levels within an organization and the promotion of effective communication.
4. The resulting change should be controlled and monitored by top management as a continuing exercise so that the organization develops and maintains a positive focus on safety issues – another important aspect of safety culture. In this way, management will be seen to be committed to safety, including the reduction of human errors which occur through its own decision-making processes.

For managers wishing to take the management of human error seriously, Lourens (1989) recommends the following steps for instituting a programme for safety:

1. create a human factors database on incidents and accidents;
2. reassess operators' performance regularly;
3. study operators' habits during routine activity;
4. introduce computer-based displays of information to provide unambiguous signs;
5. in group tasks, be aware of risk-enhancing factors in interaction (e.g. 'risky shift' and groupthink – chapter 7, pp. 189–92).

---

organization which has a tradition of seeking disciplinary measures as a response to what are frequently labelled as 'human error failures', but is essential for organizational learning in health and safety (and in other areas) to occur. Change in this area may not happen rapidly, especially where there is a legacy of mistrust to overcome. However, the success of those organizations which achieve accident rates significantly below their industry averages shows what can be achieved over time.

It is unsurprising to an extent that organizations seek to allocate blame to individuals for making errors when typically we often make comparable judgements in respect of our own errors, thinking ourselves as 'careless' or 'stupid' for having made mistakes. Individual factors in error liability are considered next.

Individual differences in error liability

It is worth considering human error within the context of some individual factors discussed in earlier chapters, particularly in chapters 6 (on personality) and 8 (on stress). For example, could there be an error-prone personality? Broadbent et al. (1982), using their Cognitive Failures Questionnaire (CFQ), report evidence to indicate that liability for absent-minded errors (e.g. opening the wrong door) is a feature of the make up of some individuals. Where it exists, it is likely to be associated with, for example memory lapses (e.g. forgetting where you left something) and lack of attention (e.g. not noticing something). Reason and Mycielska (1982) report studies which indicate a link between error-proneness and the obsessionality personality trait (as measured by a version of the Middlesex Hospital Questionnaire – an instrument developed for primary use in clinical settings to measure various personality traits) – which could be related to the conscientiousness dimension of the 'big five' (chapter 6, pp. 147–9). Thus, the more obsessive an individual is, the lower is their propensity to make errors. There are also reported links between greater error rates and trait anxiety and neuroticism (chapter 6, pp. 140–9 and 155–61) as well as with external locus of control (chapter 8, pp. 223–4).

Broadbent et al. (1982) also note that general vulnerability to stress is related to error-proneness, and it is known that high levels of stress can increase the likelihood of human error (e.g. Marshall, 1978). That there is an association between individual proneness to cognitive failures and increased vulnerability to stress is accepted (Broadbent et al., 1986; Reason, 1988). However, Reason (1990) argues that it is not so much that stress induces a high cognitive failure rate, but rather that certain cognitive styles can lead to **both** absent-mindedness **and** inappropriate matching of coping strategies to stressful situations. Reason and Mycielska (1982) consider that this is also related to the amount of attentional capacity which we have available to deal with stress after other matters have been dealt with.

Thus, there is strong evidence for individual differences in error proneness, which could be a new factor or dimension associated with one or more existing personality traits. First, it is known that there are stable individual differences in minor cognitive failures. Second, a high incidence of slips and lapses is associated with increased vulnerability to stress. It seems that the same general control factor which determines error liability is also involved in coping with adverse effects of stress (chapter 8, pp. 219–24).

Reason and Mycielska (1982) consider that coping strategies which are based upon increasing our capacity to pay attention through focusing upon the relaxation response can reduce errors as well as alleviate stress. For example, meditation could be an antidote both to stress and to mental predisposition to errors, such as lapses, lack of attention and absent-mindedness. An alternative is hypnosis, which like meditation, involves controlling our attention and physical relaxation (see chapter 8, pp. 224–32).

HUMAN FACTORS

Ergonomic principles

The subject which addresses issues of the human–system interface is ergonomics – also known as human factors or human engineering. Major writers in the area consider human factors and ergonomics to be synonymous (e.g. Salvendy, 1987; Sanders and McCormick, 1987). Oborne (1994) describes human factors as a 'sister discipline' to ergonomics and considers ergonomics to be a way of looking at the world. In this section (and in the book as a whole), 'human factors' and 'ergonomics' are used interchangeably.

In addition to considering the human–system interface, ergonomics is also concerned with the study of:

- human dimensions (anthropometry) and other characteristics (cognitive – e.g. spatial ability, as well as physical – e.g. height);
- the working environment and its effects upon humans;
- effects of systems of work upon humans.

In its applications, ergonomics (or human factors) seeks to:

- design equipment and the working environment so as to match human capabilities to ensure effective operation and to optimize working and living conditions;
- enhance the effectiveness and efficiency of work and other activities, for example by increasing convenience, reducing errors and increasing productivity;
- design work systems so that requirements for human physical and mental well-being are sustained;
- enhance certain desirable human values, for example safety, reduce fatigue and stress, and increase comfort, user acceptance, job satisfaction and quality of life (Sanders and McCormick, 1987).

Failure to apply these principles successfully in workplace design has consequences both for the system and for individuals. The work system will become less efficient over time and individuals are likely to suffer health impairments such as psychological stress (chapter 8).

Successful application of ergonomic principles, as well as improving efficiency and productivity, is a primary means of reducing workplace risks arising from hazards to health and safety. This is essentially done by reducing or eliminating opportunities for human operators to produce error within the work system, while retaining the necessary degree of control to overcome system errors should they occur. Thus, appropriate delegation of function to people and machines is a fundamental aspect of ergonomic design. The basic question to ask is: 'Should a person or a machine be doing this job? This issue is addressed next.

Human and machine performance

To help designers to answer questions about 'who does what' within systems, ergonomists have considered **allocation of function.** An early attempt to identify key aspects of the respective performances of human beings and machines was postulated by Fitts (1951). This was later amended by Singleton (1971), as shown in summary text 9.8.

Summary text 9.8 shows that there are some aspects of performance that human beings are best at and other things in which machines (e.g. computers) are superior. When designing systems, the ideal is to allocate to humans those activities which they perform best (e.g. problem-solving) and to assign to machines the things which they are best at (e.g. computational speed). Other

---

Summary text 9.8 Comparison of human and machine capabilities for allocation of function (Fitts' list, amended by Singleton, 1971)

Property	Human capacity	Machine capacity
Speed	Inferior	Superior
Power	Two horse power for ten seconds	Consistent at any level
Consistency	Not reliable, needs to learn, subject to fatigue	Ideal for: routine, repetition, precision
Complex activity	Single channel, low throughput	Multi-channel
Memory	Large store, multiple access, best for principles, strategy	Best for literal reproduction and short-term storage
Reasoning	Good inductive, easy to re-program	Good deductive, tedious to re-program
Computation	Slow, subject to error, good at error correction	Fast, accurate, poor at error correction
Input	Wide range and variety of stimuli dealt with by one unit (e.g. eye); affected by: heat, cold, noise, vibration, etc.; good: pattern detection, very low signals, signal in noise	Some outside human senses (e.g. radioactivity); insensitive to extraneous stimuli; poor pattern detection
Overload	Graceful degradation	Sudden breakdown
Intelligence	Can adapt, anticipate, deal with unpredicted/unpredictable	None, cannot switch goals or strategies without direction
Dexterity	Great versatility and mobility	Specific

ergonomists have produced similar types of lists (see for example Chapanis, 1961; Bekey, 1970; Murrell, 1971; Kantowitz and Sorkin, 1987 and, for an evaluation of the potential of such lists, Price, 1985). Chapanis (1965) cautions using such lists, regarding them as generalizations. He argues for considering the system as a whole, including issues such as cost-effectiveness and trade-offs (e.g. in design). It has been argued that when designing a system, it is more useful to think in terms of **complementarity** and to consider the best combination of human and machine in the light of criteria such as flexibility and consistency (see for example Meister, 1985; Kantowitz and Sorkin, 1987). Sanders and McCormick (1987) also argue that allocation of function is not straightforward, and outline a general strategy which includes a team approach to discussing human factors in system design, so as to take account of different viewpoints – an approach already espoused in chapter 7 (pp. 189–92). Their guidelines are shown in summary text 9.9.

In applying the principles underlying allocation of function, it is important to recognize that machines or computers should not be employed simply to deskill human tasks but, in line with ergonomic principles, to support and enhance human capabilities. Thus, as increasing numbers of routine, repetitive and dangerous jobs become automated, this should be seized upon as an opportunity to release people not only for the tasks and jobs for which their strengths suit them (e.g. decision-making, problem-solving) but also for those which are more psychologically fulfilling.

In considering the 'ironies of automation', Bainbridge (1987) notes that while machines may be used to replace unreliable and inefficient human operators, designers' errors also make a significant contribution to accidents (pp. 246–60 on latent errors). In automated plant, operators have to monitor events, despite the fact that humans are poor at this type of function (summary text 9.9) and thus alarms are needed – i.e. more automation. Bainbridge (1987) points out that while humans are very good at long-term decision making and problem-solving, they do not perform these functions well under stress.

It is interesting and instructive to compare characteristics of human performance with those of automated systems. Summary text 9.8 and summary text 9.9 show general characteristics of human behaviour, but within such general human limitations, there are considerable variations in performance. For example, while most adults require seven to eight hours' sleep per night, some individuals require at least nine or even ten hours' sleep, while others can manage on five or fewer hours. Over a lifetime, these individual differences can make a considerable difference in performance capacity. Chapter 6 reviews individual differences in personality, while humans also differ in a wide range of other characteristics. Age and experience are often highly correlated in respect of job or task activity, so it is usually difficult to separate out the effects of one or another of these variables, for example as they relate to accident involvement. However, studies which have investigated this issue (e.g. Hale and Hale, 1986) have on balance concluded that it is lack of experience (on a particular job or task) which is the more important factor. Thus,

---

Summary text 9.9 Allocation of function (after Sanders and McCormick, 1987, p. 526)

Humans are generally better at:
- sensing very low levels of stimuli – e.g. visual, auditory, tactile, olfactory, taste;
- detecting stimuli against high-noise level backgrounds – e.g. blips on DSE displays with poor reception;
- recognizing complex patterns of stimuli which may vary between presentations – e.g. objects in aerial photographs, speech sounds;
- remembering (storing) large amounts of information over long periods – better for remembering principles and strategies than a lot of detailed information;
- retrieving relevant information from memory (recall) frequently retrieving many related items (but low recall reliability);
- drawing upon varied experience in making decisions and adapting decisions to situational requirements; acting in emergencies (don't require re-programming);
- selecting alternative modes of operation if certain modes fail;
- reasoning inductively and generalizing from observations;
- applying principles to solutions of varied problems;
- making subjective estimates and evaluations;
- developing entirely new solutions;
- concentrating upon the most important activities when required to by overload conditions;
- adapting physical responses to variations in operational requirements (within reasonable limits).

Machines are generally better at:
- sensing stimuli outside the normal range of human sensitivity – e.g. x-rays, radar wavelengths, ultrasonic vibrations;
- applying deductive reasoning – e.g. recognizing stimuli as belonging to a general class;
- monitoring for prescribed events, especially infrequent ones;
- storing encoded information quickly and in substantial quantity;
- retrieving coded information quickly and accurately;
- processing quantitative information when so programmed;
- performing repetitive actions reliably;
- exerting considerable physical force in a highly controlled manner;
- maintaining performance over extended periods;
- counting or measuring physical quantities;
- performing several programmed activities simultaneously;
- maintaining efficient operations under conditions of heavy load and distractions.

---

there are important implications in this finding for training and supervision of inexperienced workers.

Experienced workers also make errors and have accidents, but the type of errors which they make tend to be different from those of novices and different strategies therefore need to be applied to their safety – for example, in respect of training as outlined in summary text 2.12. Novice workers are more likely to make errors because of a lack of knowledge of a task, procedure or process (e.g. that one should not add sodium to water, that there is a requirement to use a registered ladder to carry out a job or that a certain period of time has to elapse before a decontaminated building can be entered). Experienced workers on the other hand, generally know these sorts of things but remain liable to errors which relate to exercising their skills. For example, a skilled fitter or electrician is still liable to slips and lapses (pp. 244–61), while other factors such as fatigue or stress resulting from pressure to complete work on time (a factor in the Clapham rail crash – see Department of Transport, 1989 and summary text 9.10 for a brief summary of the human factors aspects) may also result in errors. Occasionally, these will culminate in fatal accidents. Individuals to a certain extent adapt to adverse physical environments such as temperature extremes or high noise levels, but such physical stressors nevertheless take their toll in respect of long-term deterioration in individual physical and psychological health.

Effects of stress on performance were outlined in chapter 8 (summary text 8.4). Disruptive stress can increase the probability of error by a factor of between two and five (Swain and Guttman, 1983) while higher levels of stress can result in even more degradation. Stress may be imported from other environments – for example the home (e.g. ambulance drivers – see Glendon and Glendon, 1992). It is known that people whose jobs involve driving (e.g.

Summary text 9.10 Clapham rail crash

A collision occurred between the 18.18 Basingstoke to Waterloo train, the 06.14 Poole to Waterloo train and a train of empty coaches south west of Clapham Junction Station at about 08.10 on 12 December 1988. Thirty-five people were killed and many others injured.

A new signal had malfunctioned, so that the second train was not prevented from occupying the same track as the earlier one and failing to stop the front of the second from running into the back of the first. The driver of the first train had seen the signal change from green to red as he passed it, and was obliged to stop and report the SPAD. He could not have known that the signal was faulty and that following trains had not also been stopped.

The immediate cause of the faulty signal was false feed of current from an old wire in the Clapham Junction relay room. This situation was the result of electrical work done on two separate occasions within the previous two weeks. On the first occasion, the senior technician responsible for the work made basic errors in not cutting back the old wire but merely bending it away. His work was not inspected by the supervisor, who was involved in other work. The second job, undertaken coincidentally by the same senior technician, compounded the initial error as the old wire reverted to its original position when a new relay was being installed.

However, the inquiry also identified responsibility among many other parties who had allowed a situation in which such errors could be made and remain undetected when such work was inspected, tested and commissioned back into service. The supervision and monitoring of poor working practices was criticized for its inadequacy. Malpractice was found to be widespread, indicating a lack of adequate staff training. Management were criticized for 'incompetence, ineptitude, inefficiency and failure' (p. 73). Lessons from previous incidents had not been learned and it was concluded that 'concern for safety was permitted to co-exist with working practices which ...Were positively dangerous'. This unhappy coexistence was never detected by management and so the bad practices were never eradicated' (p. 163). Ninety-three separate recommendations were made.

Source: Department of Transport, 1989.

HGV or PSV drivers) – already a potentially stressful type of work activity – may be subject to additional stress from domestic and other problems (see for example, Selzer and Vinokur, 1974; Gulian *et al.*, 1990). Financial worries or other concerns may also impact adversely upon work activities, particularly if support is not readily available.

INTERFACE DESIGN

The fundamentals of interface design may be identified as:

- take account of human limitations;
- fit the task to the human operator;
- reduce/eliminate possibilities for human error.

The human–machine interface may be represented in diagrammatic form, as in figure 9.3. Figure 9.3 shows that the display elements, representing 'communication' from machine to the human and the control elements – 'communication' from operator to machine – are part of a rapid feedback loop. Human limitations which need to be taken account of by the ergonomic designer are outlined in summary text 9.11.

Fitting tasks to human operators

Although human beings are extremely flexible and often willing to endure adverse working conditions, there is a price to pay in terms of health and safety – either long-term or short-term – for not insisting that the starting point for any design process should be human limitations – such as those outlined in summary text 9.11. For example, in designing machinery, physical operation of the machine as well as systems of work, potential for operator

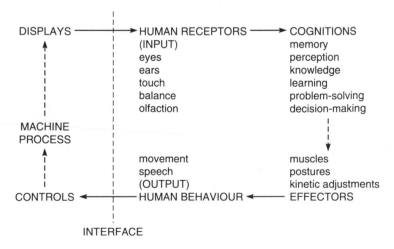

Figure 9.3 The human–machine interface (after Mackay and Whittington, 1983).

Summary text 9.11 Human limitations to be taken account of by designers

- **Sense organs** (receptors) – e.g. vision – the operator should be able to read easily controls, instruments and displays to prevent fatigue.
- **Interpretation** – information received must be organized so that the human information processing system can easily understand it – e.g. it must not overload the operator's short-term capacity or make undue attentional demands.
- **Posture** – all work processes and systems of work should be designed to allow postures to remain comfortable and to minimize strain; siting and position of controls and displays is important here.
- **Layout** – of the working area should allow adequate movement between operating positions, safe access and egress and unhindered oral and visual communication with others.
- **Comfort** – environmental factors, particularly lighting, ventilation and relative humidity, should provide for maximum operator comfort.
- **Workrate** – movements which are too fast or too slow induce fatigue, repetitive movements are particularly liable to produce adverse physical effects (e.g. WRULD); there should be variety in work rate; if people are working under stress imposed by time constraints, emergency conditions or other pressures, then they are more likely to make mistakes.
- **Fatigue** – design should take account of operator fatigue and the likelihood of mistakes being made; although humans can adapt their performance to compensate for fatigue, errors and accidents are more likely towards the end of a work shift or work period.
- **Stress** – may be physical (as a result of noise, vibration, temperature extremes, etc.) or psychological (e.g. resulting from unrealistic deadlines and other work pressures) – see also chapter 8, summary text 8.21.

---

error and routine maintenance must be considered (Morgan *et al.*, 1963). A starting point might be to consider principal causes of injury associated with machinery operation – see Booth *et al.*, 1988 and summary text 9.12.

The ergonomics of machinery design should take account of:

- procedures for job loading and removal;
- systems for changing tools;
- safe removal of scrap and waste material;
- routine maintenance procedures;
- emergency breakdown procedures;
- potential unexpected movement, failure or start-up;
- safe access to and egress from the area;
- operating space;
- risks to others passing through the area.

Because humans do not have the physical or cognitive capacity to resist the variety of risks from operating machinery, the accepted way of protecting them is from a range of appropriate guards or safety devices – summary text 9.13.

Summary text 9.12 Summary of principal causes of injury associated with machinery

- **Entrapment** – especially from in-running nips where a moving belt or chain meets a roller or toothed wheel or where revolving gears/toothed wheels, rollers or drums meet. Other entrapment hazards are reciprocating traps – encountered in the vertical and horizontal motion of machines like presses, and shearing traps – resulting from transverse movement as in a guillotine effect.
- **Entanglement** – (of loose clothing, hair, limbs, jewellery, etc.) risk may exist wherever there are unguarded rotating shafts, drills, chucks, or other rotating parts.
- **Direct contact** – with either fixed or moving parts of machinery – e.g. protruding parts, sharp corners, hot surfaces, jagged or sharp edges.
- **Ejected material** – particularly flying particles such as metal or plastic, but also larger projectiles such as machine parts or even grinding wheels.

Source: BS5304: 1988 Code of practice for safety of machinery.

Summary text 9.13 Types of machine guards and safety devices

Guard types – designed to prevent access to operators and others
- **Fixed** – preventing access to the danger, such as belt drives or other transmission machinery.
- **Adjustable** – for different operations, for example sawing or planing.
- **Distance** – to keep the hazard out of reach – e.g. barriers or tunnel guards.
- **Interlock** – having a movable part connected with the machine controls so that the dangerous parts cannot be set in motion until the guard is closed, the power is switched off and the motion braked before the guard can be opened so as to allow access to the dangerous part. Access to the danger point is denied while the danger exists.
- **Automatic** – associated with and dependent upon the machinery mechanism, operating to remove physically from the danger any part of the human operator – e.g. power presses.

Machinery safety devices – protective appliances designed to reduce or eliminate danger prior to human access
- **Trips** – designed to prevent or minimize injury – the device (which may be mechanical, photo-electrical, ultrasonic or pressure sensitive) actuates on an approach by a person beyond the safe limit of working machinery and stops the machine.
- **Two-handed controls** – require both hands to operate the machine controls, providing protection from danger to the operator's limbs.
- **Overruns** – used in conjunction with a guard to prevent access to parts which move by their own inertia after the power supply has been interrupted. The principle may be based either on rotation sensing or braking.
- **Mechanical restraint** – applying mechanical restraint to dangerous machinery which has been set in motion owing to the failure of machine controls or other parts (examples include pressure die-casting machines).

Source: BS5304: 1988 Code of practice for safety of machinery.

Ergonomic applications to reduce human error potential

Because there is potential for human error at different points in the human–machine interaction process, different considerations will apply in the task of reducing the potential for human error as a component of accident causation. Using figure 9.3 as a basis for error-reduction strategies, the remainder of this section identifies the points at which errors are possible and outlines guidelines for reducing the likelihood of such errors.

1. *The display/human receptor interface.*   This is one aspect of the traditional 'knobs and dials' aspect of ergonomics on which much research has been undertaken. Common requirements in interface design are likely to involve correct choice of a particular type of machine display – for example, as in a display panel, which should be based upon its function as far as the human operator is concerned and the nature of the task which is to be performed. Different types of displays are best suited to different tasks, as shown in figure 9.4 and summary text 9.14.

From figure 9.4, it may be seen that if precision is the most important feature of the task, then a digital scale would be used, whereas if rate of change is more important, then a moving pointer (analogue) scale would be best. In many cases, a trade-off has to be made because there is more than one requirement – perhaps one for error minimization and a different one for efficiency, in which case a compromise might be the moving scale. There are also non-quantitative aspects of tasks which require different types of displays. These are summarized in summary text 9.15. Other factors which are important in control design are shown in summary text 9.16.

Pertinent information about certain features of a person's immediate environment is provided by visual displays. For example, there are several displays in a car which provide the driver with information. The windscreen is an example of a real-time display from which the driver obtains visual information concerning the speed of the car on the road and positions of other vehicles. One reason why drivers fail to adjust their speed in foggy conditions is that they lose much of this visual information and thus, valuable feedback on their performance (chapter 2, pp. 15–23). Another display is the instrument panel which provides information about the internal functioning of

Display	Reading ease.	Precision.	Detect rate of change.	Set to reading.
Digital	+ + +	+ + +	–	+
Moving pointer	+	+	+ + +	+ + +
Moving scale	+	+	+	+

+ + + very good; + adequate; – poor

Figure 9.4 Acceptability of quantitative displays (after Grandjean, 1980).

Summary text 9.14 Respective merits of analogue and digital displays

Function	Analogue display	Digital display
Quantitative readings	Best if precise reading is not required or if task has predictive or checking components	Best for accurate reading of slow changing values; poor if task includes predictive or checking components
Qualitative readings	Best for warnings, checking and prediction; useful to have visually coded areas	Poor
Setting and tracking	Best	Poor

Summary text 9.15 Functional characteristics of qualitative displays (after Grandjean, 1980)

Display	Functional characteristic
Auditory	Attract immediate attention – as in an alarm
Visual	Represent a number of states, e.g. using different colours
Representational	To provide the operator with a model of the system – best for showing spatial or temporal relationships between system elements

---

Summary text 9.16 Factors important in control design (after Murrell, 1971; Oborne, 1994)

- **feedback** – e.g. to body or sense organs;
- **resistance** – to guard against inadvertent operation of control;
- **size** – relative to force required for operation;
- **weight** – relative to operator's position;
- **texture** – issues of slip, grip and glare;
- **coding** – e.g. colour, up to a maximum of about eleven;
- **coding by shape** – simple forms better than complex ones;
- **coding by texture** – e.g. coins, need to have many distinguishing features;
- **coding by size** – minimum 20% difference between each – shape or texture usually better;
- **coding by colour** – needs to be **seen** by the operator;
- **location** – e.g. foot pedals in a car;
- **nature of task** – e.g. design of instruments and displays;
- **compatibility** – e.g. spatial, between displays and controls.

the car, as well as its relationship with the road environment. A moving pointer has been found to be most suitable for showing speedometer readings (Feldman, 1971).

Integrating audible sounds with visual displays can improve performance monitoring, particularly when visual displays only were used previously. An auditory display acts as a warning device which conveys qualitative information. For example, a smoke detector emits an audible sound when there is smoke in the vicinity or a wheel bearing in a machine is deteriorating and the sound emitted tells an operator that something mechanically is wrong.

In contrast, quantitative information, such as a numerical reading telling us the speed at which a car is travelling, is normally associated with a visual display. However, quantitative information can also be communicated through the auditory mode (e.g. clock chimes or Morse code), while a visual display can provide low order qualitative information – for example a temperature gauge which gives a 'hot' or 'cold' reading.

2. *Human cognitions.*   We are now in the realm of cognitive ergonomics – that branch of ergonomics which is concerned with the representation of systems in the human mind and human understanding of those systems. Systems design therefore needs to go beyond the traditional 'knobs and dials' aspects and consider cognitive processes in relation to understanding machine or process inputs. Different cognitions require different approaches, depending upon where the potential for misunderstanding and error is likely to occur. This might be:

- **knowledge** – dependent upon experience and education and therefore cannot readily be improved in the short-term; a lengthy induction period required;
- **problem-solving ability** – to an extent associated with knowledge and experience, but can be trained for specific types of problems, e.g. those that are rule-based;
- **memory** – related to experience but can be massively compensated for by provision of information in appropriate format – e.g. log files on a computer, print-outs of previous system states, etc. as required;
- **perception** – related to understanding the system and having an accurate representation of it (chapter 5), can be trained (chapter 2);
- **decision-making ability** – combines the above cognitions and is dependent upon experience and judgement.

Notwithstanding the advantages already noted (summary text 9.8 and summary text 9.9) of humans making decisions, they are still subject to a number of biases, analogous with attributional biases reviewed in chapter 3 (pp. 189–92) and of groupthink, discussed in chapter 7 (pp. 48–56). Biases relevant to decision making were identified by Wickens (1984) and are shown in summary text 9.17.

Because of individual differences in the range of cognitive abilities outlined above, selection procedures may play a part in increasing the chances that a

---

Summary text 9.17 Biases in decision-making (after Wickens, 1984)

- Greater weight given to early compared with later information (primacy effect);
- Less information is extracted from sources than should be;
- Subjective odds for two alternatives are poorly assessed;
- More information makes people more confident but not necessarily more accurate;
- We tend to seek more information than we can absorb adequately;
- We tend to treat all information as equally reliable – it isn't;
- We are only able to consider a maximum of three or four hypotheses at a time;
- We tend to focus upon a few critical attributes and choices at a time;
- We tend to seek information supporting chosen actions and to avoid testing or disconfirming evidence;
- A potential loss is seen as having greater consequences than a gain of the same magnitude and thus exerts more influence on decision-making;
- We have an optimistic bias which favours less extreme outcomes. This results in the order of perceived likelihood of outcomes shown below:

Most likely   *Least likely*
mildly +ve;   highly +ve;   mildly –ve;   highly –ve

---

suitable person will be obtained. In deciding whether to select or to train for a particular job, the decision sequence shown in chapter 2 (summary text 2.2) may be of use. Principles of training were considered in chapter 2 (pp. 15–23), while some aspects of selection were briefly reviewed in chapter 6 (pp. 149–55).

3. *Carrying out the required movements.*   Here a wide range of human movements may be required in an almost infinite variety of combinations. In seeking to reduce human error, design factors need to take account of:

- **muscle fatigue** – either from continuous strain, cold, over-exertion or repetitive movement, any of which can lead to error;
- **awkward postures** – the possibility of unnatural postures should be designed out of the system;
- **kinetic adjustments** – some skilled jobs require these to a fine degree (e.g. 'shoe makers' dance' – attributed to complex movements required to operate shoe-making machinery), even life-preserving in the case of lumberjacks and some other jobs (chapter 5, pp. 110–11 gives a description of the kinaesthetic sense); generally, design of machines and processes should allow for a solid base for the human operator;
- **skills limitations** – resulting from innate abilities, personal disposition and training received.

4. *The display/control interface.*   In reading displays or operating controls, an important consideration is expectation or stereotype (inbuilt expectation). For example, in the UK people expect a switch in the 'up' position to mean 'off', while in the USA the 'up' position means 'on'. Similarly, we normally

turn knobs clockwise to increase power, light, current, etc. An insightful and occasionally amusing account of people's ways of approaching and thinking about everyday things is given by Norman (1988). Summary text 9.18 shows directions of movement stereotypes for controls. However, stereotypes or movement compatibilities do not always apply (Petropoulos and Brebner, 1981). For example, in releasing fluid (e.g. water, gas) under force, we turn taps anticlockwise to increase the flow. Violations of our expectations of what should happen increases the chances of errors being made. Under the stress of an emergency, poor design could increase the probability of an error by up to 1000 times (MacKay and Whittington, 1983). Common deficiencies in interface design are identified in summary text 9.19.

Research has shown that different types of controls are better for different types of activities or tasks. MacKay and Whittington (1983) summarize much of the work in this area and figure 9.5 is derived from their summary.

As with display devices, there may be design trade-offs in controls for a given system. However, functions, expectations and performance characteristics should be a good guide to ergonomic principles of control design. Taking controls and displays together, probably the most important single critical aspect is compatibility between these system components. Compatibility refers to the extent to which relationships are consistent with

---

Summary text 9.18 Direction of movement stereotypes for controls

Function	Control movements
On	Down, right
Off	Up, left
Right	Clockwise, right
Left	Anticlockwise, left
Up	Up, rearwards
Down	Down, forwards
Retract	Rearwards, pull, anticlockwise, up
Extend	Forwards, push, clockwise, down
Increase	Right, up, forwards
Decrease	Left, down, rearwards

Summary text 9.19 Common deficiencies in interface design

For displays	For controls
Not there!	Inaccessible
Give correct information	Too difficult to operate
Unreliable (therefore ignored)	Operable accidentally
Not (readily) visible	Contrary to convention/stereotype
Not legible (e.g. poorly illuminated)	Incompatible with displays
Contrary to convention/stereotype	Inadequately differentiated (confusing)
Inadequately differentiated	
Information irrelevant (causes confusion)	
Incompatible with controls	

Control type	Performance characteristics rating for:			
	Speed	Accuracy	Force	Range
Push button (hand)	+ +	0	– –	– –
Toggle switch	+ +	0	– –	– –
Select switch	+	+	0	+
Knob	– –	+ +	0	+
Thumbwheel	– –	+ +	0	+
Small crank	+ +	–	– –	+
Large crank	+ +	– –	+ +	+ +
Handwheel	–	+ +	+	+
Horizontal lever	+ +	–	–	–
Vertical lever	+ +	+	+ +	+ +
Keyboard	+ +	+	0	–
Push button (foot)	+	0	– –	– –
Foot pedal	+ +	–	+ +	– –

+ + good; + moderate; – poor; – – very poor; 0 not applicable

Figure 9.5 Performance characteristics of different types of controls (after Mackay and Whittington, 1983).

human expectations. In systems which are compatible, learning and reaction time is faster, fewer errors are made and user satisfaction is higher (Oborne, 1994). However, some compatibilities are stronger than others – i.e. some expectations are shared by a higher percentage of the population than others. Thus, it may be necessary to violate one compatibility relationship in order to take advantage of another (Bergum and Bergum, 1981). Relationships between displays and controls should be standardized where possible, and be logical and explicable. If there are no standards or obvious relationships, then empirical work should be conducted to match user expectations. A summary of compatibilities is given in summary text 9.20.

To conclude this overview of ergonomic applications, Pheasant's five ergonomic fallacies (Pheasant, 1988) are a reminder of the problems that those seeking good ergonomic design features may encounter:

- design is OK for me and therefore OK for everybody;
- design is OK for 'average' and therefore OK for everybody;
- people are adaptable and variable so need not/cannot cater for this in design;

Summary text 9.20 Compatibilities between displays and controls (after Oborne, 1994)

- **spatial** – e.g. control knobs and display dials lined up;
- **movement** – e.g. clockwise rotation of knob to increase something;
- **cognitive** – what is expected from the user in terms of what can be done – e.g. linguistic, memory, perceptual;
- **mobility** – better to use auditory presentations and vocal response for vocal task; for spatial task, better to use visual presentation and manual response (Wickens *et al.*, 1983);
- **conceptual** – e.g. does the symbol seem to represent something we are already aware of – e.g. an outline airplane to represent an airport.

- purchases are made on the basis of style not design, so ignore expensive ergonomic applications;
- ergonomics is intuitive/common sense, so data are not needed.

TECHNIQUES FOR REDUCING HUMAN ERROR/INCREASING HUMAN RELIABILITY

This section considers a small sample of techniques which have been used in various types of workplaces to reduce human error and to increase human reliability. In this section, we shall first consider task analysis as the basis for many human error reduction approaches, before proceeding to consider three techniques based upon task analysis: Task Analysis For Error Identification, Predictive Human Error Analysis and Quantitative Human Reliability Assessment.

Task analysis

Task analysis is a formal methodology, derived from systems analysis, which describes and analyses performance demands made upon humans in the system. The goal is to achieve integration of human and machine components of the system (see earlier discussion on allocation of function on pp. 262–4). There are a number of texts on task analysis (see for example: Annett and Duncan, 1967; Annett *et al.*, 1971; McCormick; 1976a; Patrick *et al.*, 1980; Drury, 1983; Shepherd, 1985; Drury *et al.*, 1987; Kirwan and Ainsworth, 1992). Many varieties of task analysis exist – over 80 are listed by Astley (1991). Figure 9.6 gives a general overview of typical stages in the process of using task analysis.

While task analysis itself is not a technique for reducing human error or for improving human reliability, some form of task analysis is the basis for many other techniques which have this aim. Therefore, it is appropriate to devote some space to describe a major task analysis technique and to give an example of its use.

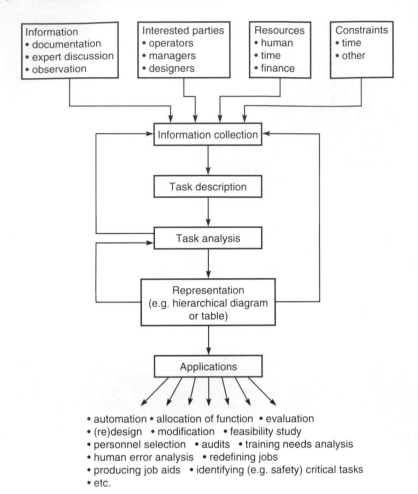

Figure 9.6 Stages in task analysis.

Task analysis is based upon the principle that the task is the basic unit of behaviour at work (or elsewhere). Task performance is described in terms of its goals and the plans needed to achieve these goals. One of the most commonly used forms of task analysis is Hierarchical Task Analysis (HTA). HTA begins with a statement about the overall goal of the task and at each level these goals are analysed in more detail, forming a hierarchical structure. Tasks are represented by operational statements indicating that an action (or a series of actions) is carried out to achieve the task goal.

The main operation is broken down into its constituent sub-tasks or subordinate operations, typically between two and six. The process continues until each task is broken down into its component sub-tasks until the level of detail required is reached. In deciding upon a suitable criterion for stopping the task breakdown process, reference is made to the application(s) planned for the task analysis – see figure 9.6 for examples of some of these. For example, in using task analysis as a basis for defining errors with the aim of finding ways of reducing these, the analysis would proceed to the point at which separate human actions could be identified at which errors were possible – see example of the HTA in figure 9.7.

In the task analysis, all tasks are uniquely numbered for identification, using hierarchical serial numbers. As an illustration of a hierarchical task analysis, figure 9.7 shows part of a task analysis for a high voltage switching operation. Plans indicate the sequencing of operations as well as other features, for example constraints, alternatives and conditions. Plans are specified for each superordinate task which is broken down into sub-tasks. Sub-tasks which require no further breakdown are underlined to indicate this. Many variations and enhancements on this basic approach are possible, including the use of a tabular format.

HTA is the basis for both qualitative and quantitative forms of human reliability assessment (HRA). Examples of qualitative HRA – Task Analysis for Error Identification and Predictive Human Error Analysis – are described in the next two sub-sections. A generic form of quantitative HRA is considered in the third sub-section.

Task Analysis for Error Identification (TAFEI)

The Task Analysis for Error Identification (TAFEI) technique takes a systematic approach to human error occurrences in relation to particular operational sequences. The method, developed by Baber and Stanton (in press), extends the psychological approach to human error (e.g. Reason and Mycielska, 1982; Reason, 1990) into the applications area. TAFEI treats the human in the system as an active (cognitive) interpreter of stimuli and uses the notion of 'affordances' – in which the appearance of an object defines its use. For example, a handle is for pulling, a plate (e.g. on a door) is for pushing and a knob is for turning. Baber and Stanton's approach is an ergonomic one in that design (of machines, layout, etc.) is seen as the key to producing clarity in respect of the correct procedure to perform. It is appropriate to use TAFEI in closed systems where humans interact with equipment which has a finite number of possible states which can all be defined.

Like practically all attempts to deal with human error from a human factors perspective, TAFEI is based upon task analysis, in this case hierarchical task analysis (HTA). TAFEI can be used when humans operate within systems in a relatively fixed location – for example an individual operating a piece of equipment or machinery. The TAFEI methodology has five stages:

1. define components and media;
2a. describe the human components using HTA;
2b. describe other system components using a system state diagram (SSD);
3. map 2a onto 2b to define 'legal' transitions;
4. define 'illegal' transitions as possible or impossible and in terms of error types;
5. (re)design systems to reduce errors.

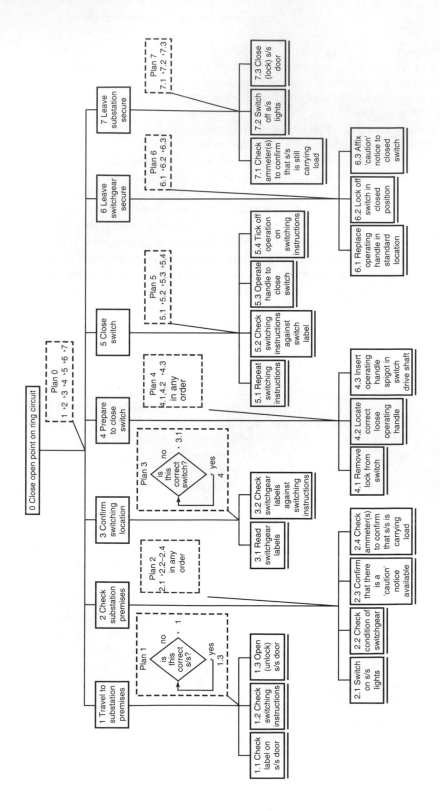

Figure 9.7 Hierarchical task analysis of part of a high voltage switching sequence.

To show how TAFEI could be used, we shall continue with the high voltage switchgear task sequence example described in figure 9.7. Figure 9.8 shows the system state diagram (SSD) corresponding with the operations described in figure 9.7. The SSD shows the state of the system corresponding with each of the first 6 main steps in the task analysis shown in figure 9.7. Also shown on the SSD (figure 9.8) is the expected next action – indicated by a line (called a transition) from one system to the next.

From the SSD, it is possible to derive a transition matrix (figure 9.9), showing the six stages represented by the SSD, indicating which transitions are impossible (e.g. because of forcing functions or other system features) and which are possible. Of those that are possible, some will be 'legal' transitions – i.e. following the laid down procedure or acceptable versions of it. The remainder will be 'illegal' transitions because while they are possible, they are undesirable because they would cause the system to malfunction – i.e. would be classed as errors. At least some of the illegal transitions will be violations, although the TAFEI analysis may reveal other illegal transitions which had not previously been considered by the system designers or operators.

The transition matrix shown in figure 9.9 reveals that it is possible to go directly from stages two to either of stages four or five and that other moves also represent 'illegal' transitions. Thus, these transitions would represent the potential for error at this human–machine interface. The complete list of possible errors, based upon the transition matrix in figure 9.9, is shown in figure 9.10. Such an analysis allows these potential errors to be identified as a first step to redesigning the system to eliminate them or to reduce either their likelihood or occurrence or their consequences should they occur – i.e. to reduce the risk from human error.

The TAFEI technique can thus provide a useful picture of interactions between human operators and machine components within a system in respect of possible actions and possible errors. From the information gleaned from such an analysis, possible errors which are critical to the safe and efficient operation of the system may be tackled, usually by redesign of the system – e.g. equipment and/or rules and procedures.

Predictive human error analysis

This technique, developed by Embrey (1994), typifies a systematic approach to the identification and reduction of human–error potential in systems in line with a risk management approach, effectively taking the form of a human error risk assessment. The purpose of Predictive Human Error Analysis (PHEA) is to identify human interactions within a system that are likely to give rise to human errors with potentially serious consequences. Four main objectives may be identified:

- representing operations performed by people in human–machine systems;
- determining what can go wrong;
- assessing consequences for the system;
- generating strategies to prevent error or to reduce the impact of error.

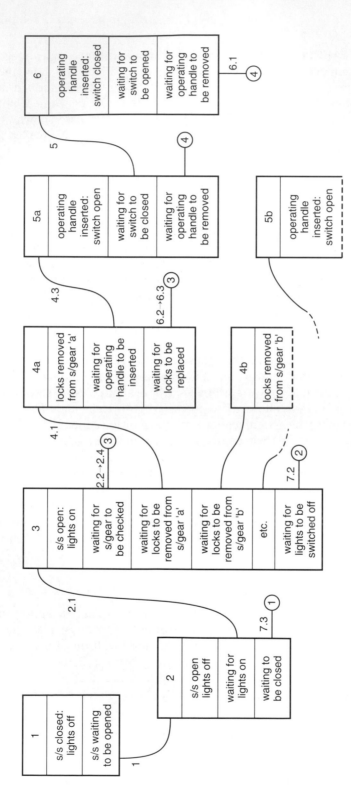

Figures on lines refer to the HTA activities in figure 9.7. Figures in circles indicate that when the activity has been completed, the system returns to the state number indicated by the figure.

Figure 9.8 System State Diagram (SSD) for switchgear operations in a substation.

Steps in the task analysis (figure 9.7) which also
correspond with the stages in the SSD (figure 9.8)
are shown on both axes of the transition matrix

States to

States from		1	2	3	4a	4b	5a	5b	6a	6b
	1		L	—	—	—	—	—	—	—
	2	L		L	I	I	—	—	—	—
	3	I	L	(I)	L	L	—	—	—	—
	4a	I	I	L		I	L	—	—	—
	4b	I	I	L	I		—	L	—	—
	5a	I	I	I	I	I		—	L	—
	5b	I	I	I	I	I	—		—	L
	6a	I	I	I	L	I	I	—		—
	6b	I	I	I	I	L	—	I	—	

L legal transitions;   I illegal transitions;   — impossible transitions

Figure 9.9 Transition matrix for TAFEI.

PHEA can be used in the design of new products and systems so that human
machine mismatches which are likely to lead to errors are identified and eliminated at the design stage. It can also be used in risk assessments in which the
prediction of human intentions and actions which may initiate, compound or
resolve a critical system state is vital. PHEA can also be used in accident
investigation, where the cause(s) of human error(s) need to be determined so
that effective error reduction strategies can be devised and implemented.

The PHEA technique has five main stages:

1. problem definition;
2. task analysis;
3. human error analysis;
4. consequence analysis;
5. development of error reduction strategies.

The problem definition stage requires consideration of types of human
interactions within a system which could lead to accidents or incidents. These
could be either active or latent failures and include:

- maintenance/testing errors affecting safety system availability;
- operator errors initiating an incident;
- recovery actions by operators which can terminate an incident;
- errors by operators which can prolong or aggravate an incident;
- actions by which operators can restore unavailable systems.

No.	Transition	Error description
1	2–4a	Remove lock from s/gear 'a' without putting light on
2	2–4b	Remove lock from s/gear 'b' without putting light on
3	3–1	Leave light on in substation
4	3–3	Recursive activity – could forget to check s/gear
5	4a–1	Leave substation without replacing locks
6	4a–2	Leave substation without replacing locks
7	4a–4b	Remove lock from wrong switchgear
8	4b–1	Leave substation without replacing locks
9	4b–2	Leave substation without replacing locks
10	4b–4a	Remove lock from wrong switchgear
11	5a–1	Leave s/s with handle still inserted and switch open
12	5a–2	Leave s/s with handle still inserted and switch open
13	5a–3	Leave handle still inserted and switch open
14	5a–4a	Remove handle before closing switch
15	5a–4b	Remove lock from wrong switchgear
16	5b–1	Leave s/s with handle still inserted and switch open
17	5b–2	Leave s/s with handle still inserted and switch open
18	5b–3	Leave handle still inserted and switch open
19	5b–4a	Remove lock from wrong switchgear
20	5b–4b	Remove handle without closing switch
21	6a–1	Leave substation with handle still inserted
22	6a–2	Leave substation with handle still inserted
23	6a–3	Leave handle still inserted
24	6a–4b	Open lock on other switchgear before locking off
25	6a–5a	Open switch again
26	6b–1	Leave substation with handle still inserted
27	6b–2	Leave substation with handle still inserted
28	6b–3	Leave handle still inserted
29	6b–4a	Open lock on other switchgear before locking off
30	6b–5b	Open switch again

Figure 9.10 Errors identified from TAFEI.

The task analysis stage uses HTA, as described above and illustrated in figure 9.7. The human error analysis stage takes the output from the task analysis and uses it as a basis for determining the types of error which could occur at each point. This stage uses a classification system based upon six categories of errors, shown in summary text 9.21. The classification is applied to each task step in turn and feasible errors identified.

Consequence analysis requires detailed knowledge of the system and its functioning and seeks to determine system consequence of human errors identified at the previous stage. Where consequences are negligible, there is no requirement to proceed further with the analysis, but where they are unacceptable the information goes forward to the next stage. At this stage also, the possibility of errors being recovered at future task steps is considered. For a task step where no recovery is possible and severe consequences are likely, particular attention needs to be given to the possibility of an error (low, medium or high – on the basis of empirical data on incidents, near misses or accidents for example, or from expert judgement). The error can then be classified as critical or non-critical. Critical errors with a high probability require high priority attention. An example of one step from the

Summary text 9.21 Human error analysis – error categories

Planning errors – associated with performing a sequence of actions:
• plan preconditions ignored,
• incorrect plan executed,
• correct but inappropriate plan executed,
• correct plan executed too soon/too late,
• correct plan executed in wrong order.

Action errors – associated with performing observable actions:
• operation too long/too short,
• operation mistimed,
• operation in wrong direction,
• operation too little/too much,
• misalignment,
• right operation on wrong object,
• wrong operation on right object,
• wrong operation on wrong object,
• operation mistimed,
• operation incomplete.

Checking errors – associated with performance checks:
• check omitted,
• check incomplete,
• right check on wrong object,
• wrong check on right object,
• wrong check on wrong object,
• check mistimed.

Retrieval errors – associated with retrieval of information from memory, paper or screen:
• information not obtained,
• wrong information obtained,
• information retrieval incomplete.

Information communication errors – associated with communicating information to, or receiving information from, other parties:
• information not communicated,
• wrong information communicated,
• information communication incomplete.

Selection errors – associated with a selection from alternatives:
• selection omitted,
• wrong selection made.

task analysis shown in figure 9.7 being subjected to a human error analysis is shown in summary text 9.22.

A further analysis may also be undertaken of 'performance influencing factors' (PIFs) – more commonly called 'performance shaping factors'. These are factors which increase or decrease the likelihood of human errors, and include:

Summary text 9.22 Human error analysis example (step 5.2 of task analysis in figure 9.12)

Task step	Error made	Description	Consequences	P	C	Recovery	Remedy
5.2 Check switching instructions against switch label	Wrong check on wrong object	Checking against wrong label	If on wrong switch incorrect switching could occur	M	!	None	Final check of switch label against instruction(p) Reinforce sequence during training(t) Improved labelling(d)

The first column, *Task step,* is taken from the task analysis.

Column 2, *Error mode,* refers to the error from the list given in summary text 9.21.

The *Description* column indicates the precise nature of the error in this particular case.

The *Consequences* column indicates what could happen as a result of the error.

The *P* column indicates the probability of such an error occurring (L = low; M = medium, as in this case; H = high).

The *C* column is left blank unless the error is critical, in which case – as here – an exclamation mark is inserted to indicate that the error is critical. Critical errors are defined according to system characteristics – in this case, if the probability is at least medium, the outcome is serious and there is no possibility of recovery at any future step, as shown in the *Recovery* column.

The final column – *Remedy* – indicates the remedies which are available to deal with this particular error. In this case, there are procedural (p), training (t) and design (d) remedies identified, these being the main three categories of interventions in respect of human error correction.

- corporate factors (e.g. management, financial pressure, safety audits – chapter 10);
- process factors (e.g. technology, workplace hazards);
- machine interface factors (e.g. controls, displays, compatibilities – pp. 269–71);
- environmental factors (e.g. work patterns, physical conditions);
- equipment factors (e.g. PPE, tools, plant);
- individual factors (e.g. experience, knowledge, personality, health).

The above are all factors which can affect human performance, some external to the individual (e.g. equipment design, work environment, rules and procedures) and others internal (e.g. skills, motivation, experience). Information from the PIF analysis can be used to determine which errors are most likely and help in the development of error reduction strategies. In a study of performance shaping factors affecting errors in high-voltage switching, Glendon *et al.* (1994) found a total of eleven factors affecting performance. The most important factor was 'work pressure', followed by 'procedures' and 'work relationships'.

Quantified human reliability assessment

Reliability is the probability of successful performance. Human reliability and machine reliability together comprise system reliability. Human reliability is the complement of human error, and has recently received increased attention from researchers and practitioners. Reviews of the field include those by Meister (1984), Williams (1985), Humphreys (1988), Health and Safety Commission (1991) and Kirwan (1994). This attention is unsurprising, given the importance of human beings in many complex systems.

Quantified Human Reliability Assessment (HRA) attempts to quantify the probability of human errors occurring in specific operations, but without any theory of why such errors occur – i.e. it is a behavioural rather than a cognitive approach to human error. HRA draws upon a wealth of experience and expertise using expert judgement and quantified analysis in making predictions about human error potential. The various HRA techniques use different combinations of expert judgement and database material to assess human reliability in situations where the probability of an error may be small but where the consequences of such errors could be catastrophic and expensive. Examples of industries where HRA may be appropriate include: power generation and distribution, chemical and other process industries and other sectors involving high risk (e.g. mass transport systems or places where large numbers of people are exposed, as at mass leisure events).

HRA is analogous with Probabalistic Risk Assessment (PRA), used to assess hardware reliability. The objective of HRA, like PRA, is to arrive at a risk assessment which can be used as a basis for control measures to be implemented which will reduce either or both the probability of human errors occurring, or if such errors do occur, to mitigate their consequences. HRA models task sequences which are then combined mathematically to determine the error probability of the whole task. It is a useful diagnostic tool in assessing detrimental effects of humans on systems, involving the following steps:

- task analysis;
- estimation of number of errors – from empirical and/or expert judgement data;
- combine the above with error probabilities for machinery and equipment, for example in a fault tree or an event tree.

The methodology of HRA involves identifying points in a sequence of tasks or operations at which human error could lead to loss – either in the form of life or limb or material damage – usually on a large scale, for example of nuclear power plant. A commonly used HRA technique – Technique for Human Error Rate Prediction (THERP) – was developed mainly to assist in determining human reliability in nuclear power plants. THERP uses detailed procedures for analysing a task and applying tables of human reliability estimates to determine the overall reliability of the task. For descriptions of THERP and other HRA techniques, see Swain and Guttman (1983), Miller and Swain (1987), Health and Safety Commission (1991), Kirwan (1992a,b).

Summary text 9.23 Illustrative performance shaping factors (PSFs) (after Miller and Swain, 1987)

Internal PSFs

Emotional state	Skill level
Intelligence	Social factors
Motivation/attitude	Strength/endurance
Perceptual abilities	Stress level
Physical condition	Task knowledge
Sex differences	Training/experience

External PSFs
Inadequate workspace and layout
Poor environmental conditions
Inadequate design
Inadequate training and job aids
Poor supervision

The next stage is to assign probabilities to each of the identified potential errors, either on the basis of empirical data or whatever other evidence is available – past events, expert judgement, etc. This aspect of HRA is the most problematic because probability judgements often have to be made on inadequate data. Other aspects of the risk equation are then considered – numbers at risk, exposure time and potential consequences (worst possible case). These are weighted and combined with the probability ratings for the various possible errors to arrive at a risk rating for each task or operation. These may then be rank ordered to produce a list of items requiring control measures. The resulting scale, if reasonably valid for the tasks being considered, will provide a good measure of the **relative** importance of the risks and hence of the priorities for action.

It is important that the control measures component of the risk management sequence are implemented as part of the HRA approach. Control measures may be categorized as being either ergonomic – relating to workplace layout, the environment or to the human machine interface for example; procedural – relating to work system elements, including management and organizational factors (chapter 10); or individual – relating to the people undertaking those tasks or operations. These latter are sometimes referred to as 'performance shaping factors' (PSFs) – very much the same as the performance influencing factors (PIFs) used in the PHEA technique described above. Examples of PSFs are shown in summary text 9.23. According to Miller and Swain (1987), PSFs include any factor that influences human performance. PSFs may be internal to the individual or external – relating to the environment. Of these two types, external factors are considered to have the greater impact (Miller and Swain, 1987). Most of the PSFs listed in summary text 9.23 are discussed in various places in this book.

To reduce errors using HRA techniques, as well as training, supervision, selection and design control measures, it is important to use employee participation – this is true for all the techniques described. Those who work with the equipment and who commit the errors are most likely to have ideas about preventing them. It is important to conduct such analyses in a blame-free environment, accepting worker representatives as part of a quality team.

There have been criticisms of the human reliability approach, for example that:

- human behaviour is so variable that a single estimate cannot be assigned to it (Meister, 1985) and thus an illusory level of precision is given to human variability;
- not all errors result in failure (Adams, 1982);
- it is inappropriate for continuous tasks such as monitoring and tracking (Regulinski, 1971);
- despite being based upon expert judgement, it is a subjective approach requiring interpretation (Sanders and McCormick, 1987).

Like most of the techniques in the human reliability field, HRA is still in its infancy and requires more testing and experience before it is widely accepted and used as a tool for assessing human reliability in complex systems. Nevertheless, it can provide useful data for guiding decision-making on risk (Meister, 1985).

CONCLUSIONS

Because of its evolutionary function, human error is a natural and all-pervasive component of our being. While a small proportion of errors may result from unconscious needs or motives, the overwhelming basis for error-related behaviour is cognitive. An important task for safety and risk professionals, and other parties such as line managers, is to control the worst effects of human error upon workplace losses through ergonomic, managerial and human resource applications.

Errors are essential for learning because of the feedback that they provide. There is evidence that we learn best if we are allowed to make errors. The same principle applies to organizations – we should not blame people for making errors, but accept these as a natural human feature and develop systems to learn from them.

Many accidents and incidents are attributed to 'human error'. However, if a large proportion (say 80% or 90%) are so attributed, the term becomes little more than a convenient label – which may actually serve to hinder attempts to investigate a complete range of factors associated with accidents.

Through research and applications, understanding of human error and its control is rapidly increasing and is amenable to workplace implementation. One of the main barriers to this implementation, which is also one of the potentially damaging forms of human error, is that which resides within systems. Forms which it might take include: poor rules and procedures, inability of an organization to learn from its own and others' mistakes and inadequate management decision-making.

A first step is to categorize types of human error – ideally a generic classification is needed so as to be relevant to the widest possible range of situations

– that derived from skills-, rules- and knowledge-based performance levels has been shown to be valid and useful. However, empirically-based classifications derived from particular environments (e.g. different forms of transport) should also be used as these are likely to reflect actual problems encountered in that environment.

Major catastrophes are very difficult to guard against because they typically involve a combination of factors, any one of which by itself would probably not cause a serious problem. It is necessary to address underlying factors, in particular latent failures and 'resident pathogens' in systems. These relate to organizational structures, high-level decision making and features which could trigger a major accident.

Humans will continue to be needed as monitors of complex systems (despite their poor monitoring capacity compared with machines) because they are very good at detecting errors and at taking effective action to resolve problems. A basic principle is to ensure that humans and machines monitor one anothers' actions. In the allocation of functions between people and machines, it is important to consider not only the respective advantages of the performance of each type of system component, but also the nature of the total system design and the fact that humans require work which will be personally fulfilling.

There is strong evidence for stable individual differences in error propensity which seem to be linked to cognitive style. This incorporates coping with stress and appears to be to do with self-control. (chapter 8, pp. 224–32) and attentional spare capacity.

There is a variety of techniques available for human error reduction, based upon task analysis and systematic approaches to identifying potential sources of human error and its correction.

PART FOUR
Directions For Action

10 MANAGING HUMAN RISKS

❏ This chapter opens the final part of the book and provides a context for managing features of human behaviour discussed in earlier chapters. A broad framework is provided in the consideration of safety management systems, followed by a discussion of safety culture. Attention turns next to the measurement of management performance in health and safety, before a detailed review of one type of measurement – safety auditing and briefer reviews of some other techniques. The topic of risk management is then addressed before a final strategic overview through a human resource management perspective.

INTRODUCTION

It is frequently stated that management should manage health and safety risks with the effectiveness and commitment with which they manage other functions. For example, the HSE (1991) consider that safety management is part of sound management. It could be argued that such risks should be managed **better** than other functions. This chapter overviews selected components of managing health and safety which are included within risk management, a topic which encompasses broad principles and criteria (for example, Bamber, 1990). In selecting topics for inclusion in this chapter, we have considered the book's primary orientation towards managing human, rather than technical aspects of risk, as well as featuring emergent aspects of managing such risks. Thus, for example considerable space is devoted to the topics of safety auditing and risk assessment as these are central components of managing risks related to human activities. For more comprehensive reviews of risk management and risk analysis, the interested reader is invited to refer to Cox and Tait (1991) or Dickson (1991).

Managing human risks is one component of managing all risks, for which an integrated strategy is required. From a broadly strategic perspective, this chapter considers the topics of: safety management systems, safety culture, measuring management performance in health and safety, safety auditing and other techniques, risk assessment and human resource management. The first two topics of this chapter – safety management systems and safety culture – set the scene for the next four sections which are concerned with measuring and evaluating risk in various ways. The penultimate section on human resource management offers a possible framework for managing risks arising from human activity.

SAFETY MANAGEMENT SYSTEMS

Wright (1994) considers a safety management system (SMS) to be the 'means by which the organization controls risk through the management process'. The Health and Safety Commission (1993b) consider that the SMS refers collectively to 'those elements in the management system which are particularly concerned with health and safety performance and legal compliance, as well as with loss control' (p. 101). The importance of an adequate SMS to effective organizational functioning on safety has been recognized in reports of disasters such as those at Clapham Junction (Department of Transport, 1989) and Piper Alpha (Department of Energy, 1990). It is increasingly likely that the notion of an adequate SMS will become enshrined in legislation. An SMS is a mechanism for setting safety goals. The role of an external agency would be to verify the goals as being appropriate (e.g. using a validation audit – pp. 298–312) and to establish that safety goals are being pursued by appropriate systems (e.g. using a verification audit – pp. 298–312).

Wright (1994) identifies three distinct approaches to SMSs. The first, exemplified by HSE (1991), is based upon a traditional systems approach and is described in this section. The second focuses upon the concept of safety culture and attitudes, as described for example in Hale *et al.* (1991) and in Pidgeon *et al.* (1991), and is developed in pp. 291–5. The third approach is based upon 'best practice', typified by safety auditing, described in pp. 298–312, and developed from practices in the petrochemical and other process industries. The auditing approach, based upon expert opinion, is more a set of practices than a system of management and relates elements of an audit to such management functions as: planning, organizing, implementing and controlling, as well as accountability.

All three approaches bring together human and managerial aspects of risk and emphasize such features as:

- the importance of top management commitment;
- setting clear safety objectives;
- communicating required information adequately.

However, an integrated SMS approach poses many challenges and most have only been partially evaluated or else validation of their utility has produced conflicting results (Wright, 1994). The issue of measurement is specifically addressed in pp. 296–8.

A systems approach

A systems approach to safety is described by Waring (1989, 1991). A system comprises:

- structural elements
- processes
- interconnections
- external influences
- sub-systems.

Structural elements are relatively enduring system components such as: key posts, reporting relationships, committees and other groups, safety documentation. Processes tend to be more changing aspects, including: action, decision-making, problem-solving, information provision and communication. Interconnections between system elements and processes include feedback loops and provide a framework for the system.

The HSE (1991) approach to safety management has six elements:

- policy
- organizing
- planning and implementing
- measuring performance
- reviewing performance
- auditing.

These elements are supported by processes such as employee involvement, continuous improvement, resource provision and risk control and there are interconnections between them which include feedback loops.

External influences include government, legislation, the economy, the state of technology, rate of change and public opinion (see for example, chapter 5, pp. 132–7 and figure 5.5). More complex systems are likely to include sub-systems, perhaps nested like Russian Matreshka dolls. Examples of sub-systems include:

- control – decision-making, policy, strategic planning;
- monitoring – systematic checking of safety performance;
- executive – operational sub-systems (e.g. maintenance, production);
- communication – transmission via one or more channels (e.g. chapter 5 summary text 5.6).

Waring (1991) argues that the conditions necessary for effective SMSs are both functional – involving management control, monitoring, executive and communications sub-systems and human – involving leadership, political and safety culture sub-systems. Thus, political will and top management commitment need to be reinforced with a common set of safety beliefs, values and behaviours from all those within the organization – comprising the safety culture.

SAFETY CULTURE: WHAT IS IT AND WHY IS IT IMPORTANT?

The importance of safety attitudes and culture was heavily underlined by both the Chief Inspector of Factories, HSE, and the Director of the Accident

Prevention Advisory Unit, HSE, in separate articles in the June 1994 edition of *Safety Management.*

The concept of safety culture emerged from earlier ideas of organizational climate, organizational culture and safety climate. Safety culture can be described as the embodiment of a set of principles which loosely define what an organization is like in terms of health and safety.

As an illustration, the ten aspects of organizational life shown in summary text 10.1 were suggested many years ago as a measure of how good the organizational 'climate' is within an organization.

Cultural features are complex, shared characteristics of a group dynamic, relating to a system (e.g. group, community, race, nation, religion). These include: beliefs, values, attitudes, opinions, motivation, meanings, ideas, expectations, linguistic features, actions, rituals, ceremonies, quirks, symbols and responses. More tangible aspects are: buildings, uniforms, documents, liveries, logos, equipment and designs.

More recent expositions of organizational culture or climate include that of Rousseau (1988, 1990), who considers that culture may be expressed at five levels:

- artefacts – observable (e.g. company logo);
- patterns of behaviour – observable actions;
- behavioural norms – can be inferred from observed behaviour;
- values – as expressed consciously by organization members;
- fundamental assumptions – core values, may not be articulated.

From the notion of organizational climate came the idea that this general measure could be disaggregated into measures of different aspects of organizational life – including health and safety. Thus, around the early 1980s a number of studies (e.g. Glennon, 1980, 1982; Zohar, 1980a) sought to identify key elements of a good health and safety climate within an organization. Based upon the work of Zohar (1980a), Cooper and Phillips (1994) developed a safety culture measure and found seven factors which affected employee perceptions of safety climate. These were:

- management attitudes towards safety;
- perceived level of risk;

Summary text 10.1 Ten features of organizational climate

- Is there mutual trust between management and employees?
- Is management interested in staff?
- Is there management understanding of subordinates' problems?
- Is training, assistance and advice generally available?
- Is a problem-solving approach frequently adopted?
- Is there adequate support from physical resources?
- Is information available to staff generally adequate?
- Is there general use of employees' ideas?
- Is management approachable?
- Is credit and recognition generally given?

- effects of work pace;
- management actions towards safety;
- status of safety adviser and safety committee;
- importance of health and safety training;
- social status of safety and promotion.

Thus, these appeared to be important features of safety climate. Typically, safety culture or climate is measured by surveying workforce attitudes and key elements are then extracted to establish which attitudes are important – i.e. which predict changes or differences in accident rates. Thus, safety culture within an organization is closely linked to attitudes (discussed more generally in chapter 4) in respect of safety. Donald and Canter (1993) identify three major elements in respect of safety attitudes:

- organizational rules – perceptions of others' attitudes, in particular those of workmates, supervisors, higher management and safety representatives;
- safety object of attitudes – both passive e.g. checking equipment, wearing appropriate PPE, housekeeping; and active, e.g. finding out results of safety inspections, making suggestions, seeking safety information;
- behaviour in respect of safety.

Donald and Canter (1993) found that a number of these safety attitudes were related to accident rates within a steelworks, for example in relation to:

- management support and encouragement;
- employee training;
- employee satisfaction;
- management support for meetings.

However, in a study to determine whether there had been any changes in British Rail safety culture following the Clapham Junction rail crash (chapter 9, summary text 9.10) which might have been associated with accident rates, Guest *et al.* (1994) found only some differences in safety attitudes and perceptions between permanent way staff in gangs with high and low accident rates, indicating that a unified safety culture had not yet emerged. Furthermore, despite a perception among BR employees that the safety culture was improving and that accident rates were reducing, these perceptions were not reflected in lost time accidents reported, nor in aspects of safety culture which they measured. Guest *et al.* (1994) caution against system improvements which reduce employees' personal control of safety when seeking to change safety culture.

The term 'safety culture' is generally taken to be more embracing than that of 'safety climate' although the meanings of the two terms are quite similar. 'Culture' also implies a notion of residing within an organization, whereas 'climate' has more passive connotations of being subject to the external environment. The ACSNI study group (HSC, 1993a) propose the following definition:

The safety culture of an organization is the product of individual and group values, attitudes, perceptions, competencies, and patterns of behaviour that determine the commitment to, and the style and proficiency of, an organization's health and safety management.

Organizations with a positive safety culture are characterized by communications founded on mutual trust, by shared perceptions of the importance of safety and by confidence in the efficacy of preventive measures.

In the CBI's (1990) report on safety culture, similar themes emerge, namely:

- the critical importance of leadership and commitment of the chief executive;
- the executive safety role of line management;
- involvement of all employees;
- openness of communication;
- demonstration of care and concern for all those affected by the business.

Thus, a reasonable degree of consensus is emerging in respect of what constitutes safety culture. Studies carried out in the US nuclear industry (Ryan, 1991), identified four critical indicators of safety culture:

- effective **communication**, leading to commonly understood goals and means to achieve them at all levels;
- good organizational **learning**, whereby organizations are able to identify and respond appropriately to change;
- organizational **focus** upon health and safety – essentially how much time and attention is paid to health and safety issues;
- **external** factors, including the financial health of the organization, the prevailing economic climate and the impact of regulation and how well these are managed.

The ACSNI Human Factors Study Group (HSC, 1993a) concluded that effective provision for health and safety depends as much upon organizational culture generally – as reflected in such aspects as communication and learning – as it does upon specific attention to health and safety matters.

Given the progress which has been made in respect of describing and defining safety culture, it would be expected that within a fairly short time there will be an audit (or several) available for measuring the safety culture of an organization. The ACSNI Study Group provide a draft audit of safety culture – called 'A safety culture prompt-list'. The 90 or so questions comprising this relatively brief audit emphasize critical aspects of organizational functioning, including: leadership, management style, communication, policy, planning, risk assessment, risk management, perceptions, stress, training, monitoring and regulation.

As far as safety auditing (pp. 298–312) in the general sense is concerned, the safety culture of an organization will be critical in the following ways:

- whether management are willing to entertain the prospect of safety auditing in the first place;
- whether management are willing to devote adequate resources to the safety auditing process (e.g. auditor training and time);

- involvement of line management and employee representatives in the auditing process;
- implementation of findings from audits carried out;
- long-term commitment to auditing.

The Institution of Occupational Safety and Health (IOSH, 1994) maintains that organizations with a positive safety culture have competent people, strongly committed to safety who put their values into practice. This reinforces the view that a positive safety culture is central to health and safety management and is increasingly used as an indication of an organization's determination and competence to control dangers at work. The IOSH policy statement on safety training (IOSH, 1992) also recognizes that safety training (chapter 2) should be designed to create a positive safety culture. IOSH (1994) urges management to consider safety culture when developing or reviewing SMSs, but cautions that safety culture cannot necessarily be improved prescriptively, a point also made by Beer *et al.* (1990) and Toft (1992a).

Features deemed to be required for the development and maintenance of a strong safety culture include:

- continual variation in approach (IOSH, 1994);
- mutual trust and confidence between management and workforce (HSC, 1993a);
- recognize variety of perceptions among different groups (Royal Society, 1992);
- organizational learning (Toft, 1992b; Waring, 1992).

Organizational learning is the process whereby those in an organization learn to change their characteristic ways of thinking and acting as a result of shared experience, addressing problems mutually and sharing in the life of the organization. Organizational learning is not only critical to safety culture, but to all aspects of organizational life. As Senge (1990) notes: 'learning disabilities are tragic in children, but they are fatal in organizations. Because of them, few corporations live even half as long as the person – most die before they reach the age of forty.' Thus organizational learning is not an option for those organizations desiring to survive. Turner (1992) proposes a new model of organizational learning directed at safety and risk management which extends beyond rationally conceived models.

A feature of any culture is its high resistance to change, such that attempts to change culture may only serve to reinforce pre-existing beliefs (Turner, 1992). Thus, attempts to change aspects of organizational culture, including safety culture, may be perceived as a threat by many within the organization – resulting in resistance to proposed changes. Toft (1992) notes the inappropriateness of a traditional engineering model in respect of safety culture, and argues that a holistic approach is required to change safety culture, involving:

- sustained management commitment;
- sound safety policy;

- visible management support;
- allocation of sufficient resources;
- use of appropriate safety management techniques;
- continuous motivation of all staff;
- safety training provision;
- fostering a 'no blame' culture;
- organizational learning;
- persistence of purpose.

The critical role of power relations within an organization and their effect upon risk perceptions, decision-making and action also needs to be addressed (Waring, 1993, 1994). For further information on the important role of power relations in safety culture, risk assessments and SMSs, the interested reader is referred to Waring's (1994) power model of risk behaviour.

MEASURING MANAGEMENT PERFORMANCE IN HEALTH AND SAFETY

Drucker's maxim, 'what gets measured, gets done' is a reminder of the importance of measuring performance if useful safety objectives are to be achieved. It could be added that 'what get's done should be measured' – as a basis for further action.

This section considers some essential principles of measurement and relates them to measuring management performance in health and safety. Health and safety audits, considered in the next section, are one of a variety of measures of management performance in health and safety. Health and safety performance measures which can be used include those shown in summary text 10.2.

Summary text 10.2 briefly describes some of the many ways in which health and safety performance can be measured. A more comprehensive range of measures which might be used, is shown in summary text 10.3. Summary text 10.3 shows that there is a considerable number of possible measures of health and safety performance that might be used by management. Meanings of the dimension descriptions in summary text 10.3 are:

- **objective** – measures which are essentially detached from an assessor's judgement – i.e. judged against an independent standard;
- **subjective** – measures which are subject to influence or bias from an assessor (the person doing the measuring); this is not to decry the usefulness of subjective measures but merely to qualify the results which are obtained;
- **quantitative** – measures which can be calculated on some sort of a scale – i.e. **quantifiable** in some way;
- **qualitative** – measures which cannot be scaled but which may be readily seen to be present or absent.

In summary text 10.3 the allocation of certain measures to particular cells of the matrix may be debated. However, the essential point to note is that

Summary text 10.2 Management health and safety performance measures

- **Workplace inspections** – concerned essentially with what can be observed or inferred from observations on a site (pp. 314–15);
- **Safety tours** – systematic or ad hoc reviews of a plant, for example on a 'walk through' basis;
- **Safety sampling** – involves reviewing specific aspects of health and safety on a random basis;
- **Behaviour sampling** – assesses workers' behaviour on a systematic sampling basis to establish the proportion of unsafe work behaviours which might require correction, for example by training or design improvements (pp. 313–14);
- **Probabilistic risk assessments** – such as fault tree analysis, failure mode and effects analysis and event tree analysis, which assign probabilities to foreseen occurrences as a prelude to risk reduction programmes;
- **HAZOPs/HAZAN techniques** – represent experts' contingency-based assessments of plant, particularly process plant, as part of a risk assessment programme (e.g. Dickson (1991) gives a descriptive account of HAZOP);
- **Analysis of accident/ill-health/damage data** – evaluates specified past events with a view to prevent recurrences;
- **Analysis of near miss data** – a more proactive version of the above in which events which **might** have led to accidents or unwanted incidents are evaluated with a view to prevent more serious outcomes (van der Schaaf *et al.,* 1991);
- **Management Oversight and Risk Tree (MORT)** – uses a logic tree to analyse organizational functions required in the safe management of high risk technologies; also used to gain insights during accident investigations, near miss reviews and safety audits (Johnson, 1980; Knox and Eischer, 1992);
- **Job Safety Analysis (JSA)** – a semi-formal hazard analysis which evolved from work study techniques and which uses task analysis to identify accident potential within a job (e.g. Bamber, 1990).

Summary text 10.3 Measures of health and safety performance

Objective	*Subjective*
Quantitative	
• calibrated instrument measures (e.g. air, noise)	• attitude surveys
• hazard analysis using formal system	• prosecutions, notices, etc.
	• unverified quantified audit
• verified quantified audit	• motivation surveys
• behaviour sampling	• unverified accident/disease/ damage etc. occurrences
• verified accident/disease/ damage etc. occurrences	
• structured interviews/surveys	
Qualitative	
• workplace inspections	• ad hoc observations
• health and safety adviser employed?	• status of health and safety adviser
• accident investigations	• ad hoc safety tours
• documentary analysis	• health and safety consultation
• extent of health and safety training	• effectiveness of training
• diary monitoring	• unverified expert judgement
	• in-depth interviews

attempts to measure management performance in health and safety should use a variety of measures or techniques – for example, at least one from each quadrant.

Desirable characteristics of measures

Because of the variety and range of potential measures of health and safety performance, there are five important issues to be addressed when deciding upon which measure(s) to use in assessing management performance in health and safety. These are described in summary text 10.4.

The reason that we have devoted space to reviewing some of the principles of measurement in summary text 10.4 is that it is important when measuring anything to know:

- what the ultimate objective (criterion) is;
- how valid the indicators (measures) being used are;
- what is the appropriate scale to measure on;
- what combination of measures will best improve the validity of the overall assessment.

Because the scope and extent of performance measurement in this area has not yet been developed sufficiently to answer this final question, it will rest upon professional judgement as to how many and what combination of methods are used to assess management performance in health and safety. In other fields (e.g. personnel selection) there has been a considerable amount of research to establish what combination of selection or assessment methods should be used in the selection process to achieve an optimum result (selecting the right people for the right jobs) – chapter 6, pp. 149–55. In the future, it may be predicted that performance measurement in health and safety will reach higher levels of certainty.

Types of safety auditing

Safety auditing is considered in more detail in the next section, but is considered here as an example of measurement of management performance in health and safety. The term 'safety auditing' means different things to different people. Some have treated it as being almost synonymous with workplace inspection, although as already indicated, auditing is a much more detailed review of procedures beyond what can merely be observed in a workplace. Saunders (1992) uses a very broad definition, implying that safety auditing encompasses virtually all safety management activities. Greeno *et al.* (1988) and Kase and Wiese (1990) adopt more focused technical approaches. The HSE (1991) consider (safety) auditing to be a crucial part of the feedback process in safety management systems and define it as: 'the structured process of collecting independent information on the efficiency, effectiveness and reliability of the total safety management system and drawing up plans for corrective action'.

Summary text 10.4 Issues to be addressed in measuring management performance

1. **Reliability** – this describes the extent to which a measure will give the same result on successive occasions of use. This assumes that what is being measured stays the same. For example, a measure of housekeeping in a workplace (e.g. an observation checklist) might be reliable even though it gave different results each time. This could be because the housekeeping was changing over time. One way of establishing the reliability of an instrument is to get different people to use it at the same time (called **inter-rater reliability**).

For example, the same safety audit checklist is completed by two independent assessors in the same workplace. If they obtain the same, or almost the same result, then the chances are that this is a reliable checklist (for this particular workplace). If their respective results differ widely then it is unlikely that this is a reliable measure. Measures which are unreliable will remain subjective, even though the results may be quantifiable. The results may still be important, however. For example, if the two people completing an audit checklist are the plant manager and the safety representative and they get widely differing results (it has happened!), then this is an important indication that someone's perceptions (perhaps those of both parties) are partly wrong. This finding may lead to vital changes in health and safety provision – both technical and organizational aspects.

2. **Validity** – This refers to whether the indicator being used really is a good measure of what is being measured. For example, asking whether accident data are a valid measure of management performance in health and safety is really just asking whether they are a **good** (in the sense of adequate or satisfactory) measure (summary text 10.6 provides comments on this point). Similarly, we may ask whether safety audits are a valid way of measuring health and safety performance.

To answer this question, it is necessary to know what our ultimate objective is. Our objective is sometimes called a **criterion** measure – because it is the criterion against which something is assessed. Generally, for health and safety, the criterion (or ultimate objective) is a significant reduction in reported instances of accidents or ill-health. Thus, to establish the validity of safety auditing as a performance measure, we would correlate (i.e. establish whether there is an association between) safety audit scores over a period of time – which could be several years – with accident rates (or with whatever criterion or outcome measure we selected). A high correlation (say in the order of 0.7 or above) would indicate a reasonably valid measure, while a low correlation (say less than 0.2) would suggest that our indicator (the audit scores) was not very valid. For a description of a published study which has investigated this issue, see Eisner and Leger (1988).

If a particular criterion is used as an objective – e.g. reducing reports of accidents or ill health – it cannot also be used as an indicator. This is because they are one and the same measure and are thus not independent. This is simply a matter of logic. Thus, logically, if we use accident or disease data as a measure, we need to set some **other** criterion or objective that we are using accident rates as an indicator of. This might be difficult, although we might suggest for example that production quality, profitability through cost reduction, efficiency and effectiveness or managerial excellence would be candidates.

3. **Triangulation** – This term originates from the geographical sciences when it is usually used to denote the practice of taking a minimum of two different measures to gauge the true height of a point above sea level. This practice has been taken up by a number of other disciplines and translates into the principle of not relying upon a **single** measure to assess something but rather to use a **combination** of measures (or methods or data) to evaluate for example the effectiveness of a management practice. Thus, if management's health and safety performance is being evaluated, it will be

Summary text 10.4 (continued)

necessary to use a number of **different** measures in order to gain a good (i.e. a **valid**) assessment of that performance. In practical terms, this might mean using at least one measure from each of the cells of the matrix shown in summary text 10.3. This would provide a much better overall assessment of management performance than relying upon any single measure.

4. **Accuracy and completeness** – These are relatively straightforward principles – that whatever measures (whether as indicators or criterion measures) are used, should be accurate and complete. Measures which are inaccurate or incomplete can be neither valid nor reliable (although accuracy and completeness alone of course are not enough). Thus, the accuracy and completeness of all data should be systematically checked.

5. **Measurement scales** – There are three basic types of scales which may be used when anything is measured. First, **nominal** (or **categorical**) scales simply measure **qualitative** differences between things. For example, Company A has carried out a risk assessment while Company B has not. That is a qualitative difference – which could also be a valid measure of safety performance.

Second, **ordinal** (or **rank-order**) scales can be used to determine the ranking of different items. For example, three plants in a company carry out safety audits. Plant A achieves a score of 66%, Plant B has a score of 50%, while Plant C ends up with 33%. These data, assuming they are verified, tell us that Plant A is better than Plant B, which in turn is better than Plant C. However they do **not** tell us **how much** better Plant B is than Plant C nor how much better Plant A is than Plant B. Thus, for example just because Plant A's score is twice that of Plant C, we cannot validly draw the conclusion that Plant A's health and safety performance is twice as good as that of Plant C (only that is certainly is better, given that the measure is valid).

The key is how the instrument is scaled – or calibrated. Thus, for example it may be relatively 'easy' to achieve a score of 50% on this audit and with a little bit of effort, Plant C could bring itself up to Plant B's level. However, thereafter it many become increasingly difficult to achieve higher scores so that 66% is really quite good. The point is that from the scores alone, we have no way of knowing and thus can only draw the conclusion that the rank order is correct but we cannot talk about the relative difference between the three plants in terms of a ratio. It is therefore important not to rely exclusively upon numerical data when making comparisons between workplace audit scores, but also to consider for example historical data and information about management and safety culture.

Finally, **interval** (or **ratio** if there is a zero start point) scales do enable us to state how much of a difference there is between two things. This is because an interval scale is calibrated so that a difference of one point means the same irrespective of where we are on the scale. For example, because accident rates (frequency or incidence) are calculated on the basis of a ratio (i.e. per hours worked or people employed) then we know that an increase from 0 to 1 represents the same interval as an increase of 1 to 2 – or from 99 to 100. However, interval scales will not be widely found in measures of management performance in health and safety. This is because for the most part we are measuring things which cannot be quantified to the degree necessary to construct an interval scale. Thus, for the most part, measures in this area will be qualitative – i.e. nominal, or at best ordinal.

In this section a distinction is made between proactive and reactive monitoring as well as between different types of proactive monitoring. The essential difference between reactive monitoring and proactive monitoring is that the former is concerned with reacting to events – e.g. accidents and dangerous occurrences – while the latter attempts to institute practices which will prevent or mitigate the worst consequences of those events. Sometimes, reactive data are known as **outcome** data (what management react to) while **audit** data are an example of data for proactive monitoring (gathered by management as a prevention tool).

Reactive (outcome) data

An 'accident' may be described as an unplanned event which usually results in loss of some sort. Accidents are an example of **outcomes** which are undesired because they cost money, time and suffering. Other forms of losses from an organization which are examples of outcome data are briefly described in summary text 10.5.

It is essential to collect outcome data because these are what safety and risk

---

Summary text 10.5 Examples of outcome data from organizations

- **accident injuries** – all personal injuries resulting from accidents;
- **lost-time accidents** – generally when at least one work shift is lost by a person as a result of an accident injury (other periods of time might be used);
- **non lost-time accident injury** – usually an accident resulting in injury which does not involve the loss of time beyond the work shift in which it occurs (other periods of time may be used);
- **first aid accident injury** – an injury which results from an accident and which requires only first aid treatment before the person returns to work;
- **major injury** – legally defined in RIDDOR;
- **dangerous occurrence** – legally defined in RIDDOR;
- **serious incident** – a general category of events which have the potential for loss (e.g. of time, production, materials, etc. through accident or damage);
- **damage only incidents** (accidents) – incidents (accidents) involving no personal injury but which result in damage to property (e.g. plant, vehicles);
- **operational incidents** – incidents (accidents) which result in some loss (e.g. of production) and in which there may also be personal injury;
- **sickness absence** – employee absences which are certificated as resulting from illness;
- **non-sickness absence** – employee absences which are not certificated according to regulations and which may be due to other factors;
- **fires** – perhaps associated with one or more of the above, resulting in plant damage and/or personal injury and production loss;
- **theft** – of products, plant, equipment or material by employees or others;
- **spoiled work** – e.g. due to faulty plant/equipment or to poor materials/employee skills or motivation;
- **downtime** – production ceases (e.g. due to breakdowns, lack of components/ supplies, industrial action);
- **poor timekeeping** – e.g. due to poor employee motivation or supervision.

professionals are trying to prevent. In other words, these are our criterion measures – our objective is to minimize such sources of loss to the organization. Therefore, they must be measured as criteria for long-term success.

As far as possible, outcome data should be quantified, for example expressed as numbers or rates so that they can be compared over time. It should also be possible to translate these losses into monetary terms – this can act as a powerful motivator for senior management. Such an exercise also makes it possible to balance the costs of losses which are occurring with expenditure on measures designed to control the losses. This is a component of the economic reason for safety auditing – setting actual or projected losses from accidents and other losses against the costs of auditing. Some studies have shown that safety auditing can have other benefits for an organization (Gaunt, 1989; IAPA, 1990), although these studies can be criticized on methodological grounds (Glendon, 1993).

However, outcome data are not suitable as an exclusive monitoring device, for reasons given above and also because they cannot validly be used in personal appraisal systems for managers and other staff. This is because it is unreasonable to expect line managers, for example, to be able to control all the causes of such losses. If a manager does not have effective control or authority over the losses, then he or she cannot reasonably be held accountable or responsible for them.

To illustrate further the problems with outcome data, summary text 10.6 identifies some reasons why one type of data – that from accidents – is unlikely to be a valid management performance measure. Similar sets of problems would arise in using the other types of outcome data (e.g. sickness absence, first aid treatments, damage incidents, fires).

A conclusion from this section is that there must be alternative means of monitoring management performance in health and safety which do not rely upon the collection and analysis of various sorts of outcome data. A number of proactive measures of health and safety management are available – some of the main ones were outlined in summary text 10.1. Summary text 10.4 introduced the principle of triangulation – using a variety of measures to ascertain the 'true' value of something. Extending this principle to measuring management performance in health and safety, it is necessary to develop an integrated combination of measures which will provide rewards to management and employees in their attempts to improve health and safety performance and to build a positive safety culture (see pp. 291–5). The same principle was identified in chapter 6 (pp. 149–55) in respect of using a variety of measures in the selection process. It is thus important that management implement a suitable **range** of health and safety performance measures. The next section is concerned with one that has already been widely introduced – safety auditing.

Summary text 10.6 Why accident data are a poor measure of safety performance

1. **Insufficiently sensitive:**
   • statistically sound only for large samples (say a minimum of 50 accidents or one million person-hours worked);
   • serious (e.g. fatal) injuries are fortunately rare events and often result from unusual or 'freak' factors;
   • a single (unusual) event can greatly influence rate calculations (e.g. the fires and explosions which occurred at Flixborough in 1974 and on the oil rig Piper Alpha in 1988);
   • large fluctuations are possible – what are seen as 'trends' are often only random movements about a mean value (there are statistical tests available for determining this);
   • affected by many factors which are outside management control (e.g. personal, social, economic);
   • small firms or units tend to have few, if any, accidents and thus this measure is unavailable for them;
   • safety changes take time to show up in the accident data – making it a poor measure in the short term.

2. **Dubious accuracy:**
   • under-reporting (or occasionally over-reporting, e.g. back injuries sustained elsewhere) – industries differ in this respect;
   • cheating – people 'massage' accident data, perhaps because of pressure to maintain a 'good' record;
   • cultural differences between regions – this makes comparisons problematic;
   • individual differences – some people report all trivial injuries while at the other extreme some may not even report very serious ones.

3. **After the event:**
   • because they are what safety and risk professionals are trying to prevent, they should not be used as a performance measure.

4. **Ignore risk exposure:**
   • the main correlate of accidents is the amount of work done, yet this fact is usually overlooked;
   • there are different risks inherent in different jobs, tasks, etc. – again often overlooked;
   • hours of exposure is not equivalent to risk because of the above, yet rate calculations ignore this.

SAFETY AUDITING

In this section, the term 'safety auditing' is deemed to be synonymous with 'health and safety auditing', the two terms being used interchangeably. While a validated audit for measuring risks from human behaviour has still to be developed, a checklist of human factors items was produced by HSE (1989). A comprehensive list of human factors was developed by Embrey (1994) as 'performance influencing factors' (PIFs) which could influence human performance in tasks, either positively or negatively (chapter 9, pp. 283–6). However, a human factors safety audit will be subject to the same comments and principles as are described in this section.

Types of safety audit

At least six types of safety audit may be usefully be distinguished.

1. Safety audits on **specific topics**, for example human factors, hazardous substances or the environment.
2. **Plant technical audits** – involving an in-depth review of all plant and processes carried out by specialist staff, for example on a five-yearly basis.
3. The **site technical audit** covers all work of a specified type at predetermined intervals and involves both local and specialist staff. For a consideration of technical safety audits, see for example, Kase and Wiese (1990).
4. **Compliance audits** (or **verification audits**) are designed to establish whether the range of relevant health and safety legal requirements have been complied with by the organization. Verification is concerned with whether the SMS is doing what it is claimed to do in its extent and quality and whether this is adequate as operated. It is analogous with the quality approach, as exemplified by BS5750 and BS7750.
5. **Validation** audits are concerned with the scope of an audit and with its design. They focus upon such matters as whether the right kinds of subsystem and components are being adopted, whether the right kinds of monitoring are being done and whether appropriate sub-systems are in place. Together, validation and verification audits comprise the management safety audit.
6. The **management safety audit** (or **area safety audit**). This is typically carried out annually, covers general safety matters, involves local staff and perhaps specialist auditing staff as well. A management safety audit could be carried out at both strategic and operational levels. Because of the human orientation of this book, it is this type of audit which is considered in this chapter.

Rationale for measuring health and safety by auditing

The essential rationale for auditing health and safety is that management is able to measure health and safety effort and to express this in a way that can be commented upon and evaluated. It also makes possible comparison of results over time, systematic review of risks and ensures that (external) legal and (internal organizational) policy requirements are being met. A safety audit also performs the functions and features outlined in summary text 10.7. There is no 'model' audit; rather each health and safety audit should be unique and should be derived from the strategic safety and risk management needs of the organization.

Principles of management safety auditing

Within the risk management tradition, health and safety problems should be:

• identified;
• assessed or evaluated;

Summary text 10.7 Functions and features of a safety audit

- an all-embracing approach which can give both a single quantified or qualitative measure of management performance in the principal area and a disaggregated view of performance in selected areas;
- a proxy measure of risk in an organization which is proactive rather than reactive (as in the case of accident or ill health data), looks to make changes where required and which provides guidance for doing so;
- should be tailored to the requirements (risks, hazards, etc.) of each organization;
- provides an overview of the range of issues requiring attention, thereby providing a strategic perspective;
- can provide guidance not only on **what** has to be done but also on **why** (e.g. legal or efficiency requirements) and **how** to achieve it;
- enables senior management to be assured of compliance;
- offers local management the means to promote compliance;
- provides for a longitudinal approach to health and safety;
- a flexible approach to managing health and safety.

- controlled (by implementing appropriate measures);
- monitored on a continuous basis.

Safety auditing is a management tool which can assist in all these risk management components in the following ways. The process of developing an audit or conducting it for the first time can play a vital part in the **identification** of hazards. Once the audit items are weighted, answered and scored, the resultant figures (on an ordinal scale – pp. 298–300) provide an **assessment** of the risk (pp. 315–22) – provided that the audit is valid. A number of audits provide guidance on the correction of hazards and risks (CHASE and ISRS for example do) as an aid to management in **controlling** workplace risks. Finally, successive completions of the audit provide an excellent means of **monitoring** management performance in health and safety over time.

The safety audit is an expression of opinion on the validity and reliability of the effectiveness of the health and safety management system or a particular aspect of it. However, a safety audit is not a substitute for an effective safety

---

Summary text 10.8 Principles of safety auditing

- seek to be positive rather than being preoccupied with fault finding;
- identify deviations from agreed standards;
- facilitate the analysis of events which lead to those deviations;
- highlight good practices;
- be professional, impartial and objective;
- integrate auditing into safety and risk management systems;
- assess a management function or area as objectively and accurately as possible;
- provide a measure of the state of risks to health and safety;
- indicate strengths and weaknesses in key areas;
- provide clear guidelines for improvements;
- be a means for monitoring improvements in health and safety.

---

management system, but can complement the requirement to prioritize health and safety objectives. Managerial decisions on priorities will have to be made on a far more frequent basis (i.e. daily, weekly, monthly) than could be indicated by a safety audit. Summary text 10.8 outlines the principles of (management) safety auditing – hereafter safety auditing.

There are as yet no universally agreed standards for carrying out safety audits – different organizations and safety audit providers follow a variety of practices. Neither is there agreement in respect of professional requirements for auditors. Some audit providers specify 'accredited auditor' status for those who would use their systems, while for others, safety auditing is simply one component of good risk management practice. Glendon (1993) provides a brief review of some proprietary audit systems. In this section, safety audit examples are derived mainly from the CHASE family of audits as these are the audits which the first author has had direct experience of. However, this should not be taken to imply that other audit systems are not equally valid measures. For example, some audits adopt a quantitative approach, while others use a qualitative or mixed approach.

Summary text 10.9 Advantages of safety auditing over outcome (reactive) data as a measure of safety performance

1. The audit process is explicitly designed to be **preventive** – i.e. to avoid risks which lead to accidents. (Accident investigations may also be geared to preventive activities, but by definition, the damage has already been done.)
2. Involvement in a safety audit gives managers the opportunity to influence events in the workplace and thus provides them with greater **control** over things which affect safety provision.
3. Because of this control, safety audit scores can be used as a component in personal appraisal schemes – i.e. they help to promote **responsibility** and **accountability** of line management for health and safety. They also allow for more **active** involvement of managers in the safety monitoring process.
4. Safety audits are a more **transparent** measure of safety performance because they allow examination of every question and answer which make up the components of an audit as well as the overall audit score.
5. Safety audits are a more **sensitive** measure of safety performance because they are composed of many questions and thus allow for the measurement of more aspects of performance than can be possible with accidents. This also permits improvements to be made on a more **continuous** basis.
6. Safety audits are a more **complete** measure because they can sample comprehensively from all aspects of a manager's safety performance – i.e. they can help to assess those risks which have not yet led to accidents – but which could do so, as well as those which already have.
7. Safety audit data are **independent** of the criterion measure – e.g. accidents or other outcomes, and they can therefore be validated by correlating them with outcome data.
8. Safety audits can measure **success** as well as relative failure – i.e. they can identify what is being done right and thus be an aspect of positive rewards. Accidents measure only failures. Which of the two is likely to be more motivating?

The main problems of using accident data as a measure of safety performance were outlined in summary text 10.6. Advantages which safety auditing has over the use of outcome data, such as accident data are reviewed in summary text 10.9.

Thus, a safety audit is a tool for use in improving both the efficiency (doing things right) and the effectiveness (doing the right things) of management performance in designated areas (e.g. as defined in the organization's safety policy). It can be used as a means for controlling losses in many areas of management activity. Because one objective of safety auditing is to reduce the probability (likelihood) of loss through accidents, absences, damage incidents, etc., auditing can be seen as part of good business practice in general and as an important component of attempts to improve quality.

Developing safety audits

Audits are developed according to some important principles. First, the audit should suit a particular situation – e.g. organization size, industry sector, audit type (e.g. human factors) or user need. Second, specific expertise is required in the development of the appropriate structure, questions and user guidance. Piloting on relevant users is essential and the system should be clear to the user and readily usable with minimum training (say two days) for someone who is already competent in health and safety matters – e.g. a corporate member of the Institution of Occupational Safety and Health. For guidance on safety auditing, see for example, Greeno *et al.* (1988) and Kase and Wiese (1990).

Despite a minimum training requirement for audit system users, some of the issues to be dealt with will inevitably be both managerially and technically complex. These will require specialist advice both in question setting, advice provision, answering and rectifying any problems. A typical series of stages in the development of a health and safety audit is shown in summary text 10.10.

When developing safety audits, it is important to consider audit standards. Audit standards, in the form of a reference document, are concerned with every aspect of auditing and provide a framework for 'best practice'. Standards may be derived from within an organization or may be available as a national standard. At the time of writing, a British Standard on occupational health and safety management systems is being developed – projected to be available in 1995 – and this will include a standard on safety auditing. Audit standards should provide guidance on all features of safety auditing from the training and selection of audit teams, through specifying and drafting key elements, to drawing up and application of the scoring system or other type of measure.

The precise methodology employed for developing any particular safety audit will depend upon the objectives and circumstances involved. For example, CHASE I (Booth *et al.,* 1987) and CHASE II (Booth *et al.,* 1989) safety audits were developed in conjunction with a range of organizations, mainly in

Summary text 10.10 Stages in the development of a health and safety audit

1. Site(s) visit(s) and familiarization.

2. Design pilot questionnaire and scoring system and revise as necessary. This is the longest stage of the process which may take many months as the questions will need to be refined through many drafts to ensure that all aspects are covered adequately and consistently. Core topics will depend upon the nature of the audit being developed. Illustrative topics may be seen in the CHASE family of safety audits – see Booth *et al.*, 1987, 1989, 1990, 1991a,b. A scoring system usually involves weighting of questions on the basis of relevant expertise in the particular sector.

3. Audit premises and activities – sometimes referred to as the 'baseline' audit, this involves going through the audit questions and answering each one on the basis of the best evident available.

4. Verify answers and/or audit scores – for example, by taking a sample of questions which have received 'yes' answers (meaning that conditions are judged to be adequate in the area concerned) and asking for concrete evidence that this is so (e.g. demanding to **see** machine guards or people using their PPE correctly).

5. Analyse findings – for example derive summary reports or percentage scores for a number of sections or elements, write overview report or derive overall percentage or 'star rating'.

6. Determine problem areas – from low scoring sections or elements.

7. Prepare and submit report – prioritizing actions to rectify problem areas and making appropriate recommendations.

8. Implement recommendations – i.e. the control measures.

9. Monitor changes over time – usually by repeating the audit at intervals (e.g. 6 months initially and 12 months thereafter) to assess progress.

the manufacturing sector as well as using expertise from a variety of sources. The original version of ISRS was developed from a study of relevant literature describing studies which identified the factors which discriminated between good and poor firms in terms of safety management. The discriminating factors were used as the basis for the 20 elements which comprise ISRS.

Construction CHASE, a sector-specific safety audit, was developed as a specialist audit for the construction sector and was piloted in about a dozen organizations involved in construction activities (Booth *et al.*, 1990). COSHH CHASE (Booth *et al.*, 1991a) and Environment CHASE (Booth *et al.* 1991b) were both developed and tested in partnership with a large multi-site organization which had internal occupational hygiene expertise and a strong motivation to use these audits in its risk management programme.

All these audits were developed through a number of stages. Initial questions were first derived from appropriate legislation and other relevant sources. This was followed by testing for logic and preparation of a pilot manual. Sites were then piloted and the audit revised as necessary to incorporate guidance and question weightings. Thus, each audit began as a draft manual which was completed by managers at a number of sites with varying problems in the areas of the audit. From the responses, the manual versions went through a series of draftings and further site testing while guidance was incorporated to assist users. Question weightings reflect the relative importance of the questions – for example, because of the emphasis accorded to a particular issue in the relevant legislation or because of the degree of risk represented by a particular hazard if not controlled. However, the precise weightings allocated to questions is ultimately based upon professional judgement and weightings may change over time as new legislation appears or scientific knowledge reveals more about different risks. All these audits are available as manuals and as software – advantages of which are described by Glendon (1993) and by Glendon *et al.* (1992).

The audit in action: audit teams and uses of a safety audit

When considering the audit in action, a number of issues need to be addressed. The first is the extent to which a safety audit is seen to be something which is 'imposed' on one party (e.g. a line manager) by another party (e.g. one or more accredited safety auditors). This is the perspective adopted for example in the advice given by Greeno *et al.* (1988). The alternative perspective is that people whose **performance** (i.e. not them as individuals) is being audited should be involved in the auditing process. This is in keeping with the spirit of 'self-regulation' and is far more likely to result in ownership of the auditing process by those whose performance is the focus of the audit. In particular, it is important that those introducing safety auditing bring line management with them and encourage managers to consider safety auditing as a learning opportunity.

Summary text 10.11 Factors in assembling a safety audit team

- the interdisciplinary nature of the team – it should include expertise from a range of relevant backgrounds;
- how much should it be connected with the plant? – there are advantages in having a mixture of local and external knowledge;
- tenure – advantages of (semi) permanent appointments mean that a body of experience can be built up, although rolling term appointments enable that expertise to be distributed within the workplace and for 'new blood' to be introduced;
- role of members – observer status only might permit greater objectivity while executive status might ensure more practicable recommendations;
- employee representation – desirable for the same reason as management involvement and be more likely to spread ownership of the problems and responsibility for solutions;
- relative participation of safety specialists and line management – both are needed for balance.

Summary text 10.12 Valid uses of a safety audit

- as a one-off audit – i.e. on one site/area on a single occasion to measure safety performance at a moment in time;
- to verify another audit – testing the validity of a new audit against one which has been shown to be a valid measure of health and safety;
- as a starting point for developing a customized audit for the organization (likely to be the goal of most organizations which use safety audits);
- as a basis for inter-site comparisons – care should be taken to compare like with like, although managers will seek to compare safety performances across plants, sites, regions, etc.;
- for mutual (cross) auditing of sites – personnel from Site A audit Site B and personnel from Site B audit Site A;
- to compare health and safety performance of a single site over time;
- to check implementation of safety policy – items from the policy can be incorporated within the audit and the extent of compliance checked;
- to help identify safety training needs – the audit process will help to identify where line management and other functions are deficient in their knowledge by drawing attention to deficits;
- as a health and safety training or development aid – active involvement in the audit process will help line managers to gain expertise relevant to their health and safety responsibilities;
- as a means of enhancing health and safety involvement – when managers and employee representatives participate in the safety auditing process, levels of involvement in health and safety within the organization will increase;
- to help develop health and safety awareness – as people see the range and extent of items in a safety audit, their awareness of health and safety requirements will increase;
- to check accuracy of health and safety perceptions – in some cases, managers may be unaware of the state of health and safety within their area of responsibility; completing a safety audit (particularly where a safety representative completes the audit independently) can help to identify erroneous perceptions.

Whether they are from inside or outside the organization, safety auditors need to be independent. There is value in bringing a 'fresh pair of eyes' to the auditing process as this assists in the objectivity of auditing. Effective involvement and participation of managers and other parties is essential in order to maximize the impact of an audit. Because both independence and involvement are essential aspects of safety auditing, management skill is required to achieve a successful coalition of these criteria.

When assembling the team responsible for a safety audit, a number of factors need to be considered. These are outlined in summary text 10.11.

Uses of a safety audit

Up to now, our discussion of safety auditing has assumed that a safety audit will be used in one way only. However, in practice, audits are flexible enough tools to be used for a variety of purposes. Summary text 10.12 identifies a dozen valid uses of a safety audit.

The value of safety audits to different parties

Having agreed the principle of safety auditing within an organization, the issue of persuading various parties of its value needs to be considered as part of the process of 'winning hearts and minds'. As far as safety and risk professionals are concerned, their concerns are likely to include:

- a means of compiling a **priority list** of items requiring attention – a practical and important function;
- a means of getting line management to **think** about health and safety issues – relates to the awareness generating function of the safety audit referred to above;
- a means of getting line management to **own** their health and safety responsibilities – takes the mission a stage further by helping to locate responsibility where it belongs, hopefully leaving the safety and risk professional in an advisory role.

In this latter task, it is important to provide practicable guidance to line managers. Kase and Wiese (1990) offer some guidance on reporting on controls which are highlighted as being required by a safety audit:

- present both positive and negative findings;
- cite sources of all requirements and indicate current deficit;
- don't hand over problems for which solutions do not exist;
- always offer solutions, recommendations or corrective actions;
- where options exist, appeal to the manager's expertise to derive the optimum corrective action;
- give enough time for evaluation and decision-making;
- follow up.

As far as line managers are concerned, the following factors are likely to be among those which will persuade them of the value of safety auditing:

- the technique allows them to **audit themselves** rather than to have an audit imposed on them from outside – assuming that the self-regulation route is to be followed;
- it provides for a **quantitative assessment** of their health and safety performance, thus allowing them to decide how to prioritize items as a prelude to devising and implementing solutions. While quantification is not essential for assessing risks and in many cases risk assessments and decisions about priorities can be made by informed judgement, a quantified measure is still useful for monitoring progress in the longer term;
- on the first occasion, the results of the safety audit can be **confidential** to the manager so that s/he has an opportunity to improve health and safety in his or her own area of responsibility.

These benefits have an important common factor – they all increase the degree of **control** that a manager can exert in respect of health and safety in his or her area of responsibility. Participating in the control process is much more likely to be motivating than having a solution imposed exclusively from without and thus these factors are of crucial importance.

Finally, a very important group in any organization is the executive directorate. Among the arguments which could be used to persuade **directors** of the benefits of safety auditing to them within the organization for which they have ultimate responsibility are:

- safety auditing offers a way for top management to meet their health and safety **responsibilities** – for example by ensuring that all relevant legal and company policy requirements are covered by the audit;
- a way of improving health and safety on plant and premises – auditing can provide an overview of the state of health and safety across the organization as a basis for **strategic** decision-making.
- a way of **identifying potential losses** – for example by revealing where costs may be unnecessarily high;
- to **highlight deficiencies** – for example, in emergency procedures or where audit scores are low;
- as a **cost-effective tool** – being systematic and thorough can help to make a strong case for auditing.

Again, all these items have a feature in common – in this case, it is to stress the **cost-effectiveness**, **financial value** and **efficiency** of safety auditing. These are the type of arguments that will help to persuade top management of the value of safety auditing. Increasingly, top management of well-run organizations are recognizing the value of safety auditing as a vital tool in the risk management armoury. However, it may help to produce figures which detail the costs and benefits involved as there is likely to be a heavy 'front end loaded' cost of introducing a safety audit system because of the learning (and training) involved by all parties. Once an audit system is in place, costs of running the system will diminish, while expected benefits will begin to show (see for example Gaunt, 1989; IAPA, 1990).

The enforcement basis for safety auditing

While this book has generally not considered a legal perspective on safety and risk matters, it is worth reviewing briefly the current legal position on safety auditing. The HSE (1991) view is that safety auditing **alone** is unlikely to be sufficient in controlling health and safety risks at work, but that it is an important component of managing occupational risks. In assessing compliance with HSW Act 1974 and the Management of Health and Safety at Work Regulations 1992, HSE inspectors are likely to adopt this approach. The Management of Health and Safety at Work Regulations 1992 require a monitoring and review process to occur, although the way in which this should be done is not specified in the accompanying Approved Code of Practice (ACoP). In the Offshore Installations (Safety Cases) Regulations 1992 there is a requirement for safety cases to include arrangements for auditing the safety management system.

Conclusions on safety auditing

It is important to be able to evaluate the effectiveness of a safety audit. In the short term, this can be done by verifying scores obtained. In the long term, the scores should be assessed against an independent measure such as accidents or other losses. Thus, the ultimate test of a health and safety audit is whether its use is associated with **and** can be demonstrated to have influenced, declining rates of accidents, diseases and other losses. This may be difficult because when the management of an organization decides to introduce safety auditing, they usually also make other changes and it may be a combination of factors which affect accidents and other losses. Thus, it may be difficult to disentangle cause and effect. For example, a 'positive safety culture' may be said to be required for the introduction of a safety auditing system. The safety audit process is then likely to enhance the safety culture. Both together may then work to reduce accident and absence rates, and so on. This accords with the philosophy that safety auditing is only one component of a comprehensive health and safety management system.

Trying to establish precise cause and effect sequences can be difficult and perhaps not even worth while in terms of the costs and benefits involved – although from a scientific point of view it is certainly useful to know whether safety audits are a valid means of reducing accident rates (for example, Eisner and Leger, 1988; Guastello, 1991). Sometimes it is more a matter of faith than firm evidence – perceptions as much as scientific findings – which is the determining factor.

However, from a managerial standpoint the following simple requirements for success may be identified:

- commitment and support of top management – as required for any policy in any organization to succeed;
- clearly defined objectives, methods and reporting systems – to ensure that the audit system has a logical, coherent and all-embracing framework;
- careful selection of the audit team – to ensure competence, credibility and comprehensive coverage;
- prompt implementation of changes revealed as necessary by the audit – a certain way of ensuring that an audit system fails is to collect data, analyse them and then do nothing about it; the safety audit is a tool and **not** an end in itself.

OTHER TECHNIQUES

Behaviour sampling

Behaviour sampling, in contrast with HRA (discussed in chapter 9, pp. 275–86), is a human behaviour assessment technique which is used during routine, generally low-risk operations in which the probability of unsafe behaviour is quite high, although the consequences may be low, for example injury to a single person – the operator or a work colleague.

Behaviour sampling is used to determine the extent to which unsafe behaviour exists in a workplace. It necessitates making a number of observations of behaviour on random occasions. Using this technique, the percentage of workers involved in unsafe acts and the percentage of time that workers are behaving in an unsafe way can be calculated. In carrying out behaviour sampling, it is important to have a precise definition of all the examples of unsafe acts which might be observed. An observer records systematically over defined time periods (e.g. each of ten minutes' duration) all examples of safe acts and all examples of unsafe acts. Observation periods must be at random intervals with each having an equal chance of being selected.

The size of the sample is the most important factor determining the correspondence of the sample to the population from which it is drawn. Thus, the larger the sample, the greater the confidence in any analysis performed on that sample of cases. The other factor which is important in determining sample size is the proportion of observed acts which are unsafe; the smaller this is, the larger the sample needs to be. Typically, at least 600 observations are likely to be needed, although texts which explain the formulae to be used and other details should be consulted to determine the precise number at the require accuracy (e.g. Tarrants, 1980; Bensiali and Glendon, 1987; Petersen, 1989).

Two types of bias may exist in making observations from a sample of cases. The first is random bias; for example, as one is carrying out a survey there may be omissions or misinterpretations which are distributed throughout the observation periods. These will tend to 'cancel out' and providing there are not too many of them, will not affect the reliability of results unduly. The second type is systematic bias and even a small amount of this could affect the reliability of results.

Systematic bias may be inherent in the instrument being used or in the method being applied – for example through a design fault. Another possibility is bias by the person who always carries out the reporting of unsafe acts.

Systematic bias may be reduced or eliminated by:

- selecting observation times using a table of random numbers;
- training observers;
- taking expert advice;
- checking results carefully;
- using more than one observer and checking their level of agreement.

Behaviour sampling relies upon a number of assumptions being fulfilled (summary text 10.13).

Workplace inspections

Whereas HRA and behaviour sampling are tools for assessing the potential for human error or unsafe acts, workplace inspections are an important means for assessing the extent of unsafe conditions – which in turn are likely to have been the result of unsafe behaviour. Smith and Beringer (1987) note that inspections are preferred for permanent hazards that don't vary much over time.

Summary text 10.13 Assumptions for adequate behaviour sampling

1. Observations are independent (use > 1 observer);
2. Observers are able to distinguish between safe and unsafe acts;
3. Observers are familiar with the jobs studied (train observers);
4. Workers do not alter their behaviour when observed;
5. The study is properly designed, especially noting:
   - type of sampling (random or stratified),
   - randomization of observations (use random number tables),
   - accuracy and confidence level (expert advice or see texts),
   - number of observations required (expert advice or texts),
   - economic considerations (when to carry out study),
   - scheme for making observations,
   - techniques for analysis and monitoring (expert advice, texts).

Reasons for carrying out workplace inspections include the need to:

- check results against a planned health and safety programme;
- maintain interest in health and safety;
- teach health and safety by example;
- display supervisory and management commitment to health and safety;
- collect data for meetings;
- check new facilities or alterations;
- spot unsafe conditions.

Inspections should be carried out not only with respect to the workplace, but also consider methods of work, the work environment and employee facilities. Factors determining the type of inspection to be carried out include the nature and amount of information required, when it is required and the period over which it is to be gathered as well as who is inspecting. Different types of inspections are identified in summary text 10.14.

For an effective inspection to be carried out, various tasks must be completed, including spending time perusing relevant documents such as safety manuals and working instructions, spending time in the workplace itself and researching the exact nature of hazards detected. Inspecting is not an easy task and requires a high degree of skill and considerable knowledge. For comprehensive and effective hazard detection, a methodical system of inspection is required, including the use of checklists. Advantages and disadvantages of using checklists as a basis for workplace inspections are summarized by Dickson (1991). Sanders and McCormick (1987) caution against blind application of checklists, useful though these may be, while Swain and Guttman (1983) note that the reliability of using a checklist properly is about 0.5, compared with human reliability estimates of 0.99 for errors in reading analogue or digital information (chapter 9, summary text 9.14).

As with other risk management techniques, the aim of inspections is the identification of hazards which can then be evaluated and controlled. Some important principles are:

Summary text 10.14 Types of workplace inspections

1. **Formal inspections** – the most comprehensive, perhaps being carried out annually in order to ascertain the overall state of health and safety. In addition, a check should be made that previous formal inspections were carried out properly and that conditions have not changed significantly since the previous formal inspection. There is a need for such inspections to be carefully done as much future work will depend upon findings from an initial inspection.

2. **Review/repeat inspections** – may be used to monitor progress following initial detection of a specific hazard. Also used for detecting changing conditions within the workplace in between formal inspections or in relation to a method of work which might affect employees' health and safety.

3. **Hazard spotting** – essentially day to day surveying to assess the current status of workplace risks, aiming to increase the chance of detecting potential danger before it becomes actual danger.

4. **Ad hoc inspections** – specialized in terms of techniques aimed at collecting information for a specific purpose. For example, following an injury or serious damage accident, in which case the objective would be to obtain enough appropriate information for effective action to be taken to prevent recurrence of a similar incident.

HAZARDS/DANGER	Observable (e.g. physical) or predicted from knowledge (e.g. contingent)
RISK	Not directly observable – probability of harm to system elements being realized from exposure to hazards/danger over a given period of time
HARM	Damage to system elements – long-term or short-term
ACCIDENTS	Possible outcomes – observable
INJURIES	
DISEASE	
DAMAGE	

(Safety may be considered to be control of all the above elements)

Figure 10.1 Relationship between hazard, risk and related concepts (after Glendon 1987a, b).

Summary text 10.15 Examples of different types of danger

- **immediate physical** – e.g. resulting from working on a roof which is too fragile to take the weight of a person;
- **long-term physical** – e.g. repetitive strain injury (RSI) resulting from rapid continuous limb movements such as occurs among meat processing workers and many other occupations;
- **immediate chemical** – e.g. from working with substances at the extremes of the pH scale;
- **long-term chemical** – e.g. from exposure to lead;
- **immediate biological** – e.g. from cyanide compounds;
- **long-term biological** – e.g. from exposure to mouldy hay (Farmer's Lung);
- **immediate psychological** – e.g. from having to cope with the results of a serious accident to a work colleague (chapter 8, pp. 217–19 on PTSD);
- **long-term psychological** – e.g. stress resulting from job demands which exceed the individual's ability to cope (chapter 8, pp. 219–32).

- always observe and not merely look – i.e. take detailed notice of what is seen in a workplace;
- delve deep and examine everything in detail;
- take time and don't rush the inspection;
- be patient and careful;
- ask two cardinal questions: what is wrong? why is it wrong?
- ask what if such and such happened – what would it lead to?

RISK ASSESSMENT

Defining hazard, danger and risk

It is useful to distinguish between some commonly used terms. Glendon (1987a, b) suggests the relationships between risk and related concepts shown in figure 10.1.

What is observable in the risk-outcome process are events such as accident injuries, damage, incidents and diseases. These result from hazards in the environment at work or elsewhere – which are also either observable directly because of their physical presence, such as an unfenced excavation – or indirectly using instruments, such as an excess of an airborne contaminant (e.g. which is in excess of the MEL or OES) detected using a Drager tube.

Hazards or dangers may be categorized as taking various forms and these, along with examples of each are shown in summary text 10.15.

From the examples shown in summary text 10.15, it may be seen that the notion of 'danger' is almost synonymous with 'hazard', representing the degree and type of hazard involved or the potential for harm. All hazards represent the potential for some energy exchange which is above the tolerable limit for a human being or for a system. Energy interchanges which can produce harm for individuals include:

- temperature extremes;
- ionizing and non-ionizing radiations;

- gravity (falling objects or falls from heights);
- explosions;
- lighting conditions – flicker, glare, etc.;
- electricity;
- crushing.

The extent to which a person (or a system) is exposed to danger (or a hazard) represents the risk of a certain activity as a course of action. The HSE express the relationship thus: 'A hazard is something with the potential to cause harm. Risk is the likelihood of that potential being realized' (HSC, 1991, p. 41). Alternatively, hazard is the potential danger; risk is the actual danger (Scanlon, 1990). Because it is a multi-dimensional concept it is unsurprising that there are many definitions and approaches to risk. For example, Singleton and Hovden (1987) present a range of approaches to risk – from a statistical probability definition to multiple perceptions by different parties of risk. A widely accepted definition of risk is:

Risk = Probability of occurrence of an event × Consequences, for a given time period.

Even this apparently simple definition of risk begs questions about measurement of both probabilities and consequences. Rowe (1990) identifies seven other authors' definitions of risk, most of which include similar elements. When we use the expression 'taking a risk', we usually refer to a deliberate action by someone – e.g. overtaking near a blind corner or using a pneumatic drill without wearing hearing protection, although it could as easily refer to a situation where the person is unaware of the risk involved – i.e. does not have the information to calculate either the odds or possible nature of a mishap. Even where people are 'aware' of the danger of an action in a general sense, for example in extracting material jamming a packing machine, they may not have the information to calculate the risk of injury from inserting an arm to clear the blockage.

Thus, risks *per se* cannot be directly observed – they require some calculation in order to be assessed – or more usually, to estimate them. The term usually given to people's subjective appraisals is 'risk perception' (dealt with in chapter 5, pp. 121–30), while a number of techniques are available for assessing risks more objectively (e.g. HAZOP, HAZAN, PRA). Extended definitions of risk and related terms are provided by Hale and Glendon (1987).

The risk management process involves:

- identifying hazards (what are they? how many?);
- evaluating risk (how much danger? how soon? how often? who is exposed?);
- controlling risk (what methods? to what benefit?);
- monitoring controls (how do they stand up? what changes are needed?).

Thus, the essence of risk management is: first, identify risks (i.e. measure in some way), second assess potential seriousness (how important in the light of

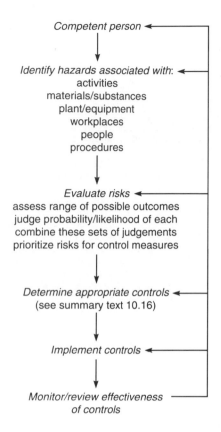

Figure 10.2 The risk management process.

other factors), third, seek to influence associated outcomes (i.e. do something about it), and finally monitor effectiveness of interventions. Identifying risk involves systematic assessment of all hazards (physical, chemical etc.) which could affect the system (human or organization). For example, under the COSHH Regulations 1988 (HSC, 1988) assessments of substances within a workplace are required. These assessments first involve determining the degree of hazard (or danger) associated with each substance. In addition to this, locations and processes in which substances are used must be identified, as must people who are exposed – or who might be exposed (i.e. visitors as well as employees or contractors).

Risk evaluation involves considering hazards associated with substances in the light of exposure of people involved in different processes. Thus, evaluating risk involves bringing together information derived from the identification process so that priorities may be assigned in respect of high-risk activities. Thus, occasions where many people are exposed to relatively high risks take precedence over occasions where small numbers of people are exposed to lower risk.

	Slightly harmful	Moderately harmful	Extremely harmful
Highly unlikely	TRIVIAL RISK	ACCEPTABLE RISK	MODERATE RISK
Unlikely	ACCEPTABLE RISK	MODERATE RISK	SUBSTANTIAL RISK
Likely	MODERATE RISK	SUBSTANTIAL RISK	INTOLERABLE RISK

RISK LEVEL	ACTION AND TIMESCALE
TRIVIAL	No action is required to deal with trivial risks, and no documentary records need be kept.
ACCEPTABLE	No further preventive action is necessary, but consideration should be given to more cost-effective solutions, or improvements that impose no additional cost burden. Monitoring is required to ensure that the controls are maintained.
MODERATE	Efforts should be made to reduce the risk, but the costs of prevention should be carefully measured and limited. Risk reduction measures should normally be implemented within three to six months, depending on the number of people exposed to the hazard. Where the moderate risk is associated with extremely harmful consequences, further risk assessment may be necessary to establish more precisely the likelihood of harm as a basis for determining the need for improved control measures.
SUBSTANTIAL	Work should not be started until the risk has been reduced. Considerable resources may have to be allocated to reduce the risk. Where the risk involves work in progress, the problem should normally be remedied within one to three months, depending on the number of people exposed to the hazard.
INTOLERABLE	Work should not be *started or continued* until the risk level has been reduced. While the control measures selected should be cost-effective, legally there is an absolute duty to reduce the risk. This means that if it is not possible to reduce the risk even with unlimited resources, then the work must not be begun, or must remain prohibited.

Figure 10.3 Simple risk estimator (after Booth 1993; reproduced with kind permission of the author).

Control of risk takes the form of implementing managerial/procedural and engineering controls which will effectively reduce or eliminate the risk. The process does not end there because these controls have to be monitored to determine both their initial and continuing effectiveness. Measuring people's exposure to hazards is one way of determining the effectiveness of control measures. This may be personal sampling in the case of implementing an LEV system to control workplace contaminants or noise measurements in the case of isolation of a noise source. Figure 10.2 represents the way in which the cycle of managing risk is carried out. Identifying and evaluating risk is the driving force within this feedback system.

Assessing risks

A number of guides to risk assessment exist (e.g. Booth, 1993; CBI, 1993; EEF, 1993; Kazer, 1993) and this discussion considers only an outline of the principles involved. The general legal basis for risk assessment in UK industry rests in Regulation 3 of the Management of Health and Safety at Work

Summary text 10.16 Hierarchy of risk control measures

Measures in rank order of preference
1. Avoid the risk by eliminating the hazardous process or substance.
2. Substitute with something less hazardous.
3. Reduce the hazard at source (i.e. use less of it).
4. Remove the person from the hazard (i.e. physical separation to reduce or minimize exposure).
5. Contain the hazard by enclosure (e.g. containment, isolation).
6. Guarding or segregation of people from the hazard.
7. Reduce exposure, e.g. by using a safe system of work that reduces the risk to an acceptable level.
8. Adapt work to the individual – e.g. design/ergonomic features.
9. Written procedures that are known and understood by those potentially exposed to the hazard.
10. Adequate supervision.
11. Training in respect of knowing and handling the risks.
12. Information and instruction – e.g. signs, notices, handouts.
13. Personal protective equipment.

General strategies
• Consider/use technological progress – e.g. to automate hazardous activities.
• A coherent policy to anticipate future requirements and the potential of new hazards so as to plan proactively.

In many cases, a suitable combination of methods may be appropriate. Note also that the amount of managerial effort required to maintain the controls is approximately in inverse rank order. For example, a design change that eliminates or considerably reduces a hazard has only to be done once, whereas options such as supervision, provision of information, training and PPE require continuous maintenance and support, which is usually costly.

Summary text 10.17 Examples of noise reduction methods

• sound absorbent material around noisy machinery;
• use of sound absorbing wall and floor materials;
• cover the source of the noise (e.g. using hoods);
• arranging plant and equipment to create screens and to reduce the level of reflected sound;
• isolating workers from the noise source;
• as a last resort provide comfortable PPE.

Regulations 1992, which requires systematic examination of hazards and the potential for the risks arising to cause harm. Other regulations also require risk assessments in specific areas (see below).

The CBI (1993) define risk assessment as 'an evaluation of the chance that harm will occur', and consider that risk control principles should link to both quality issues and to safety culture (pp. 291–5). The CBI (1993) regard risk assessment as comprising the first two stages of the risk management process – hazard identification and risk evaluation or measurement, although Kazer (1993) includes control measures as well, while the EEF (1993) include these stages plus monitoring (i.e. consider that risk assessment is synonymous with risk management). Booth (1993) describes risk assessment as 'a process where judgements are made about the harm that might arise from an activity at work, and the likelihood that harm will occur'. He explains that the main purpose of risk assessment is to determine whether planned or existing control measures (e.g. safe systems of work, physical safeguards) are adequate or need to be improved. Booth (1993) provides a prompt-list of questions that might usefully be asked when carrying out risk assessments as well as a simple risk estimator and definitions of the terms used, reproduced in figure 10.3.

Taking the risk assessment to comprise those components of the risk management process which provide the basis for determining appropriate controls, the stages in a risk assessment may be described as:

- identify all hazards (use checklist, audit, etc.);
- for each hazard, ask what is the worst outcome from that hazard, bearing in mind numbers exposed, their vulnerability (e.g. young or inexperienced workers), etc. and outcomes including fatal injury, serious injury, health damage, plant damage, environmental pollution, etc.;
- judge the probability/likelihood of harm occurring – e.g. 'likely/frequent', 'probable', 'possible', 'remote', 'improbable';
- plot outcomes against probabilities in a simple matrix (figure 10.3) to arrive at a number of different risk categories.

This last stage of the risk assessment provides a basis for ranking the risks in terms of their priorities and for determining appropriate control measures. General control measures that might be applied, in order of general preference, are shown in summary text 10.16, while an example of how these might be applied in the case of noise is shown in summary text 10.17.

At least four types of risk assessment can usefully be distinguished:

1. Assessments of large-scale complex hazard sites, such as are found in process industries, requiring quantitative risk assessment (e.g. involving fault trees, event trees, PRA, FMEA, HAZOPs) – for example Raafat (1990).
2. Risk assessments required under specific legislation – e.g. for hazardous substances (COSHH Regulations 1988), electricity (Electricity at Work Regulations 1989), pressure systems (Pressure Systems and Transportable Gas Containers Regulations 1989), noise (Noise at Work Regulations 1990) and manual handling (Manual Handling Operations Regulations 1992).
3. General assessments of the complete range of workplace risks – as required under the Management of Health and Safety at Work Regulations 1992.
4. Assessments of risk which are specific to a workplace or work process.

An example of the last type of risk assessment would be that concerning human behaviour in high hazard processes where such behaviour is critical to the safe operation of the system. The principles of carrying out human behaviour risk assessments are the same as for any other type of risk assessment. Examples of human factors risk assessments were described in chapter 9 (pp. 275–86) which considered techniques for reducing human error and increasing human reliability based upon task analysis.

It is important to recognize that risk measurement is problematic and that there are alternative ways of assessing risk. Although none can provide a definitive answer to the question 'what is an acceptable level of risk?', summary text 10.18 illustrates one method of estimating risk at work.

Summary text 10.18 A method of risk assessment at work

1. Assign a **likelihood** to an event which is a hazard, for example that fumes will escape from a fume cupboard, on a scale from 0 to 3 where 0 = highly unlikely and 3 = extremely likely.
2. Assign a set of **consequences** for the event, again on a scale from 0 to 3 where 0 = no harm or loss and 3 = severe harm (e.g. fatality) or loss (e.g. explosion).
3. Identify the **frequency** of exposure of people to the hazard, on a scale of 0 to 2 where 0 = no one is ever exposed and 2 = people are constantly exposed.
4. Identify the **number** of people exposed, where 0 = none and 2 = a large number.

The above scheme may be made more or less sophisticated depending upon the quality of data available and the accuracy with which probabilities, consequences, etc. can be specified. In some cases, probability and consequences judgements will be made on the basis of experience of the process or hazard under consideration – i.e. they will be subjective, but based upon expert knowledge. For examples of similar approaches, see Steel (1990), and Kazer (1992).

To arrive at a risk rating, the four components are multiplied together to arrive at a figure between 0 and 36. This figure gives a priority risk rating for the hazard and is a measure of the urgency with which it should be controlled. For example, if it is considered 'quite likely' that fumes will escape from the fume cupboard, then a rating of 2 might be given for likelihood. The consequences might be potentially quite serious – people could be overcome or there is the risk of fire or explosion – and thus could be rated 3. Frequency of exposure might be rated 1 on the basis that the laboratory is only staffed for certain periods, while numbers exposed is rated 1 as only a small number of people use the laboratory.

Thus, risk rating for this hazard = likelihood (probability) × (most severe possible) consequences × frequency of exposure x numbers of people exposed = 2 × 3 × 1 × 1 = 6.

By itself, the risk rating of 6 has little meaning. However, when risk ratings for all hazards in that workplace are compared, the resulting rank order will be a guide to the order in which the risks should be addressed. Alternatively, various thresholds may be identified for dealing with risks, for example any hazard which receives a risk rating of more than 20 may be deemed to be so dangerous as to merit immediate control measures. A rating of over 10 may be judged to require attention within a week and so on. Because each of the four scales which comprise the risk assessment is anchored at zero, and the final rating is the product of all four scales, a rating of zero on any of the scales results in an overall risk rating of zero. This obviates the situation in which, for example there is a high potential hazard to which no-one is exposed – for which the risk rating would be zero.

HUMAN RESOURCE MANAGEMENT

Having established the principles for measuring management performance through using assessment, auditing and other techniques, it is important to ensure that adequate provision is made for the human resources required to implement these vital components of risk management. Hence there is a need finally to consider a critical aspect of risk management, that of human resource management (HRM). The CBI (1993) note that having completed a risk assessment, management should allocate resources and responsibilities, set priorities and deadlines, ensure quality, allocate resources for controls and institute auditing procedures. These steps are the province of human resource management.

Origins and characteristics of human resource management

The term 'HRM' was first used in the 1950s and a number of lineages are identifiable. One is the human relations management tradition, originating in the 1930s, which emphasized leadership and communication (referred to in chapter 7, pp. 171–7). A second tradition is that of behavioural science within management, as seen in the work of such writers as Drucker, McGregor, Maslow, Likert, Blake and Herzberg, mentioned at various points in this book. These two strands constitute the 'soft' HRM orientation. A harder focus for HRM is derived from corporate strategy and business policy origins – with the imperative of managing human resources as part of business planning. A changing external environment demands corresponding changes in business strategy if the organization is to survive and prosper (see also pp. 291–5 on safety culture). These changes in turn drive the principles of HRM which are reflected in a variety of practices and techniques. Other influences upon modern HRM include corporate culture analysis (e.g. Peters and Waterman, 1982) and organization development.

Guest (1987) describes HRM as constituting the range of policies which have strategic significance in an organization. These may be designed to maximize organizational integration, employee commitment, flexibility and work quality. HRM includes topics traditionally within personnel management and industrial relations as well as more innovative and strategic approaches to managing people. In short, HRM is concerned with all aspects of managing people at work.

Although still used as a synonym for personnel management, HRM has wider connotations, involving qualitatively different interventions, for example to secure employee commitment (e.g. Storey, 1992). HRM thus involves a number of areas, including organizational behaviour and occupational psychology as well as personnel management and industrial relations.

'Hard' and 'soft' sides to HRM may be identified – reflecting the different origins of the subject already described. The hard site of HRM stresses the 'resources' aspect and is dispassionate and quantitative. The soft side reflects the 'human' component, more suggestive of a human relations approach. In essence, HRM is a business-oriented approach to managing people, on a par with other resource functions. It can be considered as a systematic, integrated approach, incorporating a set of tools to achieve strategic objectives.

External business environment factors shaping HRM

The overriding external factor is change, particularly the increasing rate of change. This obliges organizations to respond rapidly in order to survive and prosper. This has a number of implications for organizations. The first is pressure to derive competitive advantage, for example through high productivity, the ability to innovate quickly and to manage change quickly. Examples include responding to R&D breakthroughs, emphasizing excellence and the provision of high-quality goods and services to meet increasing customer expectations. A second feature is shorter learning cycles to increase responsiveness and finally there is greater management control, for example in respect of risk management and total preventive maintenance.

Principles of human resource management

Four basic principles of human resource management may be identified, for example from texts such as Storey (1989). These are all consistent with a strategic approach to risk management.

1. HRM is **strategy-driven**. HRM follows from addressing such basic strategic questions as: what business are we in? what do we want to do? what needs to be done? by whom? what human resources do we need to do it? HRM is proactive and oriented towards meeting business objectives such as growth and profitability.
2. Employees (and sometimes customers and suppliers as well) are a strategic resource to achieve competitive advantage (in the public sector, this might be excellence, quality and delivery). Human resources are seen as the single most important agents of the organization, which views them as an **investment** not as a cost. Thus, management's objective is to direct human resources to business needs so as to make the best of them, hence concern with performance and performance measures. There is a strong imperative to manage human resources as a business contribution; thus, low labour turnover may be one objective.
3. HRM is a **line** management function – i.e. it is part of production and other management functions. While personnel policies are a major contributor to corporate objectives, in HRM they are not a specialist function. Thus, different skills are required from those demanded of the traditional industrial relations function – for example, development of commitment as opposed to confrontational tactics. The aim for management is to foster allegiance to the organization, for example as opposed to a trade union.
4. HRM is concerned with **integration and control**. Through it, management seek a common purpose or unitary perspective (as opposed to a pluralist view in which different parties hold views which reflect their own

positions). Concordance between individual needs and organizational objectives is sought. Skills and ideas of employees are sought and used as appropriate rather than 'managerial prerogative' being imposed. Positive-sum solutions (in which all parties can gain) rather than zero-sum outcomes (where one party's gain is another's loss) to problems are demanded. Management aim to shape corporate culture as a major influence upon excellence, for example through promoting shared values, an open organizational climate and appropriate management style. Monitoring of performance and accountability of line management are important in the control function.

HRM practices and techniques

A wide range of topics has been subsumed under the HRM banner, some of the main ones being described briefly below. Where topics are addressed in this book, this is indicated.

Training and development for all employees and the development of competencies is a prime orientation of investment in human resources, reflecting its strategic orientation (chapter 2). This involves using systematic techniques such as job analysis, task analysis (chapter 9, pp. 275–7), training needs analysis and skills audits. Allied with more traditional forms of training and development is organization development (OD) involving such features as coordination, integration, teamwork, conflict management, change management and commitment – important components of risk management, which are referred to in a number of chapters.

Motivation and reward, another HRM focus which involves greater diversity of reward packages and more individual packages as well as greater integration and linking of pay to performance, are dealt with in chapter 3. The traditional personnel topic of performance appraisal is also important – for example via auditing (pp. 298–312). Along with more widespread use of appraisal techniques there has been more advanced and systematic use of selection techniques such as psychometric testing (chapter 6, pp. 149–55). Once recruited, it makes good business sense to retain and develop employees. Also traditionally part of the personnel function is industrial relations – now more likely to be called 'employee relations' (ER). The 'new industrial relations' is likely to involve such elements as no-strike agreements, single unionism and pendulum arbitration (in which an arbitrator decides for one side or another rather than 'splitting the difference'). However, such features often operate in parallel with more traditional approaches. Closely allied with ER is another HRM feature – involvement and participation. Examples include employee involvement schemes such as profit sharing and various forms of employee representation (see Glendon and Booth, 1982 for a review of safety representatives and safety committees in the UK). Elements of these themes feature in a number of chapters of this book.

On the more traditional management side, HRM features include human resource planning – defining requirements, greater flexibility (for example differentiating between 'core' and peripheral workers and an increased use of consultants) and analysis techniques such as brainstorming, force field analysis and organizational climate analysis (pp. 291–5). Also in this arena is leadership, involving for example greater emphasis upon management control and initiative as well as upon on-the-job coaching and development. The reduced span of control for line management has been matched with greater responsibility. Communication is starting to take new forms, such as team briefings, quality circles, IT and problem-solving teams (chapter 7, pp. 192–200), reflecting more open and direct communication between management and employees. During production activity, emphasis is upon greater flexibility in terms of skills, hours worked, distances travelled and working from home. Finally, the notion of performance auditing is gaining widespread acceptance for a range of evaluative measures (including safety auditing – pp. 298–312). All these features figure to some extent in this book, although not all of them have complete chapters or even sections devoted specifically to them. The are reflected more in a general awareness of the significance of the changes which are taking place under the HRM banner.

The one HRM feature which has not so far been mentioned is in essence the raison d'être for this book – the health, safety and welfare function. This has been very much the Cinderella of HRM, despite the increasing realization that through techniques of loss control and risk management, attention to such features can bring financial returns to the organization (see for example, Bird and Germain, 1990; Oxenburgh, 1991).

However, as far as HRM texts are concerned there is a yawning gap waiting to be filled. Of more than twenty HRM books published since 1988, only three have chapters on health and safety. Ironically, one of these (Armstrong, 1988) which contained a brief (4½ pages) chapter in the first edition had deleted this from the second edition (Armstrong, 1992). Where health and safety is considered as part of an HRM text, the treatment is inevitably rather superficial (e.g. Graham and Bennett, 1992), although Goss (1994) has a chapter on workplace health issues. There is considerable further scope for including safety and risk matters within an HRM framework.

CONCLUSIONS

An adequate safety management system provides the framework for considering all components of safety management and for setting clear safety objectives. Whether the term 'safety climate' or 'safety culture' is used to describe the collection of attitudes, values and behaviours which characterize health and safety within an organization, the key features of this vital context for risk management are likely to be very similar. They will include: management commitment to health and safety, adequate resourcing of the risk management function – for example in respect of training and staffing levels, employee involvement and an atmosphere of trust and caring, effective communication and good organizational learning.

When measuring management performance in health and safety, a variety of measures is available. It is important to use professional judgement in selecting from those that are available to meet criteria such as accuracy and validity. Specifically, it is important to use proactive data as a measure of management performance.

Safety auditing is a valuable risk management tool which is one of a variety of measures to be used in assessing management performance in health and safety, covering the main aspects of risk management – hazard identification, risk evaluation, identification of controls and monitoring. While a safety audit is a proactive performance measure which has many advantages over other methods, for example in terms of its scope and thoroughness, it is not an all-purpose performance measure and is best used in combination with other methods. Some of the claims which have been made in respect of safety auditing have not stood up to rigorous scrutiny. Thus, it is important to distinguish between the claims of audit producers – who have an understandable commitment to their product and associated services – and the efficacy of such an instrument in practice.

In carrying out risk assessments, it is important to distinguish between hazard (the potential for harm) and risk (the likelihood of that harm being realized in a given period of time). Risk assessment may be taken to comprise the first two stages of the risk management process – hazard identification and risk measurement.

Once the policy is in place for such features of risk management as safety culture, safety auditing and risk assessment, it is important to allocate adequate human (and other) resources to them. Human resource management (HRM) is a critical aspect of all management, including risk management. While health and safety has not yet been widely considered as an HRM topic, it is nevertheless vital to include health and safety matters within human resources planning. The most important aspect of HRM from a risk management perspective, is that it is a **strategic** approach to managing people. Thus, people, for example through selection and training processes, are considered as an investment and not as a cost. HRM is a proactive approach to management in which people are considered as a competitive advantage – and whom it thus makes good business sense to protect and to involve in organizational problem solving.

11 DIRECTIONS FOR ACTION

❏ This final chapter brings together essential features from the previous nine chapters and, for the central topic of each, sets out a prescriptive programme of action based upon current knowledge. Not only could this chapter be used as a set of guidelines for action, it could also indicate areas in which further questions are pertinent and additional work is required.

PSYCHOLOGICAL FACTORS IN SAFETY AND RISK MANAGEMENT

Considering this book as a whole, it is important to establish a degree of synthesis between the various topics, which although treated under separate chapter and section headings, require integration for the purpose of effective interventions. Therefore, this brief chapter presents selective material from earlier chapters in a way which can promote applications in this field.

Safety and risk professionals face a number of challenges in managing risks during the 1990s and beyond. The first challenge is coping adequately with environmental change – both inside and outside organizations. Those responsible for managing risks arising from human activities will increasingly be faced with changing patterns of employment in which personal choice and individual needs will be considered alongside organizational requirements such as commitment and flexibility. Skills will be required to manage people in ways which take account of these juxtaposed demands. These skills are likely to involve:

- increased knowledge and understanding of human behaviour and motivation, as well as how perceptions, attitudes and environmental factors combine to shape behaviour;
- a more strategic orientation to the management of risk in all its forms, involving a 'top down' approach to risk management, taking into account organizational factors (e.g. structure, marketing and business plans) as well as the external environment (economic, political, social and legislative factors) and changing technology.

A second challenge is the integration of risk management within the management structure of organization so that it achieves a status commensurate with more traditional functions. Reason (1990) notes that in the long-term, safety and production goals are compatible, but that given finite resources, they may conflict in the short-term. Safety and risk professionals need to promote a long-term perspective within organizations and to put into practice the message that an effective way of managing risk is by influencing key decisions at an early stage.

In pursuing these challenges, safety and risk professionals also need to reinforce the strategic human resource message that expenditure on employees, if properly targeted, constitutes investment in the long-term. Such targets might include appropriate training and selection, reducing stress and anxiety to levels where they operate positively rather than negatively, increasing motivation and building strong teams. While the effort to achieve these aims may appear as a cost in the short-term, organizations which consistently support their initial investments should reap benefits, not only in respect of risk management but also in terms of product quality and competitive advantage in their markets.

The final challenge remains as it has been for some time and that is to manage the integration of humans within systems so that they remain safe, healthy, efficient, effective and productive. This requires an understanding of the multiple facets of human cognitions and behaviour to complement legal and technical knowledge. This book has sought to portray some of the most important features which require serious consideration. The remaining sections of this chapter correspond with chapters 2–10 of the book and outline actions which derive from the contents of these chapters. They are intended as guidance in respect of action on safety and risk issues.

SAFETY TRAINING (CHAPTER 2)

Develop a strategic plan for training as part of a human resources and risk management programme. Ensure that this strategic safety training plan meets individual needs as well as organizational objectives. Ensure that top management is committed to safety training to the extent that they participate in some way.

Carry out a safety skills audit and a safety skills needs analysis. Establish whether training or selection is the most appropriate way of addressing a safety skills deficit. Establish which aspects of safe behaviour can reasonably be expected to be improved by training (and which aspects require other interventions). Set out a logical sequence for safety training involving job analysis, training needs, objectives, implementation, evaluation and monitoring. Consider using an appropriate model as a basis for safety training.

Incorporate key learning principles into your organization's safety training – specifically: motivation, feedback, positive reinforcement, overlearning (e.g. for emergency training), whole-task training and active trainee involvement. Where safety training is designed to modify behaviour, make reference to successful training interventions in this field.

Where work involves a high level of decision-making or problem-solving, ensure that related safety training involves exercises at the knowledge-based level of performance so that adequate understanding of sometimes complex systems occurs and that the training links appropriately with trainees' experience. Use appropriate data from your organization (e.g. accident injury data) in safety training.

RISK MOTIVATION (CHAPTER 3)

Inducing fear in an attempt to motivate people to be safe is likely to fail as people are more likely to reject the fear-inducing message which threatens them and assume that the message is for some other audience. Fear is most effective when it reinforces already held beliefs or behaviours (for example about smoking) or when the means of avoiding the risk are made readily available.

Fundamental human motivations which need to be addressed in any risk management programme which is directed at human resources are:

1. Individuals need to perceive that they have **control** over aspects of the environment which they consider to be important. This implies empowerment and genuine involvement in decision making in respect of management actions which affect them.
2. Individuals need to maintain their self-esteem – i.e. to defend their egos. Systems which are designed primarily to apportion blame – e.g. for accidents, incidents or other mistakes, may exhibit features of extrinsic motivation (e.g. fear of actual or anticipated consequences). This is different from intrinsic motivation (e.g. positively wanting to do a job well) which may be in line with attempts to achieve quality through excellence – reflected at an individual level in such feelings as pride in the work that they are doing and a strong desire to do a job well. Management should seek to develop systems which involve people in a problem-solving approach to work issues. Humans operate most effectively in problem-solving mode (chapter 9, pp. 262–5, especially summary text 9.8 and summary text 9.9) and least well in the operation of routine or boring tasks.
3. Each individual's motivations are unique and this should be taken account of (e.g. via assessment – chapter 6, pp. 149–55) in the design and operation of work activities, job allocation and promotions.

One reason that people are motivated to take risks is because they can thereby demonstrate their skill. To try and overcome this form of motivation to take risks, it is necessary to associate competence with taking necessary precautions.

In seeking to change behaviour which is motivated towards taking specific risks (e.g. driving fast on public roads), it is necessary to understand the rewards which the individuals concerned associate with that behaviour. Only by addressing those components of the underlying motives can we begin to formulate policies to deal with such behaviour (a model for doing this – the health belief model – is described in chapter 4, pp. 84–8, especially summary text 4.7 and figure 4.7).

If there are inconsistent or conflicting messages on safety or risk-taking, then 'actions speak louder than words'. Thus, individuals' behaviour will be based upon actual incentives (e.g. effective payment for risk-taking or turning a blind eye to safety rules and regulations) rather than to officially stated policy (e.g. in respect of safety).

Generally, incentives which are based on outcomes, (e.g. reduced accident rates) are less likely to be effective than those based upon behaviours (e.g. adhering to safe systems of work), although they may be more difficult to implement. However, there have been a number of documented studies which have shown that it is possible to change behaviour using techniques which address underlying motivations. These involve individuals in important aspects of decision-making and provide them with a vital degree of control over their own behaviour.

ATTITUDES AND BEHAVIOUR (CHAPTER 4)

When seeking to change attitudes, it is important to identify these as relating to a particular behaviour in a highly specific way. Attempting to change attitudes in a general sense is unlikely to have a measurable impact upon behaviour.

While individuals may strive for consistency between their attitudes and behaviour, it is sensible from a strategic perspective to seek to influence both attitudes **and** behaviour – for example in a safety campaign using respectively information and awareness techniques (for attitudes) and training and re-inforcement (for behaviour).

To change behaviour through addressing attitudes, it is necessary first to demonstrate effectively that benefits of the desired change are greater than the barriers or costs to the individual. Second, individuals may need to be shown that they personally are vulnerable and that there is a good opportunity for them to make a change which will benefit them.

People need to feel that they are in control of their situation before attitude and behaviour change may be affected. It may be necessary to emphasize the importance of a given behaviour when seeking to change it – e.g. by showing how it affects a person's health in the long and short term.

When seeking to reinforce a desired link between attitudes and behaviour, it is necessary first to ensure that the attitudes are part of an individual's belief system, second that the behaviour is consistent with group norms and finally, that there are sanctions for non-compliance. Seeking to impose attitude and behaviour change in the other direction is less likely to succeed.

When seeking to effect attitude (and behaviour) change it is vital to have a reliable and valid method for measuring the attitudes of the target group before and after the intervention (e.g. safety training, safety campaign).

When attempting attitude change, ensure that:

- needs and motives which are important to the audience are addressed and that they are (made to be) highly involved in the issue;
- the persuader has high credibility (e.g. perceived expertise and trust) in the eyes of the target audience, and is acceptable to the audience;

- group affiliations and individual differences (e.g. intelligence and personality) are not ignored;
- a balanced viewpoint is presented and the audience is left to draw their own conclusions – unless the topic is highly complex for the audience;
- persistent attitude and behaviour change is helped by the active participation of an audience (e.g. via role playing), reinforcement of the message and perhaps by allowing time for the message to 'sink in'.

If used, safety propaganda should be: specific, backed up by training, positive, close to the desired action, built upon existing attitudes. It should not be: based upon horror, negative, general.

RISK PERCEPTION (CHAPTER 5)

When designing work environments, it is important to be aware of the limitations of people's perceptions. For example, reduced efficiency of the visual and auditory senses in particular as a result of ageing. Colour can be used to denote different conditions (up to a maximum of about eleven different colours), but be aware of the effects of juxtaposing certain colours, colour adaptation requirements and that some individuals have restricted colour vision. Also while we can adapt to changing dark and light, this process takes some time, especially dark adaptation.

When designing auditory warning systems, pay heed to recommendations developed from experience and systematic study. Combine auditory and visual displays as appropriate. Effectiveness of warnings depends upon: timing (needs to be exactly right), audience (reaching it), and explicitness (tell them exactly what to do).

In the use of warnings such as alarms, attention needs to be paid to the way in which these are likely to be perceived (e.g. as false or irrelevant). Systematic human factors models are available to determine operators' likely reactions to alarms and other warnings. These can be used to predict behaviour as well as to collect data to improve the safety and security of systems. In designing alarm systems, it is important to minimize the number of alarms which do not mean 'danger', reinforce genuine alarms whenever possible and train and refresh personnel appropriately.

Our senses provide vital information about the world around us and require protection. Personal protective equipment reduces the effectiveness of our senses and for this reason alone is a less desirable means of protecting our sensory organs than engineered solutions which control the source of the potential damage.

Education and training is required to enhance workers' awareness of the value of information from their senses. For example, explaining the kinaesthetic sense when training in correct lifting techniques, or the vestibular sense while instructing on the avoidance of slips and falls. This approach supplements people's procedural knowledge gained from everyday experience with understanding of the nature of risk in a variety of activities (chapter 2 gives further details on this).

Safety campaigns should associate competence as a positive aspect of human functioning with safe behaviour and reinforce that link. In communicating safety messages, we may have to challenge the present views of an audience. In any communication, it is necessary to pay regard to relevant features of the sender, the message itself and the channel through which it is sent as well as the intended audience. There is a need to be aware of individual differences in perception when presenting safety messages. For example, males and females may process information differently and may have different motivations in respect of compliance.

Use windows of opportunity in presenting safety information and emphasize the control that individuals have over their own behaviour. Oblige them to assume responsibility for their own behaviour.

It is important to consider the best way of presenting information. Generally, simple messages are best portrayed visually while more complex ones are best put across in textual format. Both may be used in combination to reinforce a message providing that the result is not then too complex or confusing to be optimally effective.

Measuring perceptions (like measuring attitudes) can help to reveal prejudices which may be based upon stereotypes of other people or groups. It is important to take steps to overcome these, for example as a prelude to or concomitant with seeking behaviour change.

In guiding people's behaviour towards desired goals, perception of risk has to be considered alongside issues of attitudinal and motivational factors. Informing people – and perhaps altering the way in which they perceive situations goes hand in hand with attitude change (chapter 4, pp. 93–7). Use of case studies which are relevant to an individual's own circumstances or organization can be a potent educational tool.

People have a wide possible variety of dimensions available which they can use to perceive risk or danger. One task of communication is to tune them in to the most appropriate ones (this requires *a priori* analysis of the nature of the risk) to reduce the inevitable gap between subjective and objective risk evaluation.

Because people use heuristics (rules of thumb) in their appraisal of risk, it is vital to provide full and understandable information about the risks faced by them – including any uncertainty about the risk. If such information is withheld – for whatever reason – then we cannot expect people's perception of risk to be accurate.

PERSONALITY (CHAPTER 6)

This section suggests an approach to using personality measures which is commensurate with current knowledge in this area within a risk management framework of identifying, evaluating, controlling and monitoring risks which might arise because of mismatches between job requirements and personality factors. Thus, the points in this section are in the form of a series of logical steps.

1. Determine safety critical tasks (chapter 9, pp. 275–86 gives examples of appropriate methodologies). This involves identifying those features of a task or job that are critical to safety (e.g. attention, vigilance, resistance to distraction, routine aspects, etc.).
2. Assess whether there is any relation between these specific aspects and personality traits (studies are cited in chapter 6). Determine whether the personality of an individual performing these tasks could be a critical risk factor.
3. If this is the case, use appropriate personality tests as part of a battery of techniques to select for desirable features for the requirements of the task or to identify training needs (e.g. for control room operators, drivers, line managers in charge of safety critical systems). If there is evidence to link these critical aspects with personality traits, then it could be worth screening out applicants who score at the opposite extreme for important traits (e.g. select introverts for vigilance tasks and extraverts for complex tasks which could be subject to distraction). In selection procedures, systematically identify personality tests or measures which, in combination with other selection techniques (e.g. ability tests, biodata, work sample tests) perhaps as part of an assessment centre, can profile a range of dimensions or traits which are deemed through systematic analysis to be appropriate to the job.
4. Continue to monitor the effectiveness of this approach.

In the longer term, where necessary, develop specific tests to assess the personality dimensions or types which relate to the performance of particular jobs or tasks which are safety critical, including managerial jobs.

GROUPS AND TEAMS (CHAPTER 7)

Groups are important in the change process (along with attitudes) and when seeking to initiate change, it is vital to find out what sort of group(s) you are dealing with. This should go beyond the formal/informal categorization to determine answers to the following questions:

- What are the group's goals and objectives?
- How stable and coherent is the group?
- Are the members loyal?
- Is the group volatile or predictable?
- What are the group norms?
- How strong are the norms?

Involve groups in decisions which affect them and their members. Changes will be more readily accepted if people are able to participate in the decision-making process through their existing groups. Where two groups are in conflict and this has important implications for safety, it is vital to find a task, the completion of which has outcomes which are important for both groups, and that will also require cooperation between the groups in order for the task to be completed successfully.

Use groups to make decisions which are particularly complex, require a variety and quantity of information to be synthesized and involve making judgements. Avoid isolating groups from their environment or excluding the results of their decision-making process from critical examination. This is because groups can make very poor decisions and their decisions should always be challenged or subject to scrutiny. Institute processes to achieve this.

In decision-making groups, ensure heterogeneity of participation, especially where decision outcomes are critical to safety and risk issues. Various (not mutually exclusive) means to achieve this include:

- build in checks within the group decision-making procedures;
- ensure a mixture of cognitive styles among participants (there are tests available to measure these);
- use a combination of different team roles – this also involves using techniques to assess personal preferences for team roles and the perceptions of others to confirm (or otherwise) individual members' own perceptions.

Successful safety and risk management depends upon effective use of teams. Be proactive in building to support your work activities. Constantly be alive to the possibility of incorporating new members to your team – from inside or outside the organization and seek to maximize the contributions of each member. Don't try to act alone – use others and don't feel threatened by them. Become aware of your own strengths (and weaknesses) in a team and use these to increase your work role effectiveness.

Be prepared to allow the person with the optimum characteristics for that particular set of circumstances (task, group members, situation) to be group leader and be prepared to change the leader if the situation demands it.

STRESS MANAGEMENT (CHAPTER 8)

Individual strategies

Become aware of your personal resources (internal and external) for dealing with stress and opportunities for expanding the quality and quantity of these. For example, seek to enhance the range of coping strategies available to you, including: problem-focused, emotion-focused, avoidance (where necessary), defence mechanisms (short-term for severe crises only), cognitive strategies – e.g. rational emotive approach – involving taking responsibility for your thoughts and feelings.

Recognize that over time, significant change is possible, i.e. you are not a prisoner either of your personality or of your circumstances. Your behaviour is very much under your control and habits (e.g. relating to alcohol or nicotine consumption), diet, anger responses, etc. – can all be altered and brought under self-control.

Identification of individual stressors can aid coping. Establish features of your life which cause you stress and determine which of these you can significantly influence and how. Proceed to address each stressor. This is an example of a problem-focused coping strategy. Seek to establish a personal support network – at home, at work and in the social sphere – for example a mutual support group or a co-counselling partner.

A variety of techniques can help you to achieve greater control over your body, its responses and your life. These range from biofeedback – learned initially with instruments, but subsequently rehearsed without these, to relaxation, hypnosis (including self-hypnosis), yoga and meditation.

There is sound evidence that self-belief plays a crucial role in coping with stress – believe in yourself and that you have adequate resources to cope, and you will experience less stress. However, self-efficacy beliefs need to be based upon cognitive processes of self-persuasion using information, for example from physiological, personal and social sources – i.e. it is not enough just to **say** that you feel self-confident; the belief must be genuine.

Organizational strategies

While it is neither possible nor desirable to create a stress-free environment, there are some guiding principles for reducing harmful levels of stress, and improving individual mental health and productivity. For example:

- individuals perform optimally if they are not continually stretched to their limits – it is necessary to leave psychological 'spare capacity';
- does each individual employee fit their work environment? – the person–environment fit approach to stress;
- it can be useful to identify specific stressors which relate to particular jobs.

Develop a strategy to deal with stress arising from the work environment and ensure that this remains live. Features of such a strategy might include:

- empowering individuals to take control of changes which affect them;
- appropriate training and development programmes;
- clarification of roles and responsibilities;
- develop employee assistance programmes with a wide-ranging brief.

HUMAN ERROR (CHAPTER 9)

Learning situations, for example simulations, should whenever possible be designed to allow opportunities for trainees to make mistakes so that they can learn from them. In designing representations of complex systems, for example control rooms, it is vital to have continuous input from future users. In addition to workplace ergonomic issues, this is also because their ability to have an accurate representation of the system, particularly during emergencies, is critical.

There is a need to educate (as opposed to train) senior managers and other decision-makers in issues concerned with latent errors which could lead to failures in systems. These people will usually accept the general principles fairly readily. The problem is typically getting them to acknowledge that they apply to decisions which they personally are involved in making, and thereby effectively influencing those decision-making processes. An approach is needed which is analogous with individual debiasing (summary text 3.8 in chapter 3) to enable them to appreciate the type of scenarios and circumstances in which **their** decisions can have serious implications for safety and risk factors throughout the organization. There is a need to develop effective strategies to debias decision-makers so as to change some aspects of their behaviour. An initial step would be to increase their awareness of the effects of their decisions using dramatic demonstrations and high involvement techniques, using for example role plays and case studies.

The design approach to 'human error problems' will usually be the most cost-effective in the long term because it only has to be done once – compared for example with training or selection strategies which require continuous attention. This means devoting resources initially, for example on user acceptability trials, in the reasonable expectation that such investment will be repaid in the long term. Identification and control of error, as part of a risk management strategy, requires a near miss incident reporting system involving everyone in the organization – summary text 9.7 gives details of how such a system might operate.

There is a possibility that interventions which are designed to reduce the adverse impact of stress (e.g. relaxation techniques) could also be beneficial in respect of reducing individuals' error liability. When designing systems, we should be aware of complementarity – machines and humans supporting one another – checking and monitoring each others' actions. This is important in all ergonomic (i.e. all design) strategies to involve would-be system users.

As a critical component of risk assessment, it is vital to institute some form of systematic approach to the identification of human error in work systems. This is preferable to relying upon outcome data such as accidents or incidents. This is because such an approach is focused at the places where errors initially occur, rather than upon end events – which are subject to inherent variability – i.e. it is a matter of chance and other factors as to whether any particular error leads to an accident or incident or to no incident. Techniques in this field (e.g. TAFEI, PHEA, HRA) are typically based upon some form of task analysis (e.g. HTA).

Some large organizations may already possess the human factors skills required to tackle problems arising from human error and may need to galvanize their resources to address the problem. Other organizations may need to acquire relevant expertise externally. In either case, senior management need to get a handle on the human error problem by:

- collecting relevant data from within the organization;
- analysing this to determine causal factors;
- controlling the prime or most serious factors identified;
- establishing a system to monitor the effectiveness of those control measures.

Simply expressed, organizations should manage the risk to their operations posed by human error.

MANAGING HUMAN RISKS (CHAPTER 10)

In seeking to develop an adequate safety management system within an organization, numerous aspects of organizational functioning in relation to safety need to be addressed. Foremost among these are: top management commitment to safety, setting clear safety objectives and adequate communication. From these components, other aspects of managing human risks should follow.

In making any changes to managing human aspects of risk, it is essential to ensure that the culture – specifically the safety culture – of an organization is receptive to such changes. A simple way to assess safety culture is by the measurement of employee attitudes to safety and to its management in the organization. Such an exercise can serve as a baseline from which to measure changes in the safety culture of an organization.

When assessing any aspect of management performance, it is important to decide upon an appropriate range of valid measures – i.e. not to rely upon a single measure. While reactive measures, such as accident rates, will remain necessary, it is important to use proactive measures of performance which will serve as positive motivators of behaviour that are actively under the control of individual managers.

Notwithstanding the difficulties of conclusively demonstrating that safety audits are a means to improved control of health and safety, and therefore of better safety and risk management, a well-developed safety audit can provide a systematic and detailed review of both technical and managerial aspects of safety, as well as an opportunity to investigate specific components of health and safety, such as human factors. While there are benefits in an external auditing approach, from the point of view of commitment to and ownership of the audit process and its outcomes, it is important to involve those who are the subject of the audit, in the auditing process.

While it is a legal requirement to conduct risk assessments and to act appropriately on the findings, it has long been an accepted component of risk management to conduct hazard identification and risk measurement – together comprising risk assessment. Various methods are available for undertaking risk assessments – from detailed technical approaches to more judgemental qualitative techniques. It is important to select techniques appropriate to the risks being assessed.

It is vital to allocate adequate human and other resources to the risk management function and to be able to assess the value of the contribution made by human resources to risk management.

GLOSSARY

ACoP	Approved Code of Practice
ACSNI	Advisory Committee on the Safety of Nuclear Installations
ACTH	Adrenocorticotrophic hormone (released as part of stress response)
BHSS	British Health and Safety Society
B176	Form for reporting occupational absences to DSS
BR	British Rail
BSI	British Standards Institution
CAL	Computer assisted learning
CFQ	Cognitive Failures Questionnaire (Broadbent *et al.*, 1982)
CHASE	Complete Health And Safety Evaluation (safety audit)
CHD	Coronary heart disease
COSHH	Control of Substances Hazardous to Health (Regulations 1988)
CPA	Critical path analysis
CPR	Cardiopulmonary resuscitation
dB	Decibel
DIY	Do-it-yourself
DSE	Display screen equipment
DSS	Department of Social Security
EAP	Employee Assistance Programme
EC	European Community
EPI	Eysenck Personality Inventory
EPQ	Eysenck Personality Questionnaire
ER	Employee relations
F2508	Form for reporting accident injuries and dangerous occurrences to HSE
F2508A	Form for reporting occupational diseases to HSE
FR	Frequency rate (for accident injuries)
GEMS	Generic Error Modelling System (Reason)
HASS	Home Accident Surveillance System
HAZAN	Hazard analysis
HAZOPs	Hazard and operability studies
HBM	Health belief model
HGV	Heavy goods vehicle
HMSO	Her Majesty's Stationery Office
HP	Hearing protection
HRA	Human reliability assessment

HRM	Human resource management
HSC	Health and Safety Commission
HSE	Health and Safety Executive
HSW Act	Health and Safety at Work etc. Act 1974
HTA	Hierarchical task analysis
Hz	Hertz
IOSH	Institution of Occupational Safety and Health
IR	Incidence rate (for accident injuries)
IR	Industrial relations
ISRS	International Safety Rating System (safety audit)
IT	Information technology
Km	Kilometres
LEV	Local exhaust ventilation
LTA	Lost time accident (usually more than one shift lost)
MBTI	Myers Briggs Type Indicator
ME	Myalgic encephalomyelitis
MEL	Maximum exposure limit
MHQ	Middlesex Hospital Questionnaire
MMPI	Minnesota Multi-Phasic Personality Inventory
NACE	International Standard Industrial Classification
NASA	National Aeronautical Space Administration (US)
NEBOSH	National Examination Board in Occupational Safety and Health
NIHL	Noise induced hearing loss
OD	Organization development
OES	Occupational Exposure Standard
OPQ	Occupational Personality Questionnaire
PERT	Programme Evaluation Research Technique
pH	Scale for measuring degree of acidity/alkalinity
PHEA	Predictive Human Error Analysis
PIFs	Performance influencing factors
PPE	Personal protective equipment
PRA	Probabalistic risk assessment
PSFs	Performance shaping factors
PSV	Public service vehicle
PTSD	Post-traumatic stress disorder
PTW	Permit to work
RAF	Royal Air Force
RIDDOR	Reporting of Industrial Diseases and Dangerous Occurrences Regulations
R&D	Research and development
RM	Risk management
RTA	Road traffic accident
RSI	Repetitive strain injury (see also WRULD)
SIC	Standard Industrial Classification
s/gear	Switchgear

SMS	Safety management system
SPADs	Signals Passed at Danger
Stats 19	Police form for recording road traffic accident details
SR	Severity rate (for accident injuries)
s/s	Substation
SSD	System State Diagram
TAFEI	Task Analysis for Error Identification
THERP	Technique for Human Error Rate Prediction
TMI	Three Mile Island
TQC	Total quality control
TTS	Temporary threshold shift (temporary hearing loss)
TV	Television
UK	United Kingdom
UMIST	University of Manchester Institute of Science and Technology
USA	United States of America
VALS	Values and lifestyle (psychographic types)
VDU	Visual display unit
WHO	World Health Organization
WRULD	Work Related Upper Limb Disorder

REFERENCES

Achmon, J. (1987) *The Role of Cognitive and Physiological Personality Characteristics in Self-Regulatory Processes.* PhD Thesis, Tel Aviv University.

Adams, J. (1982) Issues in human reliability. *Human Factors,* **24,** 1–10.

Adams, J. (1990) Evaluating the effectiveness of safety measures in J. Handmer and E. Penning-Rowsell, (eds), *Hazards and the Communication of Risk,* Gower, Aldershot, pp. 173–94.

Ajzen, I. (1991) The theory of planned behavior. *Organizational Behavior and Human Decision Processes,* **50,** 179–211.

Ajzen, I. and Fishbein, M. (1977) Attitude-behaviour relations: a theoretical analysis and review of empirical research. *Psychological Bulletin,* **84,** 888–918.

Alcalay, R. and Pasick, R.J. (1983) Psychological factors and the technologies of work. *Social Science and Medicine,* **17,** 1075–84.

Alderfer, C.R. (1972) *Existence, Relatedness and Growth: Human Needs in Organizational Settings,* Free Press, New York.

Anderson, N. and Prutton, K. (1993) Occupational psychology in business: strategic response or purveyor of tests? *The Occupational Psychologist,* **20,** August, 3–10.

Anderson, N. and West, M.A. (1994) Team climate: measuring and predicting innovation in groups at work. *Occupational Psychology Conference of the British Psychological Society,* 3–5 January, Birmingham.

Anderson, V.V. (1929) *Psychiatry in Industry,* Harpers, New York.

Annett, J. and Duncan, K.D. (1967) Task analysis and training design. *Occupational Psychology,* **41,** 211–21.

Annett, J., Duncan, K.D., Stammers, R.B. and Gray, M.J. (1971) *Task Analysis,* Department of Employment Training Information Paper No 6, HMSO, London.

Argyle, M. (1988) *Bodily Communication,* 2nd edn, Methuen, London.

Armstrong, M. (1988) *A Handbook of Human Resource Management,* Kogan Page, London.

Armstrong, M. (1992) *Human Resource Management: Strategy and Action,* Kogan Page, London.

Arnold, J., Robertson, I.T. and Cooper, C.L. (1991) *Work Psychology: Understanding Human Behaviour in the Workplace,* Pitman, London.

Asch, S.E. (1958) Effects of group pressure upon the modification and distortion of judgements, in E.E. Maccoby, T.M. Newcombe and E.L. Hartley, (eds), *Readings in Social Psychology.* Holt, Rinehart and Winston, New York, pp. 174–83.

Asher, S.R. and Gottman, J.M. (1981) *The Development of Children's Friendships,* CUP, Cambridge.

Ashford, S.J. (1988) Individual strategies for coping with stress during organizational transitions. *Journal of Applied Behavioral Science,* **24,** 19–36.

Ashforth, B.E. and Mael, F. (1989) Social identity theory and the organization. *Academy of Management Review,* **14,** 20–39.

Ashton, D. (1990) *The Corporate Healthcare Revolution.* Kogan Page and Institute of Personnel Management, London.

Astley, J.A. (1991) *An Evaluation of Task Analysis Techniques for Industrial Process Control,* PhD thesis, Aston University, Birmingham.

Baber, C. and Stanton, N.A. (in press) Task analysis for error identification: a methodology for designing error tolerant products. *Ergonomics.*

Bainbridge, L. (1987) The ironies of automation, in J. Rasmussen, K.D. Duncan and J. Leplat, (eds), *New Technology and Human Error,* Wiley, London, pp. 271–83.

Bales, R.F. (1950a) *Interaction Process Analysis: a Method for the Study of Small Groups,* Addison-Wesley, Cambridge, Ma.

Bales, R.F. (1950b) A set of categories for the analysis of small group interaction. *American Sociological Review,* **15,** 257–63.

Ball, K. and Owsley, C. (1991) Identifying correlates of accident involvement for the older driver. *Human Factors, 33,* 583–5.

Bamber, L. (1990) Risk management: techniques and practices, in J. Ridley (ed.), *Safety at Work,* 3rd edn, Butterworth, London, pp. 159–92.

Bandura, A. (1977) Self-efficacy: towards a unifying theory of behavior change. *Psychological Review,* **84,** 191–225.

Bandura, A. (1989) *Self Efficacy in the Exercise of Control,* Annual Conference of the British Psychological Society, April , St Andrews.

Barrett, E.S. (1987) Impulsiveness and anxiety: information processing and electro-encephalograph topography. *Journal of Research in Personality, 21,* 453–63.

Barrick, M.R. and Mount, M.K. (1991) The big five personality measures as predictors of job performance: a meta-analysis. *Personnel Psychology, 44,* 1–26.

Bartram, D. and Dale, H.C.A. (1982) The Eysenck Personality Inventory as a selection test for military pilots. *Journal of Occupational Psychology, 55,* 287–96.

Bayne, R. (1994) The 'big five' versus the Myers-Briggs. *The Psychologist,* **7(1),** 14–16.

Beaumont, P.B., Coyle, J.R., Leopold, J.W. and Schuller, T.W. (1982) *The Determinants of Effective Joint Health and Safety Committees,* Centre for Research in Industrial Democracy and Participation, University of Glasgow.

Beck, A.T. and Emery, G. (1985) *Anxiety, Disorders and Phobias: a Cognitive Perspective,* Basic Books, New York.

Beck, K.H. (1984) The effects of risk probability, outcome severity, efficacy of protection and access to protection on decision making: a further test of protection motivation theory. *Social Behavior and Personality, 12,* 121–5.

Becker, M.H. (ed.) (1974) The health belief model and personal health behaviour. *Health Education Monographs, 2,* Winter, Slack, Thorofare, NJ, pp. 324–508.

Becker, M.H. and Janz, N.K. (1987) Behavioral science perspectives on health hazard/health risk appraisal. *Health Services Research, 22,* 537–51.

Becker, M.H. and Rosenstock, I.M. (1987) Comparing social learning theory and the health belief model, in W.B. Ward (ed.), in *Advances in Health Education and Promotion* Vol 2, JAI Press, Greenwich, Ct., pp. 245–9.

Beer, M., Eisenstat, R.A. and Spector, B. (1990) Why change programs don't produce change, *Harvard Business Review,* **68(6),** 158–66.

Bekey, G.A. (1970) The human operator in control systems, in *Systems Psychology,* K.B. de Green (ed.), McGraw-Hill, New York, pp. 248–77.

Belbin, R.M. (1981) *Management Teams: Why They Succeed of Fail,* Heinemann, London.

Belbin, R.M. (1993a) *Team Roles at Work,* Butterworth-Heinemann, Oxford.

Belbin, R.M. (1993b) A reply to the Belbin team-role self-perception inventory by Furnham, Steele and Pendleton. *Journal of Occupational and Organizational Psychology,* **66,** 259–60.

Belle, D. (1982) The stress of caring: women as providers of social support, in L. Goldberger and S. Breznitz (eds), *Handbook of Stress,* Free Press, New York.

Bem, D.J. (1967) Self-perception: an alternative interpretation of cognitive dissonance phenomena. *Psychological Review,* **74(3),** 183–200.

Bensiali, A.K. (1988) *An Expert System for the Development of a Health and Safety Policy/Risk Assessment in the Plastics Industry,* PhD thesis, Aston University, Birmingham.

Bensiali, A.K., Booth, R.T. and Glendon, A.I. (1992) Models for problem solving in health and safety. *Safety Science,* **15,** 183–205.

Bensiali, A.K. and Glendon, A.I. (1987) *Safety Inspection and Auditing,* Module RA6, Risk Assessment and Control Unit, Occupational Health and Safety, Portsmouth.

Bergum, B.D. and Bergum, J.E. (1981) Population stereotypes: an attempt to measure and define. *Proceedings of the Human Factors Society 25th Annual Meeting,* Human Factors Society, Santa Monica, Ca., pp. 662–5.

Berkman, H.W. and Gilson, C. (1986) *Consumer Behaviour: Concepts and Strategies,* 3rd edn, Kent, Boston.

Berridge, J. and Cooper, C.L. (1993) Stress and coping in US organizations: the role of the Employee Assistance Programme. *Work and Stress,* **7,** 89–102.

Billings, A.G. and Moos, R.H. (1984) Coping, stress, and social resources among adults with unipolar depression. *Journal of Personality and Social Psychology,* **46,** 877–91.

Bird, F.E. Jr and Germain, G.L. (1990) *Practical Loss Control Leadership,* revised edn, Institute Publishing, Loganville, Ga.

Blinkhorn, S. and Johnson, C. (1990) The significance of personality testing. *Nature,* **348,** 671–2.

Bloom, B.S. (1956) *The Taxonomy of Educational Objectives: Cognitive Domain,* David Mackay, New York.

Boden, L.I., Hall, J.A., Levenstein, C. and Punnett, L. (1984) The impact of health and safety committees. *Journal of Occupational Medicine,* **26,** 829–34.

Bodenhausen, G.V. (1988) Stereotypic biases in social decision-making and memory: testing process models of stereotype use. *Journal of Personality and Social Psychology,* **55,** 726–37.

Bodman, H.W. (1962) Illumination levels and visual performance. *International Lighting Review,* **13,** 41–7.

Bond, M.H. and Forgas, J.P. (1984) Linking person perception to behaviour intention across cultures. *Journal of Cross-Cultural Psychology,* **15,** 337–52.

Booth, R.T. (1990) *What Determines the Tolerability of Risk?* Annual Conference of the Institution of Occupational Safety and Health, November, Harrogate.

Booth, R.T. (1993) *Where's the Harm in It? Risk Assessment Work Book,* Monitor Training, Henley-on-Thames.

Booth, R.T., Boyle, A.J., Glendon, A.I. and Hale, A.R. (eds) (1987) *CHASE I: The Complete Health and Safety Evaluation Manual for the Smaller Organization,* Version 2.0, Health and Safety Technology and Management, Birmingham.

Booth, R.T., Boyle, A.J., Glendon, A.I., Hale, A.R. and Waring, A.E. (eds) (1989) *CHASE II: The Complete Health and Safety Evaluation Manual for the Larger Organisation,* Version 4.1, Health and Safety Technology and Management, Birmingham.

Booth, R.T., Boyle, A.J., Glendon, A.I., Lander, V.W., Lomax, J.M. and McCrossen, T.A. (eds) (1990) *Construction CHASE: Complete Health and Safety Evaluation for the Construction Industry,* Building Advisory Service, London.

Booth, R.T., Boyle, A.J., Glendon, A.I., Hale, A.R., Simmons, S. and Thomas, M.S. (eds) (1991a) *Environment Audit: a Complete Guide to Undertaking an Environmental Audit for Your Business,* Mercury, London.

Booth, R.T., Boyle, A.J., Glendon A.I., Hale, A.R., Lewis, W. and Thomas, M.S. (eds) (1991b) *COSHH Audit – Control of Substances Hazardous to Health: a Complete Guide to Undertaking a COSHH Audit for Your Business,* Mercury, London.

Booth, R.T., Raafat, H.M.N. and Waring, A.E. (1988) *Machinery and Plant Integrity,* Module ST2, Safety Technology Unit, Occupational Health and Safety, Portsmouth.

Bower, G.H. and Hilgard, E.R. (1981) *Theories of Learning,* 5th edn, Englewood Cliffs, London.

Brand, C.R. and Egan, V. (1989) The 'big five' dimensions of personality? Evidence from ipsative, adjectival self-attributions. *Personality and Individual Differences,* **10,** 1165–71.

Breckler, S.J. (1984) Empirical validation of affect, behaviour and cognition as distinct components of attitude. *Journal of Personality and Social Psychology,* **47,** 1191–205.

Bridges, W. (1992) *The Character of Organisations: Using Jungian Type in Organisational Development,* Consulting Psychologists Press, Palo Alto.

Briggs Myers, I. and Briggs Myers, P. (1980) *Gifts Differing,* Consulting Psychologists Press, Palo Alto.

Briner, R.B. (1993) Bad theory and bad practice in occupational stress. *The Occupational Psychologist,* **19,** April, 8–13.

Broadbent, D.E., Broadbent, M.H.P. and Jones, J.L. (1986) Correlates of cognitive failure. *British Journal of Clinical Psychology,* **25,** 285–99.

Broadbent, D.E., Cooper, P.F., Fitzgerald, P. and Parkes, K.R. (1982) The cognitive failures questionnaire (CFQ) and its correlates. *British Journal of Clinical Psychology,* **21,** 1–16.

Broadbent, D.E. and Gath, D. (1981) Ill-health on the line: sorting out myth from fact. *Employment Gazette,* March, 157–60.

Bruner, J.S. and Tagiuri, R. (1954) The perception of people, in G. Linzey (ed.), *Handbook of Social Psychology,* vol 2, Addison-Wesley, Camb., Ma, pp. 634–54.

Bryan, L.A. (1989) The human factor: implications for engineers and managers. *Professional Safety,* **34(11),** 15–18.

Bukowski, W.M. and Newcombe, A.F. (1984) Stability and determinants of sociometric status and friendship choice: a longitudinal perspective. *Developmental Psychology,* **20,** 941–52.

Burke, R.J. (1993) Organizational-level interventions to reduce occupational stressors. *Work and Stress,* **7,** 77–87.

Burke, R.J. and Belcourt, M.L. (1974) Managerial role stress and coping responses. *Journal of Business Administration,* **5,** 55–68.

Buros, O.K. (1970) *Personality tests and reviews,* Gryphon, Highland Park, N.J.

Byrne, B.M. (1993) The Maslach Burnout Inventory: testing for factorial validity and invariance across elementary, intermediate and secondary teachers. *Journal of Occupational and Organizational Psychology,* **66,** 197–212.

Byrne, D. (1971) *The attraction paradigm,* Academic Press, New York.

Callan, V.J. (1993) Individual and organizational strategies for coping with organizational change. *Work and Stress,* **7,** 63–75.

Calnan, M. (1988) The health locus of control: an empirical test. *Health Promotion,* **2,** 323–30.

Campbell, S.S. (1992) Effects of sleep and circadian rhythms on performance, in A.P. Smith and D.M. Jones, (eds), *Handbook of Human Performance Volume 3 State and Trait,* Academic Press, London, pp. 195–216.

Caplan, R.D., Cobb, S., French, J.R.P., Harrison, R.V. and Pinneau, S.R. (1975) *Job Demands and Worker Health,* US Department of Health, Education and Welfare, Washington, D.C.

Carter, F.A. and Corlett, E.N. (1981) *Shiftwork and Accidents,* European Foundation for the Improvement of Living and Working Conditions, Dublin.

Cassel, J. (1963) The use of medical records: opportunity for epidemiological studies. *Journal of Occupational Medicine,* **5,** 185–190.

Cassidy, T. and Lynn, R. (1989) A multi-dimensional approach to achievement motivation: the development of a comprehensive measure. *Journal of Occupational Psychology,* **62,** 301–12.

Cattell, R.B. (1965) The Scientific Analysis of Personality, Penguin, Harmondsworth.

Cattell, R.B. and Scheier, H. (1961) *The Meaning and Measurement of Neuroticism and Anxiety,* Ronald Press, New York.

Cattell, R.B., Eber, H.W. and Tatsuoka, M.M. (1970) *Handbook for the 16PF Questionnaire,* IPAT, Champaign, Il.

Chambers, D.L. and Gracely, E.J. (1989) Fear of fear and the anxiety disorders. *Cognitive Therapy and Research,* **13,** 19–20.

Chapanis, A. (1959) *Research Techniques in Human Engineering,* Johns Hopkins, Baltimore.

Chapanis, A. (1961) Men, machines and models. *American Psychologist,* **16,** 113–31.

Chapanis, A. (1963) Engineering psychology. *Annual Review of Psychology,* **14,** 285–318.

Chapanis, A. (1965) On the allocation of functions between men and machines. *Occupational Psychology,* **39,** 1–11.

Chapman, J. (1982) After the inspector's visit: when group loyalty made a mockery of accident prevention. *The Safety Representative,* March, p. 5.

Chappelow, J.W. (1989) *Remedies for Aircrew Error,* RAF Institute for Aviation Medicine, Report No 664, Farnborough, Hants.

Cherniss, C. (1980) *Staff Burnout: Job Stress in the Human Services,* Sage, London.

Chhokar, J.S. (1987) Safety at the workplace: a behavioural approach. *International Labour Review,* **126(2),** 169–78.

Christensen, D. and Rosenthal, R. (1982) Gender and nonverbal decoding skill as determinants of interpersonal expectancy effects. *Journal of Personality and Social Psychology,* **42,** 75–87.

Cobb, S. (1976) Social support as a moderator of life stress. *Psychosomatic Medicine,* **38,** 300–14.

Cohen, A., Smith, M.J. and Anger, W.K. (1979) Self-protective measures against workplace hazards. *Journal of Safety Research,* **11(3),** 121–31.

Cohen, S., Tyrrell, D.A.J. and Smith, A.P. (1991) Psychological stress and susceptibility to the common cold. *The New England Journal of Medicine,* **325,** 606–12.

Commission of the European Communities. (1990) *Social Europe: Health and Safety at Work in the European Community.* Office for Official Publications of the European Community, Luxembourg.

Confederation of British Industry. (1990) *Developing a Safety Culture – Business for Safety,* Confederation of British Industry, London.

Confederation of British Industry. (1993) *Assessing the Risk: Implementing Health and Safety Regulations,* Confederation of British Industry, London.

Connor, M. (1992) Pros and cons of social cognition models in health psychology. *Social Cognition Models in Health Psychology,* British Psychological Society Health Psychology Section Conference, 18–19 Sept, University of St Andrews.

Conoley, J.C. and Kramer, J.J. (1989) *The Tenth Mental Measurements Yearbook,* Buros Institute of Mental Measurements of the University of Nebraska, Lincoln.

Cook, M. (1988) Stress Management. *Management Services,* November, 18–21.

Cook, M. (1993) *Personnel Selection and Productivity,* 2nd edn, Wiley, Chichester.

Cooke, W.N. and Gautschi, F.H. (1981) OSHA, plant safety programs and injury reduction. *Industrial Relations,* **20,** 245–57.

Cooper, C.L. (1981) Social support at work and stress management. *Small Group Behaviour,* **12,** 285–97.

Cooper, C.L. (1984) *Psychosocial Stress and Cancer,* Wiley, New York.

Cooper, C.L. (1986) Job distress: recent research and the emerging role of the clinical occupational psychologist. *Bulletin of the British Psychological Society,* **39,** 325–31.

Cooper, C.L. (1989) Are Type As prone to heart attacks? *The Psychologist,* January, 19.

Cooper, C.L., Mallinger, M. and Kahn, R. (1978) Identifying sources of occupational stress among dentists. *Journal of Occupational Psychology,* **51,** 227–34.

Cooper, M.D. and Phillips, R.A. (1994) Validation of a safety climate measure, Occupational Psychology Conference of the British Psychological Society, 3–5 January, Birmingham.

Cooper, R. and Payne, R. (1967) Extraversion and some aspects of work behaviour. *Personnel Psychology,* **20,** 45–57.

Corcoran, D.W.J. (1972) Studies of individual differences at the Applied Psychology Unit, in V.D. Nebylitsyn and J.A. Gray, (eds) *Biological Bases of Individual Behaviour,* Academic Press, New York and London, pp. 269–90.

Costa, P.T., McCrae, R.R. and Dye, D.A. (1991) Facet scales for agreeableness and conscientiousness: a revision of the NEO personality inventory. *Personality and Individual Differences,* **12,** 887–98.

Cowling, A.G., Standworth, M.J.K., Bennett, R.D., Curran, J. and Lyons, P. (1988) *Behavioural Science for Managers,* 2nd edn., Edward Arnold, London.

Cox, S.J. and Tait, N.R.S. (1991) *Reliability, Safety and Risk Management: an Integrated Approach,* Butterworth-Heinemann, Oxford.

Cox, T. (1985) Repetitive work: occupational stress and health, in C.L. Cooper and M.J. Smith, (eds), *Job Stress and Blue-Collar Work,* Wiley, Chichester, pp. 85–112.

Cox, T. and Ferguson, E. (1991) Individual differences, stress and coping, in C.L. Cooper and R. Payne, (eds), *Personality and Stress: Individual Differences in the Stress Process,* Wiley, Chichester, pp. 7–30.

Coyle, J.R. and Leopold, J.W. (1981) Health and safety committees – how effective are they? *Occupational Safety and Health,* **11,** November, 20–2.

Craig, A. and Cooper, R.E. (1992) Acute and chronic fatigue, in A.P. Smith and D.M. Jones, (eds), *Handbook of Human Performance Volume 3: State and Trait,* Academic Press, London, pp. 289–333.

Craske, S. (1968) A study of the relation between personality and accident history. *British Journal of Medical Psychology,* **41,** 399–404.

Cronbach, L.J. (1984) *Essentials of Psychological Testing,* 4th edn, Harper & Row, New York.

Crook, M.A. and Langdon, F.J. (1974) The effects of aircraft noise in schools around London Airport, *Journal of Sound and Vibration*, **12**, 221–32.

Crouter, A.C. (1984) Participative work as an influence on human development. *Journal of Applied Developmental Psychology*, **5**, 71–90.

Crump, J.H., Cooper, C.L. and Maxwell, V.B. (1981) Stress among air traffic controllers: occupational sources of coronary heart disease risk. *Journal of Occupational Behaviour*, **2**, 293–303.

Culpin, M. and Smith, M. (1930) *The Nervous Temperament*, Industrial Health Research Board Report No 61, HMSO, London.

Cushman, W.H. (1980) Selection of filters for dark adaptation goggles in the photographic industry. *Applied Ergonomics*, **11**, 93–9.

Dale, E. and Nyland, B. (1985) *Cone of Learning*, University of Wisconsin, Eau Claire.

Davidson, M.J. and Cooper, C.L. (1981) A model of occupational stress. *Journal of Occupational Medicine*, **23**, 564–74.

Davidson, M.J. and Cooper, C.L. (1983) *Stress and the Woman Manager*, Martin Robertson, Oxford.

Davidson, R.J. (1992) Anterior cerebral asymmetry and the nature of emotion, *Brain and Cognition*, **20**, 125–51.

Davies, D.R., Matthews, G. and Wong, C.S.K. (1991) Ageing and work, in C.L. Cooper and I.T. Robertson, (eds), *International Review of Industrial and Organizational Psychology 1991*, Wiley, Chichester, pp. 149–211.

Davies, D.R. and Parasuraman, R. (1982) *The Psychology of Vigilance*, Academic Press, New York and London.

Davies, D.R., Taylor, A. and Dorn, L. (1992) Ageing and human performance in A.P. Smith and D.M. Jones, (eds), *Handbook of Human Performance Volume 3 State and Trait*, Academic Press, London, pp. 25–61.

Davies, P.R. (1983) Human factors contributing to slips, trips and falls. *Ergonomics*, **26**, 51–60.

Davis, J., Millburn, P., Murphy, T. and Woodhouse, M. (1992) *Successful Team Building: How to Create Teams that Really Work*, Kogan Page, London.

Dawson, S. (1986) The training and professional development of workplace health and safety specialists, in R. C. Clarke, (ed.), *Education and Training in Health and Safety: Current Problems and Future Priorities – Proceedings of a Conference Held by the British Health and Safety Society, London, June 1986*, BHSS, Birmingham, pp. 7–20.

Dawson, S., Poynter, P. and Stevens, D. (1984) Safety specialists in industry: roles, constraints and opportunities. *Journal of Occupational Behaviour*, **5**, 253–70.

Day, D.V. and Silverman, S.B. (1989) Personality and job performance: evidence of incremental validity. *Personnel Psychology*, **42**, 25–36.

Deary, I.J., MacLullich, A.M.J. and Mardon, J. (1991) Reporting of minor physical symptoms and family incidence of hypertension and heart disease – relationship with personality and type A behaviour. *Personality and Individual Differences*, **12**, 747–51.

Deary, I.J. and Matthews, G. (1993) Personality traits are alive and well. *The Psychologist*, **6**, 299–311.

Deatherage, B.H. (1972) Auditory and other sensory forms of information presentation, in H.P. Van Cott and J. Kinkade, (eds), *Human Engineering Guide to Equipment Design*, US Government Printing Office, Washington, D.C., pp. 123–60.

De Bono, E. (1976) *Practical Thinking*, Penguin, Harmondsworth.

Deci, E.L. (1975) *Intrinsic Motivation*, Plenum, New York.

DeJoy, D.M. (1990) Towards a comprehensive human factors model of workplace accident causation. *Professional Safety,* **35(5),** 11–16.

Della-Giustina, J.L. and Della-Giustina, D.E. (1989) Quality of work life programme through employee motivation. *Professional Safety,* **34(5),** 24–8.

Dembroski, T.M. and Costa, P.T. (1987) Coronary-prone behaviour: components of the Type A patterns and hostility. *Journal of Personality,* **55,** 211–35.

Dewe, P., Cox, T. and Ferguson, E. (1993) Individual strategies for coping with stress at work: a review. *Work and Stress,* **7,** 5–15.

Dickman, S.J. and Meyer, D.E. (1988) Impulsivity and speed-accuracy trade-offs in information processing. *Journal of Personality and Social Psychology,* **54,** 274–90.

Dickson, G.C.A. (1991) *Risk Analysis,* 2nd edn, Witherby, London.

Dixon, P., Rehling, G. and Shiwack, R. (1993) Peripheral victims of the *Herald of Free Enterprise* disaster. *British Journal of Medical Psychology,* **66,** 193–202.

Dodge, K.A. (1986) A social information processing model of social competence in children, in M. Perimutter, (ed.), *Minnesota Symposium on Child Psychology Volume 18,* Erlbaum, Hillsdale, N.J., pp. 77–125.

Donald, I. and Canter, D. (1993) Psychological factors and the accident plateau. *Health and Safety Information Bulletin,* **215,** November 5–12.

Dorcus, R.M. and Jones, M.H. (1950) *Handbook of Employee Selection,* McGraw-Hill, New York.

Drury, C.G. (1983) Task analysis methods in industry. *Applied Ergonomics,* **14,** 19–28.

Drury, C.G., Paramore, B., van Cott, H.P., Grey, S.M. and Corlett, E.N. (1987) Task analysis, in G. Salvendy, (ed.), *Handbook of Human Factors,* Wiley, New York, pp. 370–401.

Duck, S. (1988) *Relating to Others,* Open University Press, Milton Keynes.

Dunnette, M.D., Bownas, D.A. and Bosshardt, M.J. (1981) *Prediction of Inappropriate, Unreliable, or Aberrant Job Behavior in Nuclear Power Plant Settings,* Personnel Decisions Research Institute, Minneapolis.

D'Zurilla, T.J. (1986) *Problem-Solving Therapy: a Social Competence Approach to Clinical Intervention,* Springer, New York.

Edman, G., Schalling, D. and Levander, S.E. (1983) Impulsivity and speed and errors in a reaction time task: a contribution to the construct validity of the concept of impulsivity. *Acta Psychologica,* **33,** 1–8.

Eisenberg, P. and Lazarsfeld, P.F. (1938) The psychological effects of unemployment. *Psychological Bulletin,* **35,** 358–90.

Eiser, J.R. and van der Plight, J. (1982) Accentuation and perspective in attitudinal judgement. *Journal of Personality and Social Psychology,* **42,** 224–38.

Eiser, J.R. and van der Plight, J. (1988) *Attitudes and Decisions,* Routledge, London.

Eisner, H.S. and Leger, J.P. (1988) The International Safety Rating System in South African mining. *Journal of Occupational Accidents,* **10,** 141–60.

Eldridge, J.E.T. and Kaye, B.M. (1970) *Wages and Accidents: an Exploratory Paper,* Department of Sociology, University of Glasgow.

Ellis, A. (1973) *Humanistic Psychotherapy: the Rational-Emotive Approach,* McGraw-Hill, New York.

Embrey, D.E. (1994) *Guidelines for Preventing Human Error in the Chemical Processing Industry,* Centre for Chemical Process Safety, American Institute of Chemical Engineers, New York.

Endler, N.S. and Parker, J.D.A. (1990) Multi-dimensional assessment of coping: a critical evaluation. *Journal of Personality and Social Psychology,* **58,** 844–54.

Engineering Employers' Federation. (1993) *Practical Risk Assessment: Guidance for SMEs,* Engineering Employers' Federation, London.

Everett, B.E. (1989) Training techniques that work within an integrated safety program. *Professional Safety,* **34(5),** 34–7.

Eysenck, H.J. (ed.) (1964) *Experiments in Motivation,* Pergamon, Oxford.

Eysenck, H.J. (1965) *Fact and Fiction in Psychology,* Penguin, Harmondsworth.

Eysenck, H.J. (1977) *Crime and Personality,* Routledge and Kegan Paul, London.

Eysenck, H.J. (1982) *Attention and Arousal: Cognition and Performance,* Springer, New York.

Eysenck, H.J. and Eysenck, M.W. (1985) *Personality and Individual Differences: a Natural Science Approach,* Plenum, New York.

Eysenck, H.J. and Eysenck, S.B.G. (eds) (1968) *Manual for the Eysenck Personality Inventory,* Educational and Industrial Testing Service, San Diego.

Eysenck, H.J. and Fulker, D. (1983) The components of Type A behaviour and its genetic determinants. *Personality and Individual Differences,* **4,** 499–505.

Eysenck, M.W. (1981) Learning, memory and personality, in H.J. Eysenck, (ed.), *A Model for Personality,* Springer, New York.

Eysenck, S.B.G. and Eysenck, H.J. (1977) The place of impulsiveness in a dimensional system of personality description. *British Journal of Social and Clinical Psychology,* **16,** 57–68.

Fagan, L. and Little, M. (1984) *The Forsaken Families,* Penguin, Harmondsworth.

Fagerstrom, K.O. and Lisper, H.O. (1977) Effects of listening to car radio, experience, and personality of the driver on subsidiary reaction time and heart rate in a long-term driving task, in R.R. Mackie, (ed.), *Vigilance,* Plenum, New York.

Farmer, E.W. (1984) Personality factors in aviation. *International Journal of Aviation Safety,* **2,** 175–90.

Farmer, E. and Chambers, E.G. (1926) *A Psychological Study of Individual Differences in Accident Rates,* Report of the Industrial Fatigue Research Board, No 4, HMSO, London.

Farmer, R.D.T., O'Donnell, I. and Tranah, T. (1991) Suicide on the London Underground System. *International Journal of Epidemiology,* **20,** 707–11.

Farmer, R.D.T., O'Donnell, I. and Tranah, T. (1992) *Suicide on the London Underground and Its Effects on Train Drivers.* Department of Public Health and Epidemiology, Charing Cross and Westminster Medical School, London.

Fazio, R.H. (1986) How do attitudes guide behaviour? in R.M. Sorrentino and E.T. Higgins, (eds), *Handbook of Motivation and Cognition: Foundations of Social Behaviour,* Guildford, New York.

Feldman, M. (1971) *Psychology in the Industrial Environment,* Butterworth, London.

Feldman, S. (1991) Today's EAPs make the grade. *Personnel,* **68,** 3–40.

Festinger, L. (1957) *A Theory of Cognitive Dissonance,* Row Peterson, Evanston, Il.

Figley, C.R. (1988) Toward a field of traumatic stress. *Journal of Traumatic Stress,* **1,** 3–16.

Finch, D.P. and Marshall, J. (1983) The role of stress, social support, and age in survival from breast cancer. *Journal of Psychosomatic Research,* **27,** 77–83.

Fine, B.J. (1963) Introversion, extraversion and motor vehicle driver behavior. *Perceptual and Motor Skills,* **12,** 95–100.

Fischhoff, B. (1975) Hindsight does not equal foresight: the effect of outcome knowledge on judgement in uncertainty. *Journal of Experimental Psychology: Human Perception and Performance,* **1,** 288–99.

Fischhoff, B. (1976) Attribution theory and judgement under uncertainty, in N.J.

Harvey, W.J. Ickes and R.F. Kidd (eds), *New Directions in Attribution Research,* Erlbaum, Hillsdale, N.J.

Fischhoff, B., Lichtenstein, S., Slovic, P., Derby, S.L. and Keeney, R.L. (1981) *Acceptable Risk,* C.U.P., Cambridge.

Fishbein, M. and Ajzen, I. (1975) *Belief, Attitude, Intention and Behaviour: an Introduction to Theory and Research,* Addison-Wesley, Reading, Ma.

Fisher, S. (1985) Control and blue-collar work, in C.L. Cooper and M.J. Smith, (eds), *Job Stress and Blue-Collar Work,* Wiley, Chichester, pp. 19–48.

Fiske, D.W. (1949) Consistency of the factorial structures of personality ratings from different sources. *Journal of Abnormal and Social Psychology,* **44,** 329–44.

Fitts, R.M. (1951) *Human Engineering for an Effective Air-Navigation and Traffic Control System,* National Research Council, Washington, D.C.

Fleishman, J.A. (1984) Personality characteristics and coping patterns. *Journal of Health and Social Behavior,* **25,** 229–44.

Fletcher, B.C. (1993) Stress and cognitive architecture, *Annual Conference of the British Psychological Society,* April, 1993.

Folkman, S. (1984) Personal control and stress and coping processes: a theoretical analysis. *Journal of Personality and Social Psychology,* **46,** 839–52.

Folkman, S. and Lazarus, R.S. (1980) An analysis of aging in a middle aged community sample. *Journal of Health and Social Behaviour,* **21,** 219–39.

Folkman, S. and Lazarus, R.S. (1988) Coping as a mediator of emotion. *Journal of Personality and Social Psychology,* **54,** 466–75.

Folkman, S., Lazarus, R.S., Dunkel-Scheffer, C., De Longis, A. and Gruen, R. (1986) Dynamics of a stressful encounter: cognitive appraisal, coping and encounter outcomes. *Journal of Personality and Social Psychology,* **50,** 992–1003.

Foot, T. (1990) Stress management. *Management Services,* **34(9),** September, 12–14.

Fox, J.G. (1983) Industrial music, in D.J. Oborne and M.M. Gruneberg, (eds), *The Physical Environment at Work,* Wiley, Chichester, pp. 211–26.

Franke, R.H. and Kaul, J.D. (1978) The Hawthorne experiments: first statistical interpretation. *American Sociological Review,* **43,** 623–43.

Fransella, F. and Bannister, D. (1977) *A Manual for Repertory Grid Technique,* Academic Press, London.

Frese, M. and Altman, A. (1988) *The Treatment of Errors in Learning and Training,* Department of Psychology, University of Munich.

Freud, S. (1938) *The Basic Writings of Sigmund Freud,* Modern Library, New York.

Freud, S. (1975) *The Psychopathology of Everyday Life,* trans. A. Tyson, Penguin, Middlesex.

Friedman, H.S. (1990) Where is the disease-prone personality? in H.S. Friedman, (ed.) *Personality and Disease,* Wiley, Chichester.

Friedman, H.S. and Booth-Kewley, S. (1987) The 'disease-prone' personality: a meta-analytic view of the construct. *American Psychologist,* **42,** 539–53.

Friedman, M. and Rosenman, R.H. (1974) *Type A Behavior and Your Heart,* Fawcett Crest, New York.

Fryer, D. (1992a) Psychological or material deprivation: why does unemployment have mental health consequences? in E. McLaughlin, (ed.), *Understanding Unemployment,* Routledge, London, pp. 103–25.

Fryer, D. (1992b) Marienthal and beyond – 20th century research on unemployment and mental health. *Journal of Occupational Psychology,* **65(4)** (special issue – various authors), 257–358.

Fryer, D. and Payne, R. (1986) Being unemployed: a review of the literature on the psychological experience of unemployment, in C.L. Cooper and I.T. Robertson, (eds), *International Review of Industrial and Organisational Psychology*, Wiley, Chichester, pp. 235–78.

Fryer, D. and Ullah, P. (1987) *Unemployed People: Social and Psychological Perspectives*, Open University Press, Milton Keynes.

Fryer, D. and Warr, P.B. (1984) Unemployment and cognitive difficulties. *British Journal of Clinical Psychology*, **23**, 67–8.

Funder, D.C. (1987) Errors and mistakes: evaluating the accuracy of social judgement. *Psychological Review*, **101**, 75–90.

Furnham, A. (1992) *Personality at Work: the Role of Individual Differences in the Workplace*, Routledge, London.

Furnham, A., Steele, H. and Pendleton, D. (1993a) A psychometric assessment of the Belbin Team-Role Self-Perception Inventory. *Journal of Occupational and Organizational Psychology*, **66**, 245–58.

Furnham, A., Steele, H. and Pendleton, D. (1993b) A response to Dr Belbin's reply. *Journal of Occupational and Organizational Psychology*, **66**, 261.

Ganster, D.C., Mayes, B.T., Sime, W.E. and Tharp, G.D. (1982) Managing occupational stress: a field experiment. *Journal of Applied Psychology*, **67**, 533–42.

Gaunt, L.D. (1989) *The effects of the International Safety Rating System (ISRS) on organizational performance*, Center for Risk Management and Insurance Research, College of Business Administration, Georgia State University, Atlanta.

Gellatly, I.R., Paunonen, S.V., Meyer, J.P., Jackson, D.N. and Goffin, R.D. (1991) Personality, vocational interest and cognitive predictors of managerial job performance and satisfaction. *Personality and Individual Differences*, **12**, 221–31.

Gibson, E.J. and Walk, R.D. (1960) The visual cliff. *Scientific American*, **202**, 64–71.

Gill, J.J., Friedman, M., Ulmer, D. and Drews, F.R. (1985) Reduction in Type-A behaviour in healthy middle-aged military officers. *American Heart Journal*, **110**, 503–14.

Glendon, A.I. (1987a) Behavioural science applications in health and safety in A. St. John Holt, (ed.), *Health and Safety: Towards the Millennium*, IOSH, Leicester, pp. 43–8.

Glendon, A.I. (1987b) Risk cognition, in W.T. Singleton and J. Hovden, (eds), *Risks and Decisions*, Wiley, Chichester, pp. 87–107.

Glendon, A.I. (1991) Influencing behaviour: a framework for action. *Journal of Health and Safety*, **6**, (March), 23–38.

Glendon, A.I. (1993) *Safety Auditing*, Module RA6, Occupational Health and Safety Training Unit, University of Portsmouth.

Glendon, A.I. (in press) Risks and values of the world of work, in W.T. Singleton, (ed.), *The Spirit at Work*, Blackwell, Oxford.

Glendon, A.I. and Booth, R.T. (1982) Worker participation in occupational health and safety in Britain. *International Labour Review*, **121**, 399–416.

Glendon, A.I., Boyle, A.J. and Hewitt, D.M. (1992) Computerised health and safety audit systems, in M. Mattila, and W. Karwowski, (eds), *Computer Applications in Ergonomics, Occupational Safety and Health*, North-Holland, Amsterdam, pp. 241–8.

Glendon, A.I., Davies, D.R., Wong, C.S.K. and Westerman, S.J. (1994) Older workers' acquisition of word processing skills, *Occupational Psychology Conference of the British Psychological Society*, 3–5 January, Birmingham.

Glendon, A.I., Dorn, L., Matthews, G., Gulian, E., Davies, D.R. and Debney, L.M. (1993) Reliability of the driver behaviour inventory. *Ergonomics,* **36,** 719–26.

Glendon, A.I. and Glendon, S. (1992) Stress in ambulance staff, in E.J. Lovesey, (ed.), *Contemporary Ergonomics 1992: Ergonomics for Industry,* Taylor & Francis, London, pp. 174–80.

Glendon, A.I. and Hale, A.R. (1984) Taking stock of Site Safe '83. *Health and Safety at Work,* **6(8),** 19–21.

Glendon, A.I., McKenna, S.P., Blaylock, S.S. and Hunt, K. (1988) Variables affecting cardiopulmonary resuscitation skill decay. *Journal of Occupational Psychology,* **61,** 243–56.

Glendon, A.I., Stanton, N.A. and Harrison, D. (1994) Factor analysing a performance shaping concepts questionnaire, in S.A. Robertson, (ed.), *Contemporary Ergonomics 1994: Ergonomics for All,* Taylor and Francis, London, pp. 340–5.

Glennon, D.P. (1980) *The Role of Safety and Health Legislation in Optimum Organisational Safety Climates for Reducing Occupational Injuries and Diseases,* MSc thesis, Aston University, Birmingham.

Glennon, D.P. (1982) Measuring organisational safety climate. *Australian Safety News,* Jan/Feb, 23–8.

Goff, M. and Ackerman, P.L. (1992) Personality-intelligence relations: assessing typical intellectual engagement. *Journal of Educational Psychology,* **84,** 537–52.

Goldhaber, G.M. and deTurck, M.A. (1988) Effectiveness of warning signs: gender and familiarity effects. *Journal of Products Liability,* **11,** 271–84.

Goss, D. (1994) *Principles of Human Resource Management,* Routledge, London.

Gouldner, A.W. (1955) *Patterns of Industrial Democracy,* Routledge, London.

Graham, H.T. and Bennett, R. (1992) *Human Resources Management,* 7th edn, Pitman, London.

Graham, J. (1989) New VALS2 takes psychological route. *Advertising Age,* 13 February, 24.

Grandjean, E. (1980) *Fitting the Task to the Man: an Ergonomics Approach,* Taylor & Francis, London.

Gray, J.A. (1981) A critique of Eysenck's theory of personality, in (ed.), H.J. Eysenck, *A Model for Personality,* Springer, New York, pp. 246–76.

Great Britain: Department of Employment. (1990) *Labour Force Survey,* HSMO, London.

Great Britain: Department of Energy. (1973) *Accident at Markham Colliery, Derbyshire: Report on the Cause of, and Circumstances Attending, the Overwind which Occurred at Markham Colliery, Derbyshire on 30 July 1973.* By J.W. Calder, HM Chief Inspector of Mines and Quarries, Cmnd 5557, HMSO, London.

Great Britain: Department of Energy. (1990) *The Public Inquiry into the Piper Alpha Disaster,* The Hon Lord Cullen, Cm 1310, HMSO, London.

Great Britain: Department of Health. (1992) *Health of the Nation,* HMSO, London.

Great Britain: Department of Transport. (1986) *Report on an Accident at Colwich Junction, Staffs on 19 September 1986,* HMSO, London.

Great Britain: Department of Transport. (1987) *Mv Herald of Free Enterprise, Report of Court No. 8074: Formal Investigation,* HMSO, London.

Great Britain: Department of Transport. (1988) *Investigation into the King's Cross Underground Fire,* Chairman D. Fennell, HMSO, London.

Great Britain: Department of Transport. (1989) *Investigation into the Clapham Junction Railway Accident,* Anthony Hidden QC, Cm 820, HMSO, London.

Great Britain: Department of Transport. (1990) Air Accidents Investigation Branch, *Aircraft Accident Report 4/90: Report on the Accident to Boeing 737-400 G-OBME near Kegworth, Leicestershire on 8 January 1989*, HMSO, London.

Great Britain: Health and Safety Commission. (1985) *The Reporting of Injuries, Diseases and Dangerous Occurrences Regulations 1985*, HMSO, London.

Great Britain: Health and Safety Commission. (1988) *The Control of Substances Hazardous to Health Regulations 1988*, HMSO, London.

Great Britain: Health and Safety Commission. (1989a) *Electricity at Work Regulations 1989*, HMSO, London.

Great Britain: Health and Safety Commission. (1989b) *Pressure Systems and Transportable Gas Containers Regulations 1989*, HMSO, London.

Great Britain: Health and Safety Commission. (1990a) *Noise at Work Regulations 1990*, HMSO, London.

Great Britain: Health and Safety Commission. (1990b) Advisory Committee on the Safety of Nuclear Installations, ACSNI Study Group on Human Factors. *First Report on Training and Related Matters*, HMSO, London.

Great Britain: Health and Safety Commission. (1991) Advisory Committee on the Safety of Nuclear Installations, ACSNI Study Group on Human Factors. *Second Report: Human Reliability Assessment – a critical review*, HMSO, London.

Great Britain: Health and Safety Commission. (1992a) *Management of Health and Safety at Work: Approved Code of Practice – Management of Health and Safety at Work Regulations 1992*, HMSO, London.

Great Britain: Health and Safety Commission. (1992b) *Manual Handling Operations Regulations 1992*, HMSO, London.

Great Britain: Health and Safety Commission. (1992c) *Offshore (Safety Cases) Regulations 1992*, HMSO, London.

Great Britain: Health and Safety Commission. (1993a) Advisory Committee on the Safety of Nuclear Installations, ACSNI Study Group on Human Factors. *Third Report: Organising for Safety*, HMSO, London.

Great Britain: Health and Safety Commission. (1993b) *Draft proposals for the Railways (Safety Cases) Regulations: Consultative Document*, Health and Safety Executive, London.

Great Britain: Health and Safety Executive. (1988) *The Tolerability of Risk from Nuclear Power Stations*, HMSO, London.

Great Britain: Health and Safety Executive. (1989) *Human Factors in Industrial Safety*, HS(G)48, HMSO, London.

Great Britain: Health and Safety Executive. (1991) *Successful Health and Safety Management*, HS(G)65, HMSO, London.

Great Britain: Health and Safety Executive. (1992a) *Display Screen Equipment Work: Guidance on Regulations – Health and Safety (Display Screen Equipment) Regulations 1992*, HMSO, London.

Great Britain: Health and Safety Executive. (1992b) *Personal Protective Equipment at Work Regulations 1992*, HMSO, London.

Green, C. (1990) Perceived risk: past, present and future conditional, in J. Handmer and E. Penning-Rowsell, (eds), *Hazards and the Communication of Risk*, Gower, Aldershot, pp. 31–52.

Green, L.W. (1978) Determining the impact and effectiveness of health education as it relates to federal policy. *Health Education Monographs*, **6(1),** 28–66.

Greeno, J.L., Hedstrom, G.S. and DiBerto, M. (1988) *The Environmental, Health and Safety Auditor's Handbook*, Arthur D. Little, Cambridge, Ma.

Greenwood, M. and Woods, H.M. (1919) *A Report upon the Incidence of Industrial Accidents upon Individuals with Special Reference to Multiple Accidents,* British Industrial Fatigue Research Board, Report No 4, HMSO, London.

Griffin, M.J. (1992) Vibration, in A.P. Smith and D.M. Jones, (eds), *Handbook of Human Performance Volume 1: The Physical Environment,* Academic Press, London, pp. 55–78.

Griffiths, R. (1993) Personality, diet and illness. *Annual Student Conference, Welsh Branch of the British Psychological Society,* 24 April, Cardiff.

Groeger, J.A. and Brown, I.D. (1989) Assessing one's own and others' driving ability. *Accident Analysis and Prevention,* 21, 155–68.

Grosch, W.N. and Olsen, D.C. (1994) *When Helping Starts to Hurt: a New Look at Burnout Among Psychotherapists,* Norton, London.

Guastello, S.J. (1991) Some further evaluations of the International Safety Rating System. *Safety Science,* 14, 253–9.

Guest, D.E. (1987) Human resource management and industrial relations. *Journal of Management Studies,* 24(5), 503–21.

Guest, D.E., Peccei, R. and Thomas, A. (1994) Safety culture and safety performance: British Rail in the aftermath of the Clapham Junction disaster, *Occupational Psychology Conference of the British Psychological Society,* 3–5 January, Birmingham.

Gulian, E., Glendon, A.I., Debney, L.M., Davies, D.R. and Matthews, G. (1989) Dimensions of driver stress. *Ergonomics,* 32, 585–602.

Gulian, E., Glendon, A.I., Davies, D.R., Matthews, G. and Debney, L.M. (1990) The stress of driving: a diary study. *Work and Stress,* 4, 7–16.

Hackman, J.R. and Oldham, G.R. (1980) *Work Redesign,* Addison-Wesley, Reading, Ma.

Hackman, R.J. (1994) The revolutionary implications of team self-management in organisations, *Occupational Psychology Conference of the British Psychological Society,* 3–5 January, Birmingham.

Hackman, R.J. and Suttle, J.L. (eds) (1977) *Improving Life at Work: Behavioral Science Approaches to Organizational Change,* Goodyear, Santa Monica, Ca.

Hale, A.R. (1974) Motivation and propaganda. *Occupational Health,* 26(3), 92–5.

Hale, A.R. (1978) *The Role of Government Inspectors of Factories with Particular Reference to their Training Needs,* PhD thesis, Aston University, Birmingham.

Hale, A.R. (1984) Is safety training worthwhile? *Journal of Occupational Accidents,* 6, 17–33.

Hale, A.R. (1987) Subjective risk, in W.T. Singleton and J. Hovden (eds), *Risk and Decisions,* Wiley, Chichester, pp. 67–85.

Hale, A.R. and Else, D. (1984) The role of training and motivation in a successful personal protective equipment programme, in *Proceedings of the 2nd Conference on Protective Equipment, Toronto, November 1984,* Canadian Centre for Occupational Safety and Health, Hamilton.

Hale, A.R. and Glendon, A.I. (1987) *Individual Behaviour in the Control of Danger,* Elsevier, Amsterdam.

Hale, A.R. and Hale, M. (1972) *Review of the Industrial Accident Research Literature,* Research Paper 1, Committee on Safety and Health at Work, HMSO, London.

Hale, A.R., Oortman-Gerlings, P., Swuste, P. and Heimplaertzer, P. (1991) Assessing and improving safety management systems, in *Proceedings of the First International Conference on Health, Safety and Environment in Oil and Gas Exploration and Production, 11–14 November 1991,* Society of Petroleum Engineers, The Hague.

Hale, M. and Hale, A.R. (1986) *A Review of Literature Relating to the Accident Experience of Young Workers and the Relation between Accidents and Age,* Health and Safety Technology and Management, Birmingham.

Hall, E.T. (1966) *The Hidden Dimension,* Doubleday, New York.

Hall, J. and Williams, M. (1980) *Work Motivation Inventory,* Telometrics International, The Woodlands, Tx.

Hamblin, A.C. (1974) *Evaluation and Control of Training,* McGraw-Hill, London.

Hancock, P.A., Wulf, G., Thom, D.R. and Fassnacht, P. (1989) Contrasting driver behaviour during turns and straight line driving, in *Proceedings of the 33rd Annual Meeting of the Human Factors Society,* Human Factors Society, Santa Monica, Ca., pp. 918–22.

Handy, C. (1984) *The Future of Work,* Blackwell, Oxford.

Handy, C. (1989) *The Age of Unreason,* Business Books, New York.

Harrington, J.M. (1978) *Shiftwork and Health: a Critical Review of the Literature,* Health and Safety Executive, HMSO, London.

Harrison, J.A., Mullen, P.D. and Green, L.W. (1992) Social psychological analysis of smoking behaviour, in J.R. Eiser, (ed.), *Social Psychology and Behavioural Medicine,* Wiley, Chichester, pp. 179–97.

Hartshough, D. (1985) Stressors and supports for emergency workers: the emergency organization role, in National Institute of Mental Health (ed.) *Role Stressors and Supports for Emergency Workers,* Government Printing Office, Washington, D.C., pp. 48–58.

Hawkins, F.H. (1987) *Human Factors in Flight,* Gower, Aldershot.

Haynes, R.S., Pine, R.C. and Fitch, H.G. (1982) Reducing accident rates with organizational behaviour modification. *Academy of Management Journal,* **25,** 407–16.

Heider, F. (1958) *The Psychology of Interpersonal Relations,* Wiley, New York.

Held, R. and Hein, A. (1963) Movement-produced stimulation in the development of visually guided behaviour. *Journal of Comparative and Physiological Psychology,* **5,** 872–6.

Herriot, P. (1989) *Recruitment in the 90s,* Institute of Personnel Management, London.

Herzberg, F. (1966) *Work and the Nature of Man,* World Publishing, Cleveland.

Herzberg, F., Mausner, B. and Snyderman, B. (1959) *The Motivation to Work,* Wiley, New York.

Hesketh, B. and Robertson, I.T. (1993) Validating personnel selection: a process model for research and practice. *International Journal of Selection and Assessment,* **1,** 3–17.

Higbee, K.L. (1969) Fifteen years of fear arousal: research on threat appeals (1953–1968). *Psychological Bulletin,* **72(6),** 426–44.

Hill, W.F. (1980) *Learning: a Survey of Psychological Interpretations,* 3rd edn, Methuen, London.

Hinton, P.R. (1993) *The Psychology of Interpersonal Perception,* Routledge, London.

Holman, R.H. (1984) A values and lifestyles perspective on human behavior, in R.E. Pitts Jr and A.G. Woodside (eds) *Personal Values and Consumer Psychology,* Lexington Books, Lexington, Ma, pp. 35–54.

Holmes, T.H. and Rahe, R. (1967) The social readjustment rating scale. *Journal of Psychosomatic Research,* **11,** 180–213

Holohan, C.J. and Moos, R.H. (1987) Personal and contextual determinants of coping strategies. *Journal of Personality and Social Psychology,* **51,** 389–95.

Holway, A.H. and Boring, E.G. (1941) Determinants of apparent visual size with distance variant. *American Journal of Psychology,* **54,** 21–37.

Honey, P. and Mumford, A. (1986) *The Manual of Learning Styles*, P. Honey, Maidenhead.

Hopkins, B.L., Conrad, R.J., Dangel, R.F. Fitch, H.G., Smith, M.J. and Anger, W.K. (1986) Behavioral technology for reducing occupational exposures to styrene. *Journal of Applied Behavior Analysis*, **19**, 3–11.

Hough, L.M. (1992) The 'big five' personality variables – construct confusion: description versus prediction. *Human Performance*, **5**, 139–55.

Hough, L.M., Eaton, N.K., Dunnette, M.D., Kamp, J.D. and McCloy, R.A. (1990) Criterion-related validities of personality constructs and the effect of response distortion on those validities. *Journal of Applied Psychology*, **75**, 581–95.

House, J.S. and Kahn, R.L. (1985) Measures and concepts of social support, in S. Cohen and L. Syme, (eds), *Social Support and Health*, Academic Press, Orlando.

Howard, J.H., Rechnitzer, R.A. and Cunningham, D.A. (1975) Coping with job tension – effective and ineffective methods. *Public Personnel Management*, **4**, 317–26.

Hoyes, T.W. and Glendon, A.I. (1993) Risk homeostasis: issues for future research. *Safety Science*, **16**, 19–33.

Humphreys, M.S. and Revelle, W. (1984) Personality, motivation and performance: a theory of the relationship between individual differences and information processing. *Psychological Review*, **91**, 153–84.

Humphreys, P. (ed.) (1988) *Human Reliability Assessors' Guide*, RTS 88/89Q, NCSR, UKAEA, Warrington.

Industrial Accident Prevention Association. (1990) *The International Safety Rating System: an Evaluation of Effectiveness*, Industrial Accident Prevention Association, Toronto.

Institution of Occupational Safety and Health. (1992) *Policy Statement on Safety Training*, IOSH, Leicester.

Institution of Occupational Safety and Health. (1994) *Policy Statement on Health and Safety Culture*, IOSH, Leicester.

Ivancevich, J.M., Matteson, M.T., Freedman, S.M. and Phillips, J.S. (1990) Worksite stress management interventions. *American Psychologist*, **45**, 252–61.

Jackson, D. N. and Rothstein, M. (1993) Evaluating personality testing in personnel selection. *The Psychologist*, **16**, 8–11.

Jahoda, M. (1981) Work, employment, and unemployment: values theories and approaches in social research. *American Psychologist*, **36**, 184–91.

Jahoda, M. (1982) *Employment and Unemployment*, CUP, Cambridge.

Janis, I.L. (1972) *Victims of Group Think: a Psychological Study of Foreign Policy Decisions and Fiascos*, Houghton and Mifflin, Boston.

Janis, I.L. and Feshback, S. (1963) Effects of fear arousing communication. *Journal of Abnormal and Social Psychology*, **48**, 78–92.

Janz, N.K. and Becker, M.H. (1984) The health belief model: a decade later. *Health Education Quarterly*, **11**, 1–47.

Jayaratne, S. and Chess, W.A. (1984) The effects of emotional support on perceived job stress and strain. *The Journal of Applied Behavioural Science*, **20**, 141–53.

Jee, M. and Reason, E. (1988) *Action on Stress at Work*, Health Education Authority, London.

Jenkins, R. and Warman, D. (eds) (1993) *Promoting Mental Health Policies in the Workplace*, HMSO, London.

Johnson, W.G. (1980) MORT: Safety *Assurance Systems*, National Safety Council of America, Chicago.

Jones, B.M. (1974) Cognitive performance of introverts and extraverts following alcohol ingestion. *British Journal of Psychology*, **65**, 35–42.

Jones, J.G. and Hardy, L. (1990) *Stress and Performance in Sport*, Wiley, Chichester.

Jones, N.A. and Fox, N.A. (1992) EEG asymmetry during emotionally evocative films and its relation to positive and negative affectivity. *Brain and Cognition*, **20**, 280–99.

Jung, C. (1953) *The Integration of Personality*, Farrar & Ruchart, New York.

Kahneman, D., Slovic, P. and Tversky, A. (eds) (1982) *Judgement under Uncertainty: Heuristics and Biases*, CUP, Cambridge.

Kanfer, F.H. and Gaelick-Buys, L. (1991) Self-management methods, in F.H. Kanfer and A.P. Goldstein, (eds), *Helping People Change: a Textbook of Methods*, Pergamon, New York, pp. 305–60.

Kantowitz, B.H. and Sorkin, R.D. (1987) Allocation of functions, in G. Salvendy, (ed.), *Handbook of Human Factors*, Wiley, New York, pp. 355–69.

Karasek, R.A. (1979) Job demands, job decision latitude and mental strain: implications for job design. *Administrative Science Quarterly*, **24**, 285–309.

Karasek, R.A. (1990) Lower health risk with increased job control among white-collar workers. *Journal of Organisational Behaviour*, **11**, 171–85.

Karasek, R.A. and Theorell, T. (1992) *Health Work: Stress, Productivity and the Reconstruction of Working Life*, Basic Books, New York.

Kase, D.W. and Wiese, K.J. (1990) *Safety Auditing: a Management Tool*, Van Nostrand, New York.

Kasl, S.V. and Cooper, C.L. (1987) *Stress and Health: Issues in Research Methodology*, Wiley, London and New York.

Katz, D. (1960) The functional approach to the study of attitudes. *Public Opinion Quarterly*, **24**, 163–204.

Kazer, B. (1992) Risk assessment: scattergram or bullseye. *The Safety and Health Practitioner*, **10(5)**, 40–1.

Kazer, B. (1993) *Risk Assessment: a Practical Guide*, Institution of Occupational Safety and Health, Leicester.

Kellett, D., Fletcher, S., Callen, A. and Geary, B. (1994) Fair testing: the case of British Rail. *The Psychologist*, **7(1)**, 26–9.

Kellett, S. and Claytor, A. (1993) Team functioning: the application of a circumplex model, *Occupational Psychology Conference of the British Psychological Society*, 4–6 January, Liverpool.

Kello, J.E., Geller, E.S., Rice, J.C. and Bryant, S.L. (1988) Motivating auto safety belt wearing in industrial settings: from awareness to behavior change. *Journal of Organizational Behavior Management*, **9(2)**, 7–21.

Kelly, G.A. (1955) *The Psychology of Personal Constructs*, vols 1 and 2, Norton, New York.

Kelman, H.C. (1958) Compliance, identification and internalisation: three processes of attitude change. *Journal of Conflict Resolution*, **2**, 51–60.

Kemeny, J. (1979) *The Need for Change: the Legacy of TMI*, Report of the President's Commission on the Accident at Three Mile Island, Pergamon, New York.

Kendall, R. (1985) Top of the class: award winners reveal safety training and motivation strategies. *Occupational Hazards*, **47(9)**, 47–51.

Kettle, M. (1984) Disabled people and accidents at work. *Journal of Occupational Accidents*, **6**, 277–93.

Kibblewhite, J.F.J. (1988) *Microcomputer Applications in Safety Management*, J. Kibblewhite, Reading.

Kiecolt-Glaser, J.K., Fisher, B.S., Ogrocki, P., Stout, J.C., Speicher, C.E. and Glaser, R. (1987) Marital quality, marital disruption, and immune function. *Psychosomatic Medicine*, **49**, 13–33.

Kiecolt-Glaser, J.K., Kennedy, S., Malkoff, S., Fisher, L., Speicher, C.E. and Glaser, R. (1988) Marital discord and immunity in males. *Psychosomatic Medicine*, **50**, 213–29.

Kinchin, G.H. (1982) The concept of risk, in A.E. Green (ed.), *High Risk Safety Technology*, Wiley, Chichester.

Kinnersley, P. (1973) *The Hazards of Work: How to Fight Them*, Pluto Press, London.

Kirwan, B. (1992a) Human error identification in human reliability assessment – Part 1: Overview of approaches. *Applied Ergonomics*, **23**, 299–318.

Kirwan, B. (1992b) Human error identification in human reliability assessment – Part 2: Detailed comparison of techniques. *Applied Ergonomics*, **23**, 371–81.

Kirwan, B. (1994) *A Guide to Practical Human Reliability Assessment*, Taylor & Francis, London.

Kirwan, B. and Ainsworth, L.K. (eds) (1992) *A Guide to Task Analysis*, Taylor & Francis, London.

Kisch, E.S. (1985) Stressful events and the onset of diabetes mellitus. *Practical Stress Management*, **3**, pp. 356–8.

Kjellén, U. and Baneryd, K. (1983) Changing local health and safety practices at work within the explosives industry. *Ergonomics*, **26(9)**, 863–77.

Klein, H.J. (1989) An integrated control theory model of work motivation. *Academy of Management Review*, **14**, 150–72.

Kleinke, C.L. (1984) Two models for conceptualizing the attitude-behavior relationship. *Human Relations*, **37(4)**, 333–50.

Kluckholn, C.M. and Murray, H.A. (1953) Personality formation: its determinants, in C.M. Kluckholn and H.A. Murray (eds), *Personality in Nature, Society and Culture*, 2nd edn, Knopf, New York, pp. 55–67.

Knapper, C.K., Copley, A.J. and Moore, R.J. (1976) Attitudinal factors in the non-use of seat belts. *Accident Analysis and Prevention*, **8**, 241–6.

Knox, N.W. and Eischer, R.W. (1992) *The MORT Users Manual: for Use with the Management Oversight and Risk Tree Analytical Logic Diagram*, Safety System Development Center of EG&G Associates, Idaho Inc., Idaho Falls.

Kochan, T.A., Dyer, L. and Lipsky, D.B. (1977) *The Effectiveness of Union-Management Safety and Health Committees*, W.E. Upjohn Institute for Employment Research, Kalamazoo, Mich.

Koeske, G.F., Kirk, S.A. and Koeske, R.D. (1993) Coping with job stress: which strategies work best? *Journal of Occupational and Organizational Psychology*, **66**, 319–35.

Kogan, N. and Wallach, M.A. (1967) Group risk taking as a function of members' anxiety and defensiveness. *Journal of Personality*, **35**, 50–63.

Kolb, D.A. (1984) *Experiential Learning*, Prentice-Hall, Englewood Cliffs, N.J.

Komaki, J., Barwick, K.D. and Scott, J.D. (1978) A behavioral approach to occupational safety: pinpointing and reinforcing safe performance in a good manufacturing plant. *Journal of Applied Psychology*, **63**, 434–45.

Komaki, J., Heintzman, A.T. and Lawson, L. (1980) Effect of training and feedback: component analysis of a behavioral safety program. *Journal of Applied Psychology*, **65**, 261–70.

Kothandpani, V. (1971) Validation of feeling, belief, and intention to act as three components of attitude and their contribution to prediction of contraceptive behaviour. *Journal of Personality and Social Psychology*, **19**, 321–33.

Krause, N. and Stryker, S. (1984) Stress and well-being: the buffering role of locus of control beliefs. *Social Science and Medicine,* **18,** 783–90.

Krause, T.R., Hidley, J.H. and Hodson, S.J. (1990a) *The Behavior-Based Safety Process: Managing Involvement for an Injury-Free Culture,* Van Nostrand Reinhold, New York.

Krause, T.R., Hidley, J.H. and Hodson, S.J. (1990b) Broad-based changes in behavior key to improving safety culture. *Occupational Health and Safety,* July, 27–31, 50.

Kroeger O. and Theusen, M. (1988) *Type Talk,* Dell, New York.

Kroeger O. and Theusen, M. (1992) *Type Talk at Work,* Delacourt, New York.

Kroes, W. (1976) *Society's Victim – the Policeman,* Thomas, Springfield, Il.

Kroll, J. (1993) *PTSD/borderlines in Therapy: Finding the Balance,* Norton, London.

Lagerlöf, E. (1982) Accident reduction in forestry through risk identification, risk consciousness and work organisation change, in *Proceedings of the 20th International Congress of Applied Psychology,* July, Edinburgh.

Latané, B. and Darley, J. (1968) Group inhibition of bystander intervention in emergencies. *Journal of Personality and Social Psychology,* **10,** 215–21.

Lau, R.R. (1982) Origins of health locus of control beliefs. *Journal of Personality and Social Psychology,* **42,** 322–34.

Lazarus, R.S., Coyne, J.C., Kanner, A.D. and Schaefer, C. (1981) Comparison of two modes of stress measurement: daily hassles and uplifts versus major life events. *Journal of Behavioral Medicine,* **4,** 1–39.

Lazarus, R.S. and Folkman, S. (1980) An analysis of coping in a middle aged community sample. *Journal of Health and Social Behaviour,* **21,** 219–30.

Lazarus, R.S. and Folkman, S. (1984) *Stress, Appraisal and Coping,* Springer, New York.

Leary, M.R. and Kowalski, R.M. (1990) Impression management: a literature review and a two-component model. *Psychological Bulletin,* **107,** 34–47.

Leather, P.J. and Butler, A.J. (1983) *Attitudes to Safety among Construction Workers – a Pilot Survey.* Reports prepared for the Building Research Establishment, Department of the Environment, by the Department of Behaviour in Organisations, University of Lancaster.

Leopold, J.W. and Coyle, J.R. (1981) A healthy trend in safety committees. *Personnel Management,* **13(5),** 30–2.

Lerner, M.J. and Simmons, C.H. (1966) Observers' reactions to the 'innocent victim': compassion or rejection. *Journal of Personality and Social Psychology,* **2,** 203–10.

Levitt, J.J.H. (1951) Some effects of certain communication patterns on group performance. *Journal of Abnormal and Social Psychology,* **46,** 38–50.

Lewin, I. (1982) Driver training: a perceptual-motor skill approach. *Ergonomics,* **25,** 917–24.

Lewin, K. (1951) *Field Theory in Social Science,* Harper, New York.

Lewin, K. (1958) Group decision and social change, in E.E. Maccoby, T.M. Newcombe, and R.L. Hartley, (eds), *Readings in social Psychology,* 3rd edn., Holt, New York, pp. 197–211.

Lewis, C. (1985) *Employee Selection,* Hutchinson, London.

Lewis, C. and Norman, D.A. (1986) Designing for error, in D.A. Norman and S. Draper, (eds), *User Centred System Design,* Erlbaum, Hillsdale, N.J., pp. 411–32.

Lichtenstein, S., Slovic, P., Fischhoff, B., Layman, M. and Combs, B. (1978) Judged frequency of lethal events. *Journal of Experimental Psychology: Human Learning and Memory,* **4,** 551–78.

Lieberman, H.R. (1992) Caffeine, in A.P. Smith and D.M. Jones, (eds), *Handbook of Human Performance Volume 2: Health and Performance,* Academic Press, London, pp. 49–72.

Likert, R. (1961) *New Patterns of Management,* McGraw-Hill, New York.

Likert, R. (1967) *The Human Organisation,* McGraw-Hill, New York.

Lindsay, F. (1980) Accident proneness – does it exist? *Occupational Safety and Health,* **10(2),** 8–9.

Lipp, M.R. (1980) *The Bitter Pill: Doctors, Patients and Failed Expectations,* Harper & Row, New York.

Lippmann, W. (1922) *Public Opinion,* Harcourt Brace, New York.

Long, B.C. and Flood, K.R. (1993) Coping with work stress: psychological benefits of exercise. *Work and Stress,* **7,** 109–19.

Lourens, P.F. (1989) Error analysis and applications in transportation systems. *Accident Analysis and Prevention,* **21,** 419–26.

Lowenstein, A. (1991) *The Influence of Learned Resourcefulness, Locus of Control, Imagery Control, and Body Consciousness on Relaxation.* Masters thesis, Tel Aviv University.

Lupton, T. (1963) *On the Shop Floor,* Pergamon, Oxford.

Luthans, F. and Kreitner, R. (1975) *Organizational Behavior Modification,* Scott Foreman, Glenview, Il.

McAfee, R.B. and Winn, A.R. (1989) The use of incentives/feedback to enhance workplace safety: a critique of the literature. *Journal of Safety Research,* **20(1),** 7–19.

McClelland, D.C., Atkinson, J.W., Clark, R.A. and Lowell, E.L. (1953) *The Achievement Motive,* Appleton Century Crofts, New York.

McCormick, E.J. (1976a) Job and task analysis, in M.D. Dunette, (ed.), *Handbook of Industrial and Organizational Psychology,* Rand McNally, Chicago, pp. 651–96.

McCormick, E.J. (1976b) *Human Factors in Engineering and Design,* McGraw-Hill, N.J.

McCrae, R.R. and Costa, P.T. (1985) Updating Norman's 'adequate taxonomy': intelligence and personality dimensions in natural language and in questionnaires. *Journal of Personality and Social Psychology,* **49,** 710–21.

McCrae, R.R. and Costa, P.T. (1986) The structure of interpersonal traits: Wiggins's circumplex and the five factor model. *Journal of Personality and Social Psychology,* **56,** 586–95.

McCrae, R.R. and Costa, P.T. (1987) Validation of the five-factor model of personality across instruments and observers. *Journal of Personality and Social Psychology,* **52,** 81–90.

McCrae, R.R. and Costa, P.T. (1989) More reasons to adopt the five factor model. *American Psychologist,* **44,** 451–2.

McGrath, J.E. (ed.) (1970) *Social and Psychological Factors in Stress,* Holt Rinehart & Winston, New York.

McGregor, D. (1960) *The Human Side of Enterprise,* McGraw-Hill, New York.

McGuire, F.L. (1976) Personality factors in highway accidents. *Human Factors,* **18,** 433–42.

Mackay, C.J. and Cooper, C.L. (1987) Occupational stress and health: some current issues, in , C.L. Cooper and I.T. Robertson, (eds), *International Review of Industrial and Organisational Psychology,* Wiley, Chichester, pp. 167–99.

Mackay, C.J. and Cox, T. (1984) Occupational stress associated with visual display unit operation, in *Health Hazards of VDUs,* (ed. B.G. Pearce), Wiley, Chichester, pp. 137–43.

Mackay, C.J. and Whittington, C. (1983) Ergonomics and human error, in J.R. Ridley, (ed.), *Safety at Work,* Butterworth, London, pp. 449–62.

McKenna, F.P. (1991) Debiasing. Paper presented to SAFETY ON THE ROAD CONFERENCE, September, Manchester University.

McLeod, R.W. and Griffin, J. (1989) A review of the effects of translational whole-body vibration on continuous manual control performance. *Journal of Sound and Vibration,* **133,** 55–115.

McLeod, R.W. and Stansfeld, S. (1986) Aircraft noise exposure, noise sensitivity and everyday errors. *Environment and Behaviour,* **18,** 214–26.

Madge, N. (1983) Unemployment and its effects on children. *Journal of Child Psychology and Psychiatry,* **24,** 311–19.

Manuso, J.S.J. (1982) Stress management and behavioral medicine: a corporate model, in M. O'Donnell and T. Ainsworth, (eds), *Health Promotion in the Workplace,* Wiley, Chichester.

March, J.G. and Simon, H.A. (1958) *Organisations,* Wiley, New York.

Margerison, C.J. and McCann, D. (1991) *Team Management: Practical Approaches,* Mercury, London.

Margerison, C.J. and McCann, D. (1992) Team Management and work preferences. *The Occupational Psychologist,* **16,** April, 21–6.

Margolis, B.L. and Kroes, W.H. (1975) *The Human side of Accident Prevention,* Charles C. Thomas, Springfield Il.

Marks, D. (1990) Imagery, information and risk, in J. Handmer and E Penning-Rowsell (eds), *Hazards and the Communication of Risk,* Gower, Aldershot, pp. 19–29.

Marshall, S.L.A. (1978) *Men against Fire,* Peter Smith, Gloucester, Ma.

Mashour, M. (1974) *Human Factors in Signalling Systems – Specific Applications to Railway Signalling,* Wiley, New York.

Maslach, C. and Jackson, S.E. (1981) *The Maslach Burnout Inventory Manual,* Consulting Psychologists Press, Palo Alto, Ca.

Maslach, C. and Jackson, S.E. (1984) Burnout in organizational settings, in S. Oskamp, (ed.), *Applied Social Psychology in Organzational Settings,* Sage, Beverley Hills, Ca., pp. 133–53.

Maslach, C. and Jackson, S.E. (1986) *Maslach Burnout Inventory Manual,* 2nd edn, Consulting Psychologists Press, Palo Alto, Ca.

Maslow, A.H. (1954) *Motivation and Personality,* Harper, New York (2nd edn 1970; 3rd edn 1987, eds R.D. Frager and J. Fadiman).

Mason, S, (1992) Practical guidelines for improving safety through the reduction of human error. *The Safety and Health Practitioner,* **10(5),** 24–30.

Matsumoto, Y.S. (1970) Social stress and coronary heart disease in Japan: a hypothesis. *Millbank Memorial Fund Quarterly,* **48,** 9–36.

Matteson, M. and Ivancevich, J. (1987) *Controlling Work Stress: Effective Human Resource and Management Strategies,* Jossey-Bass, San Francisco.

Matthews, G. (1992a) Extraversion, in A.P. Smith and D.M. Jones, (eds), *Handbook of Human Performance Volume 3: State and Trait,* Academic Press, London, pp. 95–126.

Matthews, G. (1992b) Mood, in A.P. Smith and D.M. Jones, (eds), *Handbook of Human Performance Volume 3: State and Trait,* Academic Press, London, pp. 161–93.

Matthews, G. (1993) Personal communication.

Matthews, G., Davies, D.R. and Lees, J.L. (1990a) Arousal, extraversion, and individual differences in resource availability. *Journal of Personality and Social Psychology,* **59,** 150–68.

Matthews, G., Davies, D.R. and Holley, P.J. (1990b) Extraversion, arousal and visual sustained attention: the role of resource availability. *Personality and Individual Differences,* **11,** 1159–73.

Matthews, G., Dorn, L. and Glendon, A.I. (1991) Personality correlates of driver stress. *Personality and Individual Differences,* **12,** 551–6.

Matthews, G., Dorn, L., Hoyes, T.W., Davies, D.R., Glendon, A.I and Taylor, R.G. (1994) Driver stress and performance on a driving simulator: a transactional approach, Department of Psychology, University of Dundee (paper submitted).

Matthews, G., Jones, D.M. and Chamberlain, A.G. (1990c) Refining the measurement of mood: the UWIST mood adjective checklist. *British Journal of Psychology*, **81**, 17–42.

Matthews, G., Stanton, N.A., Graham, N.C. and Brimelow, C. (1990d) A factor analysis of the scales of the Occupational Personality Questionnaire. *Personality and Individual Differences*, **11**, 591–6.

Matthews, G., Jones, D.M. and Chamberlain, A.G. (1992) Predictors of individual differences in mail coding skills and their variation with ability level. *Journal of Applied Psychology*, **77**, 406–18.

Matthews, K.A. and Haynes, S.G. (1986) Type A behaviour pattern and coronary disease risk: update and critical evaluation. *American Journal of Epidemiology*, **123**, 923–59.

Mayer, D.L., Jones, S.F. and Laughery, K.R. (1987) Accident proneness in the industrial setting, in *Proceedings of the Human Factors Society 31st Annual Meeting*, pp. 196–9.

Megaw, E. (1992) The visual environment, in A.P. Smith and D.M. Jones, (eds), *Handbook of Human Performance Volume 1: The Physical Environment*, Academic Press, London, pp. 261–96.

Meichenbaum, D. (1977) *Cognitive-Behavior Modification: an Integrative Approach*, Plenum, New York.

Meister, D. (1984) Human reliability, in F.A. Muckler, (ed.), *Human Factors Review, 1984*, Human Factors Society, Santa Monica, Ca.

Meister, D. (1985) *Behavioral Analysis and Measurement Methods*, Wiley, New York.

Milgram, S. (1965) Some conditions of obedience and disobedience to authority. *Human Relations*, **18**, 57–76.

Miller, D.P. and Swain, A.D. (1987) Human error and human reliability, in, G. Salvendy, (ed.), *Handbook of Human Factors*, Wiley, New York, pp. 219–50.

Mills, E. (1976) Altering the social structure in coal mining: a case study. *Monthly Labor Review*, October, 3–10.

Mischel, W. (1968) *Personality and Assessment*, Wiley, New York.

Mitchell, A. (1983) *The Nine American Lifestyles*, Macmillan, New York.

Mitchell, J.T. (1985) Healing the helper, in National Institute of Mental Health, (ed.), *Role Stressors and Supports for Emergency Workers*, Government Printing Office, Washington D.C., pp. 105–18.

Monk, T.H. and Tepas, D.I. (1985) Shift work, in C.L. Cooper and M.J. Smith, (eds), *Job Stress and Blue Collar Work*, Wiley, Chichester, pp. 65–84.

Moreno, J.L. (1953) *Who Shall Survive?* Beacon House.

Morgan, C.T., Cook, J.S., Chapanis, A. and Lund, M. (1963) *Human Engineering Guide to Equipment Design*, McGraw-Hill, New York.

Mowbray, G.H. and Gebhard, J.W. (1958) *Man's Senses as Information Channels*, Report Cm-936, Applied Physics Laboratory, The Johns Hopkins University, Baltimore.

Mueller, J.H. (1992) Anxiety and performance, in A.P. Smith and D.M. Jones, (eds), *Handbook of Human Performance Volume 3: State and Trait*, Academic Press, London, pp. 127–60.

Munipov, V.M. (1991) Human engineering analysis of the Chernobyl accident, in M. Kumashiro and E.D. Megaw, (eds), *Towards Human Work: Solutions to Problems in Occupational Health and Safety*, Taylor & Francis, London, pp. 380–6.

Murphy, L.R. (1984) Occupational stress management: a review and appraisal. *Journal of Occupational Psychology,* **57,** 1–15.

Murphy, L.R. (1985) Individual coping strategies, in C.L. Cooper and M.J. Smith, (eds), *Job Stress and Blue Collar Work,* Wiley, Chichester, pp. 225–39.

Murray, H.A. (1938) *Explorations in Personality,* OUP, New York, (2nd edn, 1970).

Murrell, K.F.H. (1971) *Ergonomics: Man in his Working Environment,* Chapman & Hall, London.

Näätänen, R. and Summala, H. (1976) *Road-User Behaviour and Traffic Accidents,* North-Holland, Amsterdam.

Nachreiner, F. and Hänecke, K. (1992) Vigilance, in A.P. Smith and D.M. Jones, (eds), *Handbook of Human Performance Volume 3: State and Trait,* Academic Press, London, pp. 261–88.

Naisberg-Fennig, S. and Giora, K. (1991) Personality characteristics and proneness to burnout: a study among psychiatrists. *Stress Medicine,* **17,** 201–5.

Napoles, V. (1988) *Corporate Identity Design,* Van Nostrand Reinhold, New York.

Nash, W. (1992) Stress management and coronary rehabilitation – are 'soft' strategies effective? PROCEEDINGS OF THE COLLEGE OF OCCUPATIONAL THERAPISTS' CONFERENCE, London, May, 1992, pp. 10–13.

National Institute for Occupational Safety and Health (1976) *Shiftwork and Health: a Symposium,* US Department of Health, Education and Welfare, US Government Printing Office, Washington, D.C.

Nemecek, J. and Grandjean, E. (1973) Noise in landscaped offices. *Applied Ergonomics,* **4,** 19–22.

Newcombe, T.M. (1943) *Personality and Social Change,* Dryden, New York.

Niven, N. (1989) *Health Psychology,* Churchill Livingstone, London.

Norman, D.A. (1988) *The Psychology of Everyday Things,* Basic Books, New York.

Oborne, D.J. (1994) *Ergonomics at Work,* 3rd edn, Wiley, Chichester.

O'Brien, G.E. (1986) *Psychology of Work and Unemployment,* Wiley, Chichester.

Oppenheim, A.N. (1992) *Questionnaire Design, Interviewing and Attitude Measurement,* 2nd edn, Pinter, London.

Opren, C. (1982) The effect of social support on reactions to role ambiguity and conflict: a study of black and white clerks in South Africa, *Journal of Cross-Cultural Psychology,* **13,** 375–84.

Ormel, J. and Wohlfarth, T. (1991) How neuroticism, long-term difficulties, and life situation change influence psychological distress: a longitudinal model. *Journal of Personality and Social Psychology,* **60,** 744–55.

Ornish, D., Brown, S.E., Scherwitz, L.W., Billings, J.H., Armstrong, W.T., Ports, T.A., McLanahan, S.M., Kirkeeide, R.L., Brand, R.J. and Gould, K.L. (1990) Can lifestyle changes reverse coronary heart disease? The lifestyle heart trial. *The Lancet,* **336,** 129–33.

Osgood, C.E., Tannenbaum, P.H. and Suci, G.I. (1957) *The Measurement of Meaning,* University of Illinois Press, Urbana.

Owsley, C., Ball, K., Sloane, M.E. Roenker, D.L. and Bruni, J.R. (1991) Visual/perceptual/cognitive correlates of vehicle accidents in older drivers. *Psychology and Aging,* **6,** 403–15.

Oxenburgh, M. (1991) *Increasing Productivity and Profit through Health and Safety: Case Studies in Successful Occupational Health and Safety Practice,* CCH International, Australia.

Parasuraman, S. and Cleek, M.A. (1984) Coping behaviour and managers' affective reactions to role stressors. *Journal of Vocational Behaviour,* **24,** 179–93.

Parkes, K.R. (1984) Locus of control, cognitive appraisal and coping in stressful episodes. *Journal of Personality and Social Psychology,* **46,** 655–68.

Patrick, J. (1992) *Training: Research and Practice,* Academic Press, London.

Patrick, J., Spurgeon, P. and Shepherd, A. (1980) *A Guide to Task Analysis: Applications of Hierarchical Methods,* Occupational Services Ltd., Birmingham.

Perrow, C. (1984) *Normal Accidents: Living with High Risk Technologies,* Basic Books, New York.

Pérusse, M. (1978) Counting the near misses. *Occupational Health,* **30(3),** 123–6.

Pérusse, M. (1980) *Dimensions of Perceptions and Recognition of Danger,* PhD thesis, Aston University, Birmingham.

Pervin, L.A. (1993) *Personality: Theory and Research,* 6th edn, Wiley, New York.

Pestonjee, D.M. and Singh, U.B. (1980) Neuroticism-extraversion as correlates of accident occurrence. *Accident Analysis and Prevention,* **12,** 201–4.

Peters, T.J. and Waterman, R.H. (1982) *In Search of Excellence: Lessons from America's Best-run Companies,* Harper & Row, London.

Petersen, D. (1978) *Techniques of Safety Management,* 2nd edn, McGraw-Hill, New York.

Petersen, D. (1984) *Human-error Reduction and Safety Management,* Aloray, New York.

Petersen, D. (1989) *Safe Behavior Reinforcement,* Aloray, New York.

Petropoulos, H. and Brebner, J. (1981) Stereotypes for direction-of-movement of rotary controls associated with linear displays: the effects of scale presence and position of pointer direction, and distances between the control and the display. *Ergonomics,* **24,** 143–51.

Phares, E. (1976) *Locus of Control in Personality,* General Learning Press, Morristown, N.J.

Pheasant, S. (1988) *Bodyspace: Anthropometry, Ergonomics and Design,* Taylor & Francis, London.

Piccolino, E.B. (1966) *Depicted Threat, Realism and Specificity: Variables Governing Safety Posters' Effectiveness,* PhD thesis, Illinois Institute of Technology.

Pidgeon, N.F., Turner, B.A., Blockley, D.I. and Toft, B. (1991) Corporate safety culture: improving the management contribution to system reliability, in R.H. Mathews, (ed.), *Reliability' 91,* Elsevier, Amsterdam, pp. 682–90.

Pirani, M. and Reynolds, J. (1976) Gearing up for safety. *Personnel Management,* February, 25–9.

Porter, C.S. (1988) Accident proneness: a review of the concept, in D.J. Oborne (ed.), *International Reviews of Ergonomics: Current Trends in Human Factors Research and Practice Volume 2,* Taylor & Francis, London, pp. 177–206.

Powell, K.E., Thompson, P.D., Caspersen, C.J. and Kendrick, J.S. (1987) Physical activity and the incidence of coronary heart disease. *Annual Review of Public Health,* **8,** 253–87.

Powell, P.I., Hale, M., Martin, J. and Simon, M. (1971) *2000 Accidents: a Shop Floor Study of Their Causes,* Report 21, National Institute of Industrial Psychology, London.

Price, H.E. (1985) The allocations of functions in systems. *Human Factors,* **27,** 33–45.

Price, D.L. and Lueder, R.K. (1980) Virginia union and industry management attitudes towards safety and OSHA. *Journal of Safety Research,* **12(2),** 99–106.

Quenault, S.W. (1966) *Some Methods of Obtaining Information on Driver Behaviour.* Report 25, Road Research Laboratory, Crowthorne.

Quenault, S.W. (1967a) *Driving Behaviour of Certain Professional Drivers.* Report LR93, Road Research Laboratory, Crowthorne.

Quenault, S.W. (1967b, 1968) *Driving Behaviour: Safe and Unsafe Drivers.* Reports LR70 and 146, Road Research Laboratory, Crowthorne.

Quick, J.C. and Quick, J.D. (1984) *Organizational Stress and Preventive Management,* McGraw-Hill, New York.

Raafat, H.M.N. (1990) *Risk Assessment Methodology,* Open Learning Series, Module RA3, Occupational Health and Safety Training Unit, University of Portsmouth.

Rasmussen, J. (1980) What can be learned from human error reports? in K.D. Duncan, M. Gruneberg and D. Wallis, (eds), *Changes in Working Life,* Wiley, London.

Ratliff, J.D. (1988) Motivation and the perceived need deficiencies of secondary teachers. *High School Journal,* **72(1),** 8–16.

Reason, J.T. (1974) Style, personality and accidents. *New Society.* 21 February.

Reason, J.T. (1984) Absent-mindedness and cognitive control, in J.E. Harris and P.E. Morris, (eds), *Everyday Memory Actions and Absent-Mindedness,* Academic Press, London, pp. 113–32.

Reason, J.T. (1987) The Chernobyl errors. *Bulletin of the British Psychological Society,* **40,** 201–6.

Reason, J.T. (1988) Stress and cognitive failure, in S. Fisher and J.T. Reason, (eds), *Handbook of Life Stress, Cognition and Health,* Wiley, Chichester, pp. 405–21.

Reason, J.T. (1990) *Human Error,* CUP, Cambridge.

Reason, J.T. and Lucas, D. (1984) Using cognitive diaries to investigate naturally occurring memory blocks, in J.E. Harris and P.E. Morris, (eds), *Everyday Memory Actions and Absent-Mindedness,* Academic Press, London, pp. 53–70.

Reason, J.T., Manstead, A.S.R., Stradling, S., Baxter, J., Campbell, K. and Huyser, J. (1988) *Interim Report on the Investigation of Driver Errors and Violations,* Department of Psychology, University of Manchester.

Reason, J.T. and Mycielska, K. (1982) *Absent-minded? The Psychology of Mental Lapses and Everyday Errors,* Prentice-Hall, Englewood Cliffs, N.J.

Reber, R.A., Wallfin, J.A. and Duhon, D.L. (1989) Safety programs that work. *Personnel Administrator,* **34(9),** 66–9.

Regulinski, T. (1971) Quantification of human performance reliability research method rationale, in *Proceedings of US Navy Human Reliability Workshop 22–23 July 1970,* Rep NAVSHIPS 0967-412-4010, (ed. J. Jenkins), Naval Ship Systems Command, Washington, D.C.

ReVelle, J.B. (1980) *Safety Training Methods,* Wiley, New York.

Revelle, W. (1987) Personality and motivation: sources of inefficiency in cognitive performance. *Journal of Research in Personality,* **21,** 436–52.

Revelle, W., Anderson, K.J. and Humphreys, M.S. (1987) Empirical tests and theoretical extensions of arousal-based theories of personality, in J. Strelau and H.J. Eysenck (eds), *Personality Dimensions and Arousal,* Plenum Press, London, pp. 17–33.

Revelle, W., Humphreys, M.S., Simon, L. and Gilliland, K. (1980) The interactive effect of personality, time of day, and caffeine: a test of the arousal model. *Journal of Experimental Psychology,* **109,** 1–31.

Rippere, V. and Williams, R. (eds) (1985) *Wounded Healers: Mental Health Workers' Experiences of Depression,* Wiley, Chichester.

Roberts, H., Smith, S.J. and Lloyd, M. (1992) Safety as social value: a community approach, in S. Scott, G. Williams, S. Platt and H. Thomas (eds), *Private Risks and Public Dangers,* Avebury, Aldershot, pp. 184–200.

Robertson, I.T. and Kinder, A. (1992) *The Criterion Related Validity of Personality Variables: an Hypothesis Driven Meta Analysis,* British Psychological Society Annual Conference, April, Liverpool.

Robertson, I.T. and Smith, M. (1989) Personnel selection methods, in M. Smith and I.T. Robertson (eds), *Advances in Selection and Assessment,* Wiley, Chichester, pp. 89–112.

Rodin, J. and Salovy, P. (1989) Health psychology. *Annual Review of Psychology,* **40,** 533–79.

Roethlisberger, F.J. and Dixon, W.J. (1939) *Management and the Worker,* Harvard University Press, Cambridge, Ma.

Rogers, C.R. (1980) *A Way of Being,* Houghton Mifflin, Boston, Ma.

Rogers, R.W. and Mewborn, C.R. (1976) Fear appeals and attitude change: effects of a threat's noxiousness, probability of occurrence, and the efficiency of coping responses. *Journal of Personality and Social Psychology,* **34(1),** 54–61.

Rolls, G.W.P., Hall, R.D., Ingham, R. and McDonald, M. (1991) *Accident Risk and Behavioural Patterns of Younger Drivers,* AA Foundation for Road Safety Research, Basingstoke.

Rolls, G.W.P. and Ingham, R, (1992) *'Safe' and 'Unsafe' – a Comparative Study of Younger Male Drivers,* AA Foundation for Road Safety Research, Basingstoke.

Rosario del Grayham, D.A. (1984) Behavioural science – small work group. *The Safety Practitioner,* January, 17–22.

Rose, K.D. and Rosnow, I. (1973) Physicians who kill themselves. *Archives of General Psychiatry,* **29,** 800–5.

Rosegger, R. and Rosegger, S. (1960) Health effects of tractor driving. *Journal of Agricultural Engineering Research,* **5,** 241–75.

Rosenbaum, M. (1980) A schedule for assessing self-control behaviors: preliminary findings. *Behavior Therapy,* **11,** 109–21.

Rosenbaum, M. (1988) Learned resourcefulness, stress and self-regulation, in S. Fisher and J. Reason (eds), *Handbook of Life Stress, Cognition and Health,* Wiley, Chichester, pp. 483–96.

Rosenbaum, M. (1990) The role of learned resourcefulness in self-control of health behavior, in M. Rosenbaum (ed.), *Learned Resourcefulness: on Coping Skills, Self-Control and Adaptive Behavior,* Springer, New York, pp. 3–30.

Rosenbaum, M. (1993) The three functions of self-control behaviour: redressive, reformative and experiential. *Work and Stress,* **7,** 33–46.

Rosenberg, M.J. and Hovland, C.I. (1960) Cognitive, affective and behavioral components of attitudes, in M.J Rosenberg, C.I. Hovland, W.J. McGuire, R.P. Abelson and J.W. Brehm, (eds), *Attitude Organization and Change: an Analysis of Consistency Among Attitude Components,* Yale University Press, New Haven, Conn.

Ross, L., Lepper, M. and Hubbard, M. (1975) Perseverence in self perception and social perception in biased attributional process in the debriefing paradigm. *Journal of Personality and Social Psychology,* **32,** 880–92.

Rothschild, Lord (1978) Risk. *The Listener,* **100,** 30 November, 715–18.

Rotter, J.B. (1966) Generalized expectancies for internal versus external control of reinforcement. *Psychological Monographs,* **80,** whole No. 609.

Rousseau, D.M. (1988) The construction of climate in organization research, in C.L. Cooper and I.T. Robertson, (eds), *International Review of Industrial and Organizational Psychology,* Vol 13, Wiley, Chichester, pp. 139–58.

Rousseau, D.M. (1990) Assessing organizational culture: the case for multiple methods, in B. Schneider, *Organizational Climate and Culture,* Jossey-Bass, San Francisco.

Rowe, C.J. and Mink, W.D. (1993) *An Outline of Psychiatry,* 10th edn, WB Brown & Benchmark, Oxford.

Rowe, G. (1990) Setting safety priorities: a technical and social process. *Journal of Occupational Accidents,* **12,** 31–40.

Royal Society (1983) *Risk Assessment: Report of A Royal Society Study Group,* The Royal Society, London.

Royal Society (1992) *Risk: Analysis, Perception and Management – Report of a Royal Society Study Group,* The Royal Society, London.

Rubinsky, S. and Smith, N. (1973) Safety training by accident simulation. *Journal of Applied Psychology,* **57,** 68–73.

Rudner, H.L. (1985) Stress and coping mechanisms in a group of family practice residents. *Journal of Medical Education,* **60,** 564–6.

Rumar, K. (1985) The role of perceptual and cognitive filters in observed behaviour, in L. Evans and R.C. Schwing, (eds), *Human Behaviour and Traffic Safety,* Plenum, New York, pp. 151–65.

Ryan, T.G. (1991) *Organisational Factors Regulatory Research Briefing to the ACSNI Study Group on Human Factors and Safety,* July, London.

Saarela, K.L., Saari, J. and Aaltonen, M. (1989) The effects of an informational safety campaign in the shipbuilding industry. *Journal of Occupational Accidents,* **10,** 255–66.

Saari, J. (1990) On strategies and methods in company safety work: from informational to motivational strategies. *Journal of Occupational Accidents,* **12,** 107–17.

Saarinen, T. (1990) Improving public response to hazards through enhanced perception of risks and remedies, in J. Handmer and E. Penning-Rowsell, (eds), *Hazards and the Communication of Risk,* Gower, Aldershot, pp. 279–92.

Salvendy, G. (ed.) (1987) *Handbook of Human Factors,* Wiley, New York.

Sanders, M.G. and Hoffman, M.A. (1975) Personality aspects of involvement in pilot-error accidents. *Aviation, Space and Environmental Medicine,* **46,** pp. 186–90.

Sanders, M.G., Hoffman, M.A. and Nese, T.A. (1976) Cross validation study of the personality aspect of involvement in pilot-error accidents. *Aviation, Space and Environmental Medicine,* **47,** pp. 177–90.

Sanders, M.S. and McCormick, E.J. (1987) *Human Factors in Engineering Design,* 6th edn, McGraw-Hill, New York.

Saunders, R. (1992) *The Safety Audit: Designing Effective Strategies,* Pitman, London.

Saville and Holdsworth Ltd (1984) *Occupational Personality Questionnaires Manual,* Saville and Holdsworth, Esher, Surrey.

Saville and Holdsworth Ltd (1985) *OPQ update number 1,* Saville and Holdsworth, Esher, Surrey.

Saville and Holdsworth Ltd (1987) *OPQ Concept 4.2 Profile Chart,* Saville and Holdsworth, Esher, Surrey.

Sayles, L.R. (1958) *The Behaviour of Industrial Work Groups,* Wiley, New York.

Scanlon, J. (1990) People and warnings: so hard to convince, in J. Handmer and E. Penning-Rowsell, (eds), *Hazards and the Communication of Risk,* Gower, Aldershot, pp. 233–46.

Schank, M.J. and Lawrence, D.M. (1993) Young adult women: lifestyle and health locus of control, *Journal of Advanced Nursing,* **18,** 1235–41.

Schein, E.H. (1978) *Career Dynamics: Matching Individual and Organizational Needs,* Addison-Wesley, Reading, Ma.

Schein, E.H. (1990) *Career Anchors: Discovering your Real Values,* Pfeiffer, Holland.

Schiffman, L.G. and Kanuk, L.L. (1991) *Consumer Behavior,* 4th edn, Prentice-Hall International, Englewood Cliffs, N.J.

Schmitt, N., Gooding, R.Z., Noe, R.A. and Kirsch, M. (1984) Meta-analyses of validity studies published between 1964 and 1982 and the investigation of study characteristics. *Personnel Psychology*, **37**, 407–22.

Schottenfeld, R.S. and Cullen, M.R. (1986) Recognition of occupation induced post-traumatic stress disorders. *Journal of Occupational Medicine*, **28**, 365–9.

Schwarzer, R. (1992) Self-efficacy in the adoption and maintenance of health behaviors: theoretical approaches and a new model, in R. Schwarzer (ed.), *Self-efficacy: Thought Control of Action*, Hemisphere, London, pp. 217–43.

Secord, P.F. and Backman, C.W. (1974) *Social Psychology*, 2nd edn, McGraw-Hill, Tokyo.

Sell, R.G. (1977) What does safety propaganda do for safety? A review. *Applied Ergonomics*, **8(4)**, 203–14.

Selzer, M.L. and Vinokur, A. (1974) Life events, subjective stress and traffic accidents. *American Journal of Psychiatry*, **131**, 903–6.

Semin, G.R. and Glendon, A.I. (1973) Polarisation and the established group. *British Journal of Social and Clinical Psychology*, **12**, 113–21.

Senge, P.M. (1990) *The Fifth Discipline: the Art and Practice of the Learning Organization*, Century Business, London.

Shackleton, V.J. (1989) *How to Pick People for Jobs*, Fontana Collins, London.

Shapiro, D.A., Cheesman, M. and Wall, T.D. (1993) Secondary prevention – review of counselling and EAPS, in R. Jenkins and D. Warman, (eds), *Promoting Mental Health Policies in the Workplace*, HMSO, London, pp. 86–102.

Shaver, K.G. (1970) Defensive attribution: effects of severity and relevance on the responsibility assigned for an accident. *Journal of Personality and Social Psychology*, **14**, 101–13.

Shaw, J.B., Fields, M.W., Thacker, J.W. and Fisher, C.D. (1993) The availability of personal and external coping resources: their impact on job stress and employee attitudes during organizational restructuring. *Work and Stress*, **7**, 229–46.

Shaw, L.S and Sichel, H.S. (1971) *Accident Proneness*, Pergamon, Oxford.

Shaw, M.E. (1964) Communication networks, in L. Berkowitz (ed.), *Advances in Experimental Social Psychology vol 1*, Academic Press, New York, pp. 11–47.

Sheehy, N.P. and Chapman, A.J. (1987) Industrial accidents, in C.L. Cooper and I.T. Robertson (eds), *International Review of Industrial and Organizational Psychology*, Wiley, Chichester, pp. 201–27.

Shepherd, A. (1985) Hierarchical task analysis and training decisions. *Programmed Learning and Educational Technology*, **22**, 162–76.

Sheppard, B.H., Hartwick, J. and Warshaw, P.R. (1988) The theory of reasoned action: a meta-analysis of past research with recommendations for modifications and future research. *Journal of Consumer Research*, **15**, 325–39.

Sherif, M. (1936) *The Psychology of Social Norms*, Harper & Row, New York.

Sherif, M. (1967) *Group Conflict and Cooperation: Their Social Psychology*, Routledge and Kegan Paul, London.

Siegrist, J., Peter, R., Junge, A., Crener, P. and Seidel, D. (1990) Low status, control, high effort at work and ischaemic heart disease: prospective evidence from blue-collar men. *Social Science and Medicine*, **31**, 1127–34.

Signori, E.I. and Bowman, R.G. (1974) On the study of personality factors in research on driving behaviour. *Perceptual and Motor Skills*, **33**, 1067–76.

Singh, A.P. (1978) Neuroticism, extraversion and accidents, *India Psychological Review*, **16**, 41–5.

Singleton, W.T. (1971) Current trends towards system design. *Applied Ergonomics*, **2**, 150–8.

Singleton, W.T. and Hovden, J. (1987) *Risk and Decisions,* Wiley, Chichester.

Six, B. and Schmidt, H. (1992) Overcoming a trauma: a meta-analysis of studies on the attitude-behavior relationship, *25th International Congress of Psychology,* 19–24 July, Brussels.

Skinner, B.F. (1938) *The Behavior of Organisms,* Appleton Century Crofts, New York.

Slovic, P., Fischhoff, B. and Lichtenstein, S. (1979) Rating the risks. *Environment,* **21(3),** 14–20, 736–9.

Smith, A.P. (1992) Time of day and performance, in A.P. Smith and D.M. Jones, (eds), *Handbook of Human Performance Volume 3: State and Trait,* Academic Press, London, pp. 215–35.

Smith, A.P. and Jones, D.M. (1992) Noise and performance, in A.P. Smith and D.M. Jones (eds), *Handbook of Human Performance Volume 1: The Physical Environment,* Academic Press, London, pp. 1–28.

Smith, A.P. and Stansfield, S. (1986) Aircraft noise exposure, noise sensitivity and everyday errors. *Environment and Behaviour,* **18,** 214–16.

Smith, D.I. and Kirkham, R.W. (1981) Relationship between some personality characteristics and driving record. *British Journal of Social Psychology,* **20,** 299–331.

Smith, M. and Robertson, I.T. (eds) (1989) *Advances in Selection and Assessment,* Wiley, Chichester.

Smith, M.J., Anger, W.K. and Uslan, S.S. (1978) Behavior modification applied to occupational safety. *Journal of Safety Research,* **10(2),** 87–8.

Smith, M.J. and Beringer, D.B. (1987) Human factors in occupational injury evaluation and control, in G. Salvendy (ed.), *Handbook of Human Factors,* Wiley, New York, pp. 767–89.

Snyder, M. (1979) Self-monitoring processes, in L. Berkowitz (ed.), *Advances in Experimental Social Psychology,* vol 12, Academic Press, New York, pp. 85–128.

Snyder, M., Tanke, E.D. and Berscheid, E. (1977) Social perception and interpersonal behaviour: on the self-fulfilling nature of social stereotypes. *Journal of Personality and Social Psychology,* **35,** 656–66.

Spiegel, D. (1988) Dissociation and hypnosis in post-traumatic stress disorders. *Journal of Traumatic Stress,* **1,** 17–33.

Spielberger, C.D. (1966) Theory and research on anxiety, in C.D. Spielberger (ed.), *Anxiety and Behaviour,* Academic Press, New York and London, pp. 3–20.

Spielberger, C.D. (1983) *Manual for the State-Trait Anxiety Inventory,* Consulting Psychologists Press, Palo Alto, Ca.

Spielberger, C.D., Vagg, P.R., Baker, L.R., Donham, G.W. and Westberry, L.G. (1980) The factor structure of the state-trait anxiety inventory, in I.G. Sarason and C.D. Spielberger, (eds), *Stress and Anxiety Volume 7,* Hemisphere, Washington, D.C., pp. 95–109.

Stammers, R.B. (1987) Training and the acquisition of knowledge and skill, in P.B. Warr (ed.), *Psychology at Work,* 3rd edn, Penguin, Harmondsworth, pp. 53–72.

Stanton, N.A. (1992) *The Human Factors Aspects of Alarms in Human Supervisory Control Tasks,* PhD Thesis, Aston University, Birmingham.

Stanton, N.A., Booth, R.T. and Stammers, R.B. (1992) Alarms in human supervisory control: a human factors perspective. *International Journal of Computer Integrated Manufacturing,* **5,** 81–93.

Stanton, N.A., Matthews, G., Graham, N.C. and Brimelow, C. (1991) The OPQ and the big five. *Journal of Managerial Psychology,* **6(1),** 25–7.

Steel, C. (1990) Risk estimation. *The Safety and Health Practitioner,* **8(6),** June, 20–1.

Steffy, B.D., Jones, J.W. and Noe, A.W. (1990) The impact of health habits and life-style on the stress-strain relationship: an evaluation of three industries. *Journal of Occupational Psychology,* **63,** 217–29.

Stellman, J.M. and Daum, S.M. (1973) *Work is Dangerous to Your Health: a Handbook of Health Hazards in the Workplace and What You Can Do About Them,* Vintage Books, New York.

Sterns, L., Alexander, R.A., Barrett, G.V. and Dambrot, F.H. (1983) The relationship of extraversion and neuroticism with job preferences and job satisfaction for clerical employees. *Journal of Occupational Psychology,* **56,** 145–53.

Stone, S.V. and Costa, P.T. (1990) Disease-prone personality or distress-prone personality? in H.S. Friedman (ed.), *Personality and Disease,* Wiley, Chichester, pp. 178–200.

Stoner, J.A.F. (1961) *A Comparison of Individual and Group Decisions Involving Risk,* Unpublished Masters thesis, School of Industrial Management, MIT.

Storey, J. (ed) (1989) *New Perspectives on Human Resource Management,* Routledge, London.

Storey, J. (1992) *Developments in the Management of Human Resources,* Blackwell, Oxford.

Stubbs, D.A., Buckle, P.W., Hudson, M.P., Rivers, R.M. and Worrington, R.M. (1983) Back pain in the nursing profession, Part I Epidemiology and pilot methodology. *Ergonomics,* **26,** 755–65.

Suchman, E.A. (1965) Cultural and social factors in accident occurrence and control. *Journal of Occupational Medicine,* **7,** 487–92.

Sugarman, L. (1986) *Life-span Development,* Methuen, London.

Suls, J. and Wan, C.K. (1989) The relationship between Type A behaviour and chronic emotional distress: a meta-analysis. *Journal of Personality and Social Psychology,* **57,** 503–12.

Sulzer-Azaroff, B. (1978) Behavioral ecology and accident prevention. *Journal of Organizational Behavior Management,* **2,** 11–44.

Sulzer-Azaroff, B. (1982) Behavioral approaches to occupational health and safety, in L.W. Frederiksen (ed.), *Handbook of Organisational Management,* Wiley, New York, pp. 505–38.

Sulzer-Azaroff, B. and De Santamaria, M.C. (1980) Industrial safety hazard reduction through performance feedback. *Journal of Applied Behavior Analysis,* **13,** 287–95.

Sundström-Frisk, C. (1989) Structured group discussions about motives for unsafe behaviours: effects on risk taking behaviour and safety efforts. *Journal of Occupational Accidents,* **12,** 135–6.

Surry, J. (1969) *Industrial Accident Research: a Human Engineering Appraisal,* Department of Industrial Engineering, University of Toronto.

Sutherland, V.J. and Cooper, C.L. (1991) Personality, stress and accident involvement in the offshore oil and gas industry. *Personality and Individual Differences,* **12,** 195–204.

Sutherland, V.J. and Davidson, M.J. (1993) Using a stress audit: the construction site manager experience in the UK. *Work and Stress,* **7,** 273–86.

Sutton, S.R. (1982) Fear arousing communications: a critical examination of theory and research, in J.R. Eiser (ed.), *Social Psychology and Behavioural Medicine,* Wiley, Chichester.

Svensson, O. (1981) Are we less risky and more skilful than our fellow drivers? *Acta Psychologica,* **47,** 143–8.

Swain, A. D. and Guttman, H. (1983) *Handbook of Human Reliability Analysis with Emphasis on Nuclear Power Plant Applications: Final Report,* NUREG/CR-1278, Nuclear Regulatory Commission, Washington, D.C.

Swinburne, P. (1981) The psychological impact of unemployment on managers and professional staff. *Journal of Occupational Psychology,* **54,** 47–64.

Sykes, W. (1989) Some principles of personal and organisational change, in W.L. French, C.H. Bell and R.A. Zawacki (eds), *Organisation Development: Theory, Practice and Research,* Irwin, Homewood, Il., pp. 456–8.

Tarrants, W.E. (1980) *The Measurement of Safety Performance,* Garland, London.

Taylor, F.W. (1911) *Principles of Scientific Management,* Harper, New York.

Taylor, R.K. and Lucas, D.A. (1991) Signals passed at danger: near miss reporting from a railway perspective, in T.W. van der Schaaf, D.A. Lucas and A.R. Hale (eds), *Near Miss Reporting as a Safety Tool,* Butterworth Heinemann, Oxford, pp. 79–92.

Team Management Systems. (1992) *Putting Teams into Action: Case Studies in Outdoor Management Development volume 1,* TMS (UK) Ltd, York.

Terry, D. (1991) Coping resources and situational approaches as predictors of coping behaviour. *Personality and Individual Differences,* **12,** 1031–47.

Tetlock, P.E. and Manstead, A.S.R. (1985) Impression management versus intrapsychic explanations in social psychology: a useful dichotomy? *Psychological Review,* **92,** 59–77.

Tett, R.P., Jackson, D.N. and Rothstein, M. (1991) Personality measures as predictors of job performance: a meta-analytic review. *Personnel Psychology,* **44,** 703–42.

Thompson, R. (1992) *Mental Illness: the Fundamental Facts,* Mental Health Foundation, London.

Thorne, P. (1992) Hit squads. *International Management,* **47(2),** 56.

Tilley, A. and Brown, S. (1992) Sleep deprivation, in A.P. Smith and D.M. Jones (eds), *Handbook of Human Performance Volume 3: State and Trait,* Academic Press, London, pp. 237–59.

Tillman, W.A. and Hobbs, G.E. (1949) Accident proneness in automobile drivers. *Academic Journal of Psychiatry,* **106,** 321–31.

Toft, B. (1992a) Changing a safety culture: decree, prescription or learning. Paper presented at IRST CONFERENCE ON RISK, MANAGEMENT AND SAFETY CULTURE, 9 April 1992, London Business School.

Toft, B (1992b) Changing a safety culture: a holistic approach. Paper presented at the BRITISH ACADEMY OF MANAGEMENT 6TH ANNUAL CONFERENCE, 14–16 Sept 1992, Bradford University.

Tolman, E.C. (1959) Principles of purposive behaviourism, in S. Koch (ed.), *Psychology: a Study of Science, Study 1,2,* McGraw-Hill, London, pp. 92–157.

Travers, C.J. and Cooper, C.L. (1993) Mental health, job satisfaction and occupational stress among teachers, *Work and Stress,* **7,** 203–19.

Tupes, E.C. and Christal, R.E. (1961) Recurrent personality factors based on trait ratings, USAF ASD Technical Report, pp. 61–97.

Turner, B.A. (1992) Organizational learning and the management of risk. Paper presented at the BRITISH ACADEMY OF MANAGEMENT 6TH ANNUAL CONFERENCE, 14–16 September 1992, Bradford University.

van der Schaaf, T.W., Lucas, D.A. and Hale, A.R. (eds) (1991) *Near Miss Reporting as a Safety Tool,* Butterworth-Heinemann, Oxford.

van der Velde, W. and van der Plight, J. (1991) AIDS-related behavior: coping, protection motivation, and previous behavior. *Journal of Behavioral Medicine,* **14,** 429–51.

van Doornen, L.J.P. and de Geus, E.J.C. (1993) Stress, physical activity and coronary heart disease. *Work and Stress*, **7**, 121–39.

Veiel, H.O.F. and Baumann, U. (eds) (1992) *The Meaning and Measurement of Social Support*, Hemisphere, London.

Veith, I. (1965) *Hysteria: the History of a Disease*, University of Chicago Press, Chicago.

Venables, P. (1956) Car driving consistency and measures of personality. *Journal of Applied Psychology*, **40**, 21–4.

Voke, J. (1982) Colour vision problems at work. *Health and Safety at Work*, January, 27–8.

Vroom, V.H. (1964) *Work and Motivation*, Wiley, Chichester.

Wagenaar, W.A. and Groeneweg, J. (1987) Accidents at sea: multiple causes and impossible consequences. *International Journal of Man-Machine Studies*, **27**, 587–98.

Wahba, M.A. and Bridwell, L.B. (1976) Maslow reconsidered: a review of research on the need hierarchy. *Organizational Behavior and Human Performance*, **15**, 212–40.

Waller, R.A. (1969) Office acoustics – effects of background noise. *Applied Acoustics*, **2**, 121–30.

Wallston, B.S. and Wallston, K.A. (1978) Locus of control and health. *Health Education Monographs*, Spring, 107–15.

Warburton, R.M. (1986) Training of workpeople in health and safety, in R.C. Clarke (ed.), *Education and Training in Health and Safety: Current Problems and Future Priorities – Proceedings of a Conference held by the British Health and Safety Society, London, June, 1986*, BHSS, Birmingham, pp. 32–7.

Warg, L-E. (1990) The feedback model as a means to a change risk behaviour: experiences from a study in a slaughterhouse, in L. Harms-Ringdahl and C. Sundström-Frisk (eds), *Strategies for Occupational Accident Prevention*, Stockholm, Sweden, 21–22 Sept 1989, *Journal of Occupational Accidents*, **12**, 131.

Waring, A.E. (1989) *Systems Methods for Managers: a Practical Guide*, Blackwell Scientific Publications, Oxford.

Waring, A.E. (1990) *Safety Training*, Module RA5, Risk Assessment and Control Unit, Occupational Health and Safety, Portsmouth.

Waring, A.E. (1991) Success with safety management systems. *The Safety and Health Practitioner*, **9(9)**, 20–3.

Waring, A.E. (1992) Organisational culture, management and safety. Paper presented at the *British Academy of Management 6th Annual Conference*, 14–16 Sept 1992, Bradford University.

Waring, A.E. (1993) Power and culture – their implications for safety cases and EER. Paper presented at *1993 European Seminar on Human Factors in Offshore Safety*, 29–30 Sept 1993, Aberdeen.

Waring, A.E. (1994) Power and culture in organisations and their implications for management of risk. Paper presented at *Conference on Changing Perceptions of Risk – the Implications for Management*, 27 February–1 March, Bolton.

Warr, P.B. (1987) *Work, Unemployment and Mental Health*, Clarendon Press, Oxford.

Warr, P.B. and Jackson, P.R. (1984) Men without jobs: some correlates of age and length of unemployment. *Journal of Occupational Psychology*, **57**, 77–85.

Watson, D. and Clark, L.A. (1984) Negative affectivity: the disposition to experience aversive emotional states. *Psychological Bulletin*, **96**, 465–90.

Watson, D. and Pennebaker, J.W. (1989) Health complaints, stress and distress. *Psychological Review*, **96**, 324–54.

Watson, D., Pennebaker, J.D. and Folger, R. (1987) Beyond negative affectivity: measuring stress and satisfaction in the workplace, in J.M. Ivancevitch and D.C. Ganster (eds), *Job Stress: from Theory to Suggestion*, Haworth, London, pp. 141–57.

Watson, J.B. (1950) *Behaviorism*, Norton, New York.

Weiner, B. (1992) *Human Motivation: Metaphors, Theories and Research*, Sage, London.

Weiss, S.M., Fielding, J.E. and Baum, A. (eds) (1991) *Perspectives in Behavioral Medicine: Health at Work*, Lawrence Erlbaum, Hillsdale, N.J.

Wheale, J.L. (1984) An analysis of crew coordination problems in commercial transport aircraft. *International Journal of Aviation Safety*, **2**, 83–9.

Wickens, C.D. (1984) *Engineering Psychology and Human Performance*, Merrill, Columbus, Ohio.

Wickens, C.D., Sandry, D. and Vidulich, M. (1983) Compatibility and resource competition between modalities of input, central processing, and output. *Human Factors*, **25**, 227–48.

Wilde, G.J.S. (1982) The theory of risk homeostasis: implications for safety and health. *Risk Analysis*, **2**, 209–25.

Wilkins, L. and Patterson, P. (1990) The political amplification of risk: media coverage of disasters and hazards, in J. Handmer and E. Penning-Rowsell (eds), *Hazards and the Communication of Risk*, Gower, Aldershot, pp. 79–94.

Willett, T.C. (1964) *Criminal on the Road*, Tavistock, London.

Williams, D.E. and Page, M.M. (1989) A multi-dimensional measure of Maslow's hierarchy of needs. *Journal of Research in Personality*, **23**, 192–213.

Williams, D.R. and House, J.S. (1985) Social support and stress reduction in C.L. Cooper and M.J Smith (eds), *Job Stress and Blue Collar Work*, Wiley, Chichester, pp. 207–24.

Williams, J.C. (1985) Validation of human reliability assessment techniques. *Reliability Engineering*, **11**, 149–62.

Williams, R.S. (1994) Occupational testing: contemporary British practice. *The Psychologist*, **7(1)**, 11–13.

Wilson, D.C. and Rosenfeld, R.H. (1990) *Managing Organisations: Text, Readings and Cases*, McGraw-Hill, London.

Winchester, P. (1990) Economic power and response to risk: a case study from India, in J. Handmer and E. Penning-Rowsell (eds), *Hazards and the Communication of Risk*, Gower, Aldershot, pp. 95–109.

Wistow, D.J., Wakefield, J.A. and Goldsmith, W.M. (1990) The relationship between personality, health symptoms and disease. *Personality and Individual Differences*, **11**, 717–24.

Wong, N.D. and Reading, A.E. (1989) Personality correlates of Type A behaviour. *Personality and Individual Differences*, **11**, 991–6.

Wong, W.A. and Hobbs, B.A. (1949) Personal factors in industrial accidents: a study of accident proneness in an industrial group. *Industrial Medicine and Surgery*, **18**, 291–4.

Wright, M.S. (1994) A review of safety management system approaches to risk reduction. Paper presented at *Risk Assessment and Risk Reduction Conference*, 22 March 1994, Aston University.

Wrightsman, L. (1960) Effects of waiting for others on changes in level of felt anxiety. *Journal of Abnormal and Social Psychology*, **61**, 216–22.

Yang, K. and Bond. M.H. (1990) Exploring implicit personality theories with indigenous or imported constructs: the Chinese case. *Journal of Personality and Social Psychology*, **58**, 1087–95.

Zander, A. (1982) *Making Groups Effective,* Jossey-Bass, San Francisco.

Zimbardo, P.G. (1973) On the ethics of intervention in human psychological research: with special reference to the Stanford Prison Experiment. *Cognition,* **2,** 243–56.

Zohar, D. (1980a) Safety climate in industrial organisations: theoretical and applied implications. *Journal of Applied Psychology,* **65,** 96–102.

Zohar, D. (1980b) Promoting the use of personal protective equipment by behavior modification techniques. *Journal of Safety Research,* **12,** 78–85.

Zohar, D., Cohen, A. and Azar, N. (1980) Promoting increased use of ear protectors in noise through information feedback. *Human Factors,* **22,** 69–79.

AUTHOR INDEX

SUBJECT INDEX